PROGRESS IN CLINICAL AND BIOLOGICAL RESEARCH

Series Editors

RECENT TITLES

Vol 206: **Genetic Toxicology of the Diet,** Ib Knudsen, *Editor*

Vol 207: **Monitoring of Occupational Genotoxicants,** Marja Sorsa, Hannu Norppa, *Editors*

Vol 208: **Risk and Reason: Risk Assessment in Relation to Environmental Mutagens and Carcinogens,** Per Oftedal, Anton Brøgger, *Editors*

Vol 209: **Genetic Toxicology of Environmental Chemicals,** Claes Ramel, Bo Lambert, Jan Magnusson, *Editors.* Published in two volumes: Part A: *Basic Principles and Mechanisms of Action.* Part B: *Genetic Effects and Applied Mutagenesis*

Vol 210: **Ionic Currents in Development,** Richard Nuccitelli, *Editor*

Vol 211: **Transfusion Medicine: Recent Technological Advances,** Kris Murawski, Frans Peetoom, *Editors*

Vol 212: **Cancer Metastasis: Experimental and Clinical Strategies,** D.R. Welch, B.K. Bhuyan, L.A. Liotta, *Editors*

Vol 213: **Plant Flavonoids in Biology and Medicine: Biochemical, Pharmacological, and Structure–Activity Relationships,** Vivian Cody, Elliott Middleton, Jr., Jeffrey B. Harborne, *Editors*

Vol 214: **Ethnic Differences in Reactions to Drugs and Xenobiotics,** Werner Kalow, H. Werner Goedde, Dharam P. Agarwal, *Editors*

Vol 215: **Megakaryocyte Development and Function,** Richard F. Levine, Neil Williams, Jack Levin, Bruce L. Evatt, *Editors*

Vol 216: **Advances in Cancer Control: Health Care Financing and Research,** Lee E. Mortenson, Paul F. Engstrom, Paul N. Anderson, *Editors*

Vol 217: **Progress in Developmental Biology,** Harold C. Slavkin, *Editor.* Published in two volumes.

Vol 218: **Evolutionary Perspective and the New Genetics,** Henry Gershowitz, Donald L. Rucknagel, Richard E. Tashian, *Editors*

Vol 219: **Recent Advances in Arterial Diseases: Atherosclerosis, Hypertension, and Vasospasm,** Thomas N. Tulenko, Robert H. Cox, *Editors*

Vol 220: **Safety and Health Aspects of Organic Solvents,** Vesa Riihimäki, Ulf Ulfvarson, *Editors*

Vol 221: **Developments in Bladder Cancer,** Louis Denis, Tadao Niijima, George Prout, Jr., Fritz H. Schröder, *Editors*

Vol 222: **Dietary Fat and Cancer,** Clement Ip, Diane F. Birt, Adrianne E. Rogers, Curtis Mettlin, *Editors*

Vol 223: **Cancer Drug Resistance,** Thomas C. Hall, *Editor*

Vol 224: **Transplantation: Approaches to Graft Rejection,** Harold T. Meryman, *Editor*

Vol 225: **Gonadotropin Down-Regulation in Gynecological Practice,** Rune Rolland, Dev R. Chadha, Wim N.P. Willemsen, *Editors*

Vol 226: **Cellular Endocrinology: Hormonal Control of Embryonic and Cellular Differentiation,** Ginette Serrero, Jun Hayashi, *Editors*

Vol 227: **Advances in Chronobiology,** John E. Pauly, Lawrence E. Scheving, *Editors.* Published in two volumes.

Vol 228: **Environmental Toxicity and the Aging Processes,** Scott R. Baker, Marvin Rogul, *Editors*

Vol 229: **Animal Models: Assessing the Scope of Their Use in Biomedical Research,** Junichi Kawamata, Edward C. Melby, Jr., *Editors*

Please contact the publisher for information about previous titles in this series.

Electromagnetic Fields and Neurobehavioral Function

ELECTROMAGNETIC FIELDS AND NEUROBEHAVIORAL FUNCTION

Editors

Mary Ellen O'Connor
Department of Psychology
The University of Tulsa
Tulsa, Oklahoma

Richard H. Lovely
Neurosciences Group
Battelle, Pacific Northwest Laboratories
Richland, Washington

ALAN R. LISS, INC. • NEW YORK

Address all Inquiries to the Publisher
Alan R. Liss, Inc., 41 East 11th Street, New York, NY 10003

Copyright © 1988 Alan R. Liss, Inc.

Printed in the United States of America

Library of Congress Cataloging-in-Publication Data

Electromagnetic fields and neurobehavioral function.

(Progress in clinical and biological research ; v. 257)
Based on a conference held at Priorij Corsendonk, Belgium, Aug. 19–23, 1984.
Includes bibliographies and index.
1. Nervous system—Effect of radiation on— Congresses. 2. Brain—Effect of radiation on— Congresses. 3. Electromagnetism—Physiological effect—Congresses. 4. Electromagnetism—Toxicology— Congresses. 5. Behavioral toxicology—Congresses.
I. O'Connor, Mary Ellen. II. Series. [DNLM: 1. Electromagnetics—Congresses. 2. Neurophysiology— congresses. W1 PR668E v.257 / WL 102 E3847 1984]
QP356.5.E44 1987 612'.8 87-29698
ISBN 0-8451-5107-X

Contents

Contributors

Eleanor R. Adair, John B. Pierce Foundation and Yale University, New Haven, CT 06519 **[179]**

W. Ross Adey, Departments of Physiology and Surgery, Loma Linda University School of Medicine, Loma Linda, CA 92357 **[81]**

Ernest N. Albert, Department of Anatomy, The George Washington University Medical Center, Washington, DC 20037 **[135]**

R. Robin Baker, Reader in Zoology, University of Manchester, M13 9PL, U.K. **[63]**

Carl F. Blackman, Health Effects Research Laboratory, U.S. Environmental Protection Agency, Research Triangle Park, NC 27711 **[107]**

J.A. Bonnell, Health and Safety Division, Central Electricity Generating Board, London, England **[349]**

John A. D'Andrea, Department of Electrical Engineering, University of Utah, Salt Lake City, UT 84112; present address: Department of Bioenvironmental Sciences, Naval Aerospace Medical Research Laboratory, Pensacola, FL 32508-5700 **[289]**

J.O. de Lorge, Department of Bioenvironmental Sciences, Naval Aerospace Medical Research Laboratory, Pensacola, FL 32508-5700 **[219]**

John R. DeWitt, Department of Psychology, University of Utah, Salt Lake City, UT 84112 **[289]**

M.J. Galvin, Laboratory of Behavioral and Neurological Toxicology, NIEHS, Research Triangle Park, NC 27709 **[153]**

Om P. Gandhi, Department of Electrical Engineering, University of Utah, Salt Lake City, UT 84112 **[289]**

Hans-Arne Hansson, Institute of Neurobiology, University of Gothenburg, S-40033 Gothenburg, Sweden **[119]**

Don R. Justesen, Behavioral Radiology Laboratories, Veterans Administration Medical Center, Kansas City, MO; University of Kansas School of Medicine, Kansas City, KS 66103 **[235]**

Ad. J. Kalmijn, Scripps Institution of Oceanography, University of California, San Diego, La Jolla, CA 92093 **[23]**

The numbers in brackets are the opening page numbers of the contributors' articles.

W. Gregory Lotz, Department of Bioenvironmental Sciences, Naval Aerospace Medical Research Laboratory, Pensacola, FL 32508-5700 **[203]**

Richard H. Lovely, Neurosciences Group, Department of Biology and Chemistry, Battelle, Pacific Northwest Laboratories, Richland, WA 99352 **[xi, 327]**

M.J. Marr, Naval Aerospace Medical Research Laboratory, Pensacola, FL 32508-5700; present address: School of Psychology, Georgia Institute of Technology, Atlanta, GA 30332 **[219]**

D.I. McRee, Laboratory of Behavioral and Neurological Toxicology, NIEHS, Research Triangle Park, NC 27709 **[153]**

C.L. Mitchell, Laboratory of Behavioral and Neurological Toxicology, NIEHS, Research Triangle Park, NC 27709 **[153]**

John C. Monahan, Food and Drug Administration, Center for Devices and Radiological Health, Office of Science and Technology, Rockville, MD 20857 **[309]**

W.T. Norris, Technology, Planning, and Research Division, Central Electricity Generating Board, Leatherhead, Surrey, England KT22 7SE **[349]**

Mary Ellen O'Connor, Department of Psychology, The University of Tulsa, Tulsa, OK 74104 **[xi, 265]**

R.G. Olsen, Department of Bioenvironmental Sciences, Naval Aerospace Medical Research Laboratory, Pensacola, FL 32508-5700 **[219]**

Lupita M. Portuguez, Departments of Psychology and Electrical Engineering, University of Utah, Salt Lake City, UT 84112 **[289]**

Paul J. Rosch, American Institute of Stress, Department of Medicine and Psychiatry, New York Medical College, Valhalla, NY 10595, and Department of Medicine in Psychiatry, University of Maryland School of Medicine, Baltimore, MD 21201 **[377]**

Jack L. Saxton, Department of Bioenvironmental Sciences, Naval Aerospace Medical Research Laboratory, Pensacola, FL 32508-5700 **[203]**

Peter Semm, Department of Zoology, University of Frankfurt, Frankfurt, Federal Republic of Germany **[47]**

M.G. Shandala, A.N. Marzeev Research Institute of General and Communal Hygiene, Kiev, USSR **[367]**

Mahmoud Sherif, Department of Anatomy, The George Washington University Medical Center, Washington, DC 20037 **[135]**

M. Stanford, Department of Bioenvironmental Sciences, Naval Aerospace Medical Research Laboratory, Pensacola, FL 32508-5700 **[219]**

J. Van Bladel, Department of Engineering, The University of Ghent, Ghent, Belgium, B9000 **[1]**

Preface

The contributors to this book have research interests that range from electroreception in animals to neurotoxicology and environmental health. Such diversity of research interests coupled with differing objectives and methods has not been conducive to an active dialogue concerning what is *common* to their research: the effects of electromagnetic fields on select neural and behavioral functions. Indeed, one would be hard-pressed to find reports from so many disciplines in a single volume such as this; that is why we hope that this book will be useful to a wide spectrum of readers from these diverse fields.

To introduce readers to the field, the first chapter provides a concise introduction to the physical properties of electromagnetic stimuli. The following chapters start with well-studied adaptive specializations that some species have evolved to detect and respond to electromagnetic fields. The book continues with studies ranging from cell biology and possible mechanisms of interaction to more holistic studies examining physiological and behavioral responses in whole animals. The book concludes with occupational health studies, publication of the recently adopted Soviet microwave radiation exposure standards, and a final comment on some of the clinical implications of work in this area.

We should add that the idea for this book coincided with the organization of a conference that was held August 19–23, 1984 at Priorij Corsendonk, Belgium. Although the conference and the book share a common goal—to bridge the communication gap among scientists with common interests in electromagnetic fields and neurobehavioral function—the book is not limited to, nor is it inclusive of, the material presented at the conference. We do hope, however, that it is as successful in achieving its goal as we believe the conference was.

Mary Ellen O'Connor
Richard H. Lovely

Acknowledgments

We express our gratitude to the Environmental Protection Agency, the Office of Naval Research, and the Office of Naval Research London Branch for the financial sponsorship of the workshop. Within these respective organizations, we are particularly indebted to Dr. Joseph Elder, Dr. Michael Marron, and Dr. Thomas C. Rozzell. We also wish to thank all of the workshop participants and discussants whose thoughtful and often insightful comments were instrumental in achieving the goals of the workshop. In addition to the contributors, we thank Dr. Michael Bornhausen, Dr. Charles Ehret, Dr. Victor Laties, Dr. Richard Olsen, Dr. Richard Phillips, Dr. Thomas Rozzell, and Dr. Rutger Wever.

We also thank the many reviewers who contributed to this book. Each chapter received at least two independent reviews. The editors, as well as the authors, thank them for their efforts and many useful suggestions. We wish to acknowledge:

Eleanor Adair	Henry Lai
Jane Adams	Victor Laties
E.A. Albert	D.M. Levinson
Zoltan Annau	Li-Ming Liu
David A. Bartsch	D.I. McRee
Elsworth R. Buskirk	Diane Miller
Michel Cabanac	Stata Norton
C.K. Chou	John Osepchuk
Reynaldo S. Elizondo	Philip Sagan
Richard Frankel	G.R. Sessions
Charles Graham	Asher Shepherd
James Grier	Robert Smith
C. Craig Heller	Don E. Spiers
Ronald P. Jensch	Carl Sutton
Don R. Justesen	Tom Tenforde
W.T. Kaune	Leonard Zusne

We also appreciate the support and patience of Ms. Paulette Cohen.

Electromagnetic Fields and Neurobehavioral Function, pages 1–21
© 1988 Alan R. Liss, Inc.

THE NATURE OF ELECTROMAGNETIC STIMULI

J. Van Bladel, Ph.D.

Professor of Electrical Engineering
The University of Ghent
Ghent, Belgium, B9000

The present chapter is devoted to a condensed introduction to electromagnetism, written for neurophysiologists
with little training in electromagnetic fields. Only essential concepts are discussed, but they nevertheless cover
such a wide area that a complete bibliography would fill a
separate volume. The list of references is therefore restricted to a few fundamental titles.

1. THE ELECTROMAGNETIC PROBLEM

The general bioelectromagnetic situation involves a
target body V_1, immersed in the field of a generator described by its volume current
density $\bar{j}$ (in A m^{-2}). The
generator may be located in
free space, or lie in the
vicinity of a "deflector"
volume V_2 (Fig. 1). The deflector, e.g. the walls of a
resonant cavity, serves to
focus (or concentrate) the
fields in the biological target V_1, or in selected parts
thereof. In certain cases
deflection by nearby objects
must be strictly eliminated.
To achieve these "free space"
conditions, the source may be immersed in a room with absorbing, non-reflecting walls (Fig. 2).
Let the fields produced by the source in the absence of

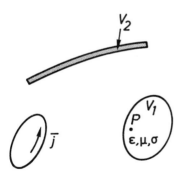

Fig. 1

target V_1 (the incident fields) be denoted by $(\overline{e}^i,\overline{h}^i)$. The presence of the target results in additional, "scattered" fields $(\overline{e}^s,\overline{h}^s)$. The total fields are now $\overline{e} = \overline{e}^i + \overline{e}^s$, $\overline{h} = \overline{h}^i + \overline{h}^s$. The bio-targets are normally extremely complex: they are strongly inhomogeneous, often nonlinear, and their characteristics are temperature sensitive. The numerical solution of the corresponding field problem is a difficult task, which is a source of joy for the professional electromagneticist. Once the fields are known in V_1, the dissipated Joule heat follows from the relationship

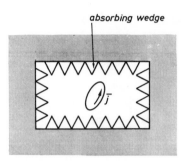

absorbing wedge

Fig. 2

$$\mathcal{P} = \sigma |\overline{e}|^2 \quad W\ m^{-3} \tag{1}$$

When this rate is expressed in $W\ kg^{-1}$ it is termed the specific absorption rate (SAR). This is a local concept, but it is also possible to define an average SAR, obtained by dividing the total power dissipated in V_1 by the mass of the body. It is evident that the distribution of the SAR throughout V_1 depends on the detailed nature of the incident fields, and not simply on a global parameter such as the incident power density.

2. MAXWELL'S EQUATIONS

The equations satisfied by the fields are, in vacuum (Van Bladel 1964),

$$\text{curl } \overline{e} = -\mu_o \frac{\partial \overline{h}}{\partial t}$$

$$\text{curl } \overline{h} = \varepsilon_o \frac{\partial \overline{e}}{\partial t} + \overline{j}$$

$$\text{div } \overline{d} = \rho \tag{2}$$

$$\text{div } \overline{b} = 0$$

The symbol ρ denotes the volume density of free charge (in $C\ m^{-3}$). The curl and div operators are collections of partial derivatives, given by

$$\text{div } \overline{a} = \frac{\partial a_x}{\partial x} + \frac{\partial a_y}{\partial y} + \frac{\partial a_z}{\partial z}$$

$$\text{curl } \overline{a} = (\frac{\partial a_z}{\partial y} - \frac{\partial a_y}{\partial z})\overline{u}_x + (\frac{\partial a_x}{\partial z} - \frac{\partial a_z}{\partial x})\overline{u}_y + (\frac{\partial a_y}{\partial x} - \frac{\partial a_x}{\partial y})\overline{u}_z \tag{3}$$

Here, $\overline{u}_i$ is a unit vector in the "i" direction. A bio-body such as V_1 can often be assumed linear and isotropic, and described by a dielectric constant $\varepsilon = \varepsilon_r\varepsilon_o$ (in F m^{-1}), a magnetic permeability $\mu = \mu_r\mu_o$ (in H m^{-1}) and a conductivity σ (in S m^{-1}). The (ε,μ,σ) parameters may be functions of position. In such a body, Maxwell's equations are

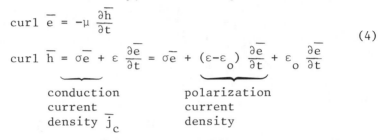

$$\text{curl } \overline{e} = -\mu \frac{\partial \overline{h}}{\partial t} \tag{4}$$

$$\text{curl } \overline{h} = \underbrace{\sigma\overline{e}}_{\substack{\text{conduction}\\\text{current}\\\text{density } \overline{j}_c}} + \varepsilon \frac{\partial \overline{e}}{\partial t} = \sigma\overline{e} + \underbrace{(\varepsilon-\varepsilon_o) \frac{\partial \overline{e}}{\partial t}}_{\substack{\text{polarization}\\\text{current}\\\text{density}}} + \varepsilon_o \frac{\partial \overline{e}}{\partial t}$$

The divergence equations are the same as in (2). In certain applications the target-body (e.g. human blood) moves with velocity $\overline{v}$ (Fig. 3). For such cases (4) holds in the rest-axes K' of V_1, and we write

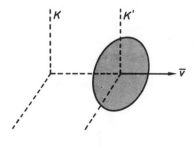

$$\overline{j}'_c = \sigma\overline{e}' \tag{5}$$

To obtain the field equations in the stationary axes K, relativistic transformations are needed (Van Bladel 1984). At low velocities (v<<c), these yield

Fig. 3

$$\overline{j}_c = \sigma(\overline{e} + \overline{v} \times \overline{b}) \tag{6}$$

To effect the solution of (2) and (4), boundary conditions at infinity and at interfaces must be taken into consideration (Van Bladel 1964,1984).

3. TIME HARMONIC PHENOMENA

The general form of a quantity with sinusoidal time-dependence is

$$v = a \cos(2\pi\nu t+\phi) = a \cos(\omega t+\phi) \qquad (7)$$

The main information, i.e. a and ϕ, can be combined economically into a complex number $V = a\, e^{j\phi}$, from which we recuperate the actual time dependence through the operation

$$v = \mathrm{Re}(Ve^{j\omega t}) = \mathrm{Re}\left[a\, e^{j\phi}\, e^{j\omega t}\right] = a \cos(\omega t+\phi) \qquad (8)$$

The complex (phasor) notation has an important property : the complex representation of $\dfrac{dv}{dt}$ is $j\omega V$.

A study of sinusoidal phenomena is important because an arbitrary time-dependent function $f(t)$ may be represented as a superposition of sinusoidal components through the Fourier integral

$$f(t) = \frac{1}{2\pi} \int_{-\infty}^{\infty} F(j\omega)e^{j\omega t}d\omega \qquad (9)$$

The Fourier spectrum is given, in amplitude and phase, by

$$F(j\omega) = \int_{-\infty}^{\infty} f(t)e^{-j\omega t}dt \qquad (10)$$

An important example is the amplitude-modulated signal

$$\cos\omega t(1+p\cos\omega' t) = \cos\omega t + \frac{p}{2}\cos(\omega+\omega')t + \frac{p}{2}\cos(\omega-\omega')t \qquad (11)$$

It is seen that this signal contains the frequencies ω, $(\omega+\omega')$ and $(\omega-\omega')$.

In many technical applications the three components of a vector (e.g. the electric field) are time-harmonic functions. We write

$$\begin{cases} e_x = A_1 \cos(\omega t+\phi_1) \\ e_y = A_2 \cos(\omega t+\phi_2) \\ e_z = A_3 \cos(\omega t+\phi_3) \end{cases} \text{or, in complex form,} \quad \begin{cases} E_x = A_1\, e^{j\phi_1} \\ E_y = A_2\, e^{j\phi_2} \\ E_z = A_3\, e^{j\phi_3} \end{cases}$$

$$(12)$$

It is appropriate to represent $\bar{e}$ by a complex vector $\bar{E}$

$$\bar{E} = E_x \bar{u}_x + E_y \bar{u}_y + E_z \bar{u}_z = A_1\, e^{j\phi_1}\bar{u}_x + A_2\, e^{j\phi_2}\bar{u}_y + A_3\, e^{j\phi_3}\bar{u}_z$$

$$(13)$$

from which $\bar{e}$ can be recuperated by the operation

$$\bar{e}(t) = \text{Re}(\bar{E}\ e^{j\omega t}) \tag{14}$$

The $\bar{e}$ vector lies in a plane. Indeed :

$$\bar{e} = (A_1 \cos\phi_1 \bar{u}_x + A_2 \cos\phi_2 \bar{u}_y + A_3 \cos\phi_3 \bar{u}_z)\cos\omega t$$

$$- (A_1 \sin\phi_1 \bar{u}_x + A_2 \sin\phi_2 \bar{u}_y + A_3 \sin\phi_3 \bar{u}_z)\sin\omega t$$

$$= \bar{\alpha} \cos\omega t - \bar{\beta} \sin\omega t \tag{15}$$

It is easy to show that the tip of this vector describes an ellipse. A time-harmonic vector is therefore said to be elliptically-polarized. When $\bar{\alpha}$ and $\bar{\beta}$ are in the same direction, the polarization is linear. When $\bar{\alpha}$ and $\bar{\beta}$ are perpendicular, and $|\bar{\alpha}| = |\bar{\beta}|$, the polarization is circular. The two rotation senses are characterized by the complex vectors $\bar{u}_x \pm j\bar{u}_y$, as shown in Fig. 4.

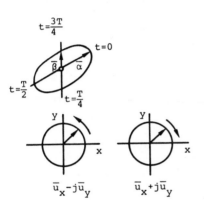

Fig. 4

Maxwell's equations (2) and (4) become, for time-harmonic fields,

$$\begin{cases} \text{div } \bar{D} = P \\ \text{div } \bar{B} = 0 \end{cases} \tag{16}$$

and

$$\begin{cases} \text{curl } \bar{E} = -j\omega\mu_o \bar{H} \\ \text{curl } \bar{H} = j\omega\varepsilon\bar{E} + \bar{J} \end{cases} \quad \text{in vacuum} \tag{17}$$

$$\begin{cases} \text{curl } \bar{E} = -j\omega\mu\bar{H} \\ \text{curl } \bar{H} = \sigma\bar{E} + j\omega\varepsilon\bar{E} \end{cases} \quad \text{in the material}$$

$$= j\omega\varepsilon_o(\varepsilon'_r - j\varepsilon''_r)\bar{E}$$

The constitutive parameters ε,μ,σ depend on the frequency. They result from
    (1) orientation of dipoles that already exist in atoms and molecules

    (2) polarization of atoms and molecules to produce
dipole moments
    (3) displacement (or drift) of conduction ("free")
electrons and ions in tissues.
The influence of the mechanisms on biophenomena (e.g.
transient or permanent alteration of nervous tissue, regulation of the cardiovascular
system, change in blood-brain
barrier permeability, ionic
motion alterations) is not within the province of the electromagneticist; it is discussed
partially in other chapters of
this book. A typical variation
of ε_r' and σ for a biomaterial
is shown in Fig. 5.

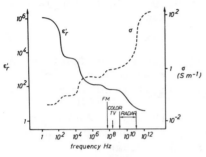

Fig. 5

4. HEAT EQUATION

From (1) it is clear that maximum electromagnetic
power is deposited at points where the electric field is
maximum. This does not necessarily mean that "hot spots"
appear at these points, as other factors, such as heat removal by blood circulation, play an important role. In
fact, the temperature T should be determined from a solution
of the heat equation

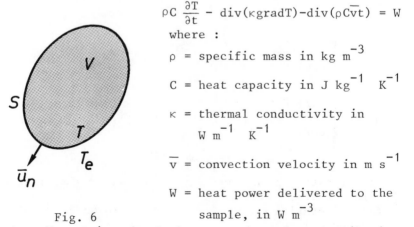

Fig. 6

$$\rho C \frac{\partial T}{\partial t} - \text{div}(\kappa\,\text{grad}T) - \text{div}(\rho C\overline{v}t) = W$$

where :

ρ = specific mass in kg m^{-3}

C = heat capacity in J kg^{-1} K^{-1}

κ = thermal conductivity in W m^{-1} K^{-1}

$\overline{v}$ = convection velocity in m s^{-1}

W = heat power delivered to the sample, in W m^{-3}

The term W contains the Joule power, but also contributions

from biological effects (e.g. metabolic heating). At the
boundary S (Fig. 6), there is an outward heat flux given by

$$-\kappa \frac{\partial T}{\partial n} = H(T-T_e) \tag{19}$$

where H is the surface heat transfer coefficient. A few
typical values for the thermal properties are, in the M.K.S.
system,

Tissue	ρ	C	κ	metabolic rate	Blood flow rate
muscle	1070	3478	0.642	0.7	$0.45\ 10^{-6}$
bone(cortical)	1790	1257	1.46		
blood	930	3897	0.506		

The complex and inhomogeneous character of biological materials turns the solution of the coupled "heat — "Maxwell"
equations into a most challenging problem. A theoretical
solution can give useful indications, but for any application
in practice, e.g. in hyperthermia, actual measurements of
the temperature are a must. Thermometry remains a difficult
problem, in particular with respect to the development of
non-invasive measurement methods.

5. SCALAR WAVES

The simplest example of a structure which can support a
one-dimensional wave is the
transmission line (Fig. 7).
The transmission line is of
importance for the bioelectromagneticist, as it is widely
used to connect components,
e.g. a microwave generator to
an applicator. The voltage on
a lossless transmission line
satisfies the one dimensional
wave equation

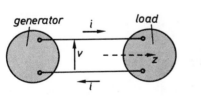

Fig. 7

$$\frac{\partial^2 v}{\partial z^2} - \frac{1}{c^2} \frac{\partial^2 v}{\partial t^2} = 0 \tag{20}$$

The general solution of this equation is

$$v = v_1(z - ct) + v_2(z + ct) \qquad (21)$$

$$\underbrace{}_{\substack{\text{wave to the}\\\text{right}\\\text{(incident)}}} \quad \underbrace{}_{\substack{\text{wave to the}\\\text{left}\\\text{(reflected)}}}$$

The first term, $v_1(z-ct)$, represents a wave to the right, because an observer moving down the z-axis with velocity c sees a constant amplitude. Also, a series of successive snapshots of the $v(z)$ curve shows a curve moving to the right with propagation velocity c (Fig. 8). A time-harmonic wave to the right, in particular, is of the general form

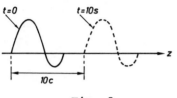

Fig. 8

$$v_1 = a \cos(\omega t - kz + \phi) \qquad (22)$$

where k is the wavenumber

$$k = \frac{\omega}{c} = \frac{2\pi}{\lambda} \qquad (23)$$

and λ is the wavelength. In complex form, (22) becomes

$$V_1 = A\, e^{-jkz} \qquad (A = a\, e^{j\phi}) \qquad (24)$$

The current on a transmission line also satisfies the wave equation (20). Its general variation is related to that of the voltage by

$$i = i_1(z-ct) + i_2(z+ct)$$

$$= \frac{1}{R_c}[\, v_1(z-ct) - v_2(z+ct)\,] \qquad (25)$$

where R_c is the characteristic impedance of the line (typical values : 50Ω, 70Ω or 300Ω). Under time-harmonic conditions :

$$V = A_1\, e^{-jkz} + A_2\, e^{jkz}$$

$$I = \frac{1}{R_c}[\, A_1\, e^{-jkz} - A_2\, e^{jkz}\,] \qquad (26)$$

The ratio $\dfrac{A_2}{A_1}$ is the <u>reflection coefficient K</u> (Fig. 9). Its

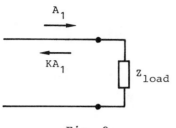

Fig. 9

value is

$$K = \frac{Z_{load} - R_c}{Z_{load} + R_c} \qquad (27)$$

When the line is terminated in a Z_{load} equal to R_c, there are no reflections, and maximum power absorption occurs. This "match" is a desirable situation, which must be realized, for example, when an applicator load is fed from a coaxial line. Matching can be obtained with the help of matching devices, e.g. stub tuners.

A form such as (21) or (_   presents a scalar wave in the z-direction (e.g. a plane acoustic wave). When the wave propagates in an arbitrary s-direction, its mathematical form becomes (Fig. 10)

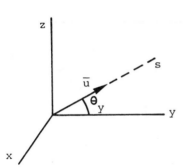

Fig. 10

$$v = a \cos(\omega t - ks + \phi) \qquad (28)$$

Complex :

$$a\, e^{j\phi} e^{-jks} = A\, e^{-jks} \qquad (29)$$

If $\bar{u}$ is the unit vector in the direction s :

$$s = \bar{u}.\bar{r} = x(\bar{u}.\bar{u}_x) + y(\bar{u}.\bar{u}_y) + z(\bar{u}.\bar{u}_z)$$

$$= x \cos\Theta_x + y \cos\Theta_y + z \cos\Theta_z \qquad (30)$$

The complex form of a wave in a direction $\bar{u}$ is therefore

$$A\, e^{-jk\bar{u}.\bar{r}} \qquad (31)$$

6. ELECTROMAGNETIC WAVES. APPLICATORS IN FREE SPACE

As every component of the electric field can be shown to satisfy the wave equation, a plane wave in vacuo can be written in complex form as

$$\overline{E} = \overline{A}_1 \, e^{-jkz} + \overline{A}_2 \, e^{jkz}$$

$$\overline{H} = \frac{1}{R_c} \left[\overline{A}_1 \, e^{-jkz} - \overline{A}_2 \, e^{jkz} \right] \tag{32}$$

Here, the $\overline{A}$'s are constant complex vectors, perpendicular to the direction of propagation z. For a general direction $\overline{u}$ we replace z by $(\overline{u}.\overline{r})$.

Plane waves are a useful model for the representation of the far-field of a current-source $\overline{j}$ (Fig. 1). To show this, let the source radiate in free space (Fig. 11). Under time-harmonic conditions the magnetic field is (Van Bladel 1964)

$$\overline{H}(\overline{r}) = \text{curl} \left[\underbrace{\frac{1}{4\pi} \iiint_V \overline{J}(\overline{r}') \, \frac{e^{-jk|\overline{r}-\overline{r}'|}}{\overline{r}-\overline{r}'} \, dV'}_{\text{vector potential}} \right] \tag{33}$$

The electric field follows from Maxwell's equation as

$$\overline{E} = \frac{1}{j\omega\varepsilon_o} (\text{curl } \overline{H} - \overline{J}) \tag{34}$$

At large distances (i.e. for $R > \frac{2d^2}{\lambda}$ and $R > \lambda$) :

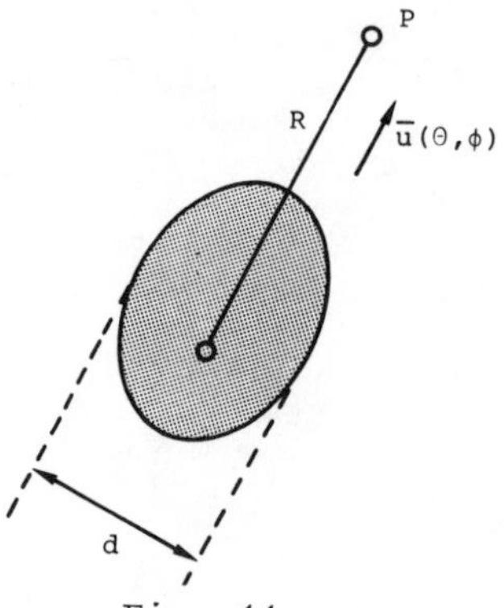

$$\overline{E} = \frac{e^{-jkR}}{R} \, \overline{F}(\theta,\phi)$$

$$\overline{H} = \frac{1}{R_c} \frac{e^{-jkR}}{R} \, \overline{u} \times \overline{F}(\theta,\phi) \tag{35}$$

where

$$R_c = \sqrt{\frac{\mu_0}{\varepsilon_0}} = 377\Omega \tag{36}$$

Fig. 11

$\overline{F}$ is the radiation vector

$$\overline{F} = j\omega\overline{u} \times (\overline{u} \times \frac{\mu_0}{4\pi} \iiint \overline{J}(\overline{r}')e^{jk\overline{u}\cdot\overline{r}'}dV') \qquad (37)$$

Clearly, the $\overline{E}$ and $\overline{H}$ fields are perpendicular to $\overline{u}$, i.e. they are transverse. Comparison with (32) shows that, in the far-field, the radiated field behaves locally like a plane wave.

The radiated field is particularly important for tele-communications applications. In bio-applications, however, the target is commonly immersed in the near-field. The transition from near to far-field can be followed with particular

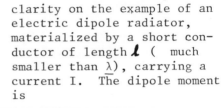

Fig. 12

clarity on the example of an electric dipole radiator, materialized by a short conductor of length l (much smaller than λ), carrying a current I. The dipole moment is

$$P_e = \frac{1}{j\omega} Il = Ql \qquad (38)$$

This source generates a magnetic field

$$H_\phi = jk\frac{Il\,\sin\Theta}{4\pi}\frac{e^{-jkR}}{R} + \frac{Il\,\sin\Theta}{4\pi}\frac{e^{-jkR}}{R^2} \qquad (39)$$

$$\underbrace{\phantom{jk\frac{Il\,\sin\Theta}{4\pi}\frac{e^{-jkR}}{R}}}_{\substack{\text{radiation or}\\\text{distant field}}} \quad \underbrace{\phantom{\frac{Il\,\sin\Theta}{4\pi}\frac{e^{-jkR}}{R^2}}}_{\substack{\text{induction or}\\\text{near field}}}$$

The induction field dominates when kR<<1, i.e. when $R \ll \frac{\lambda}{2\pi}$. The corresponding H_ϕ is $\frac{Il\,\sin\Theta}{4\pi R^2}$, which is the magneto-static value. At large distances, in the radiation field,

$$E_\Theta = -\frac{k^2}{4\pi\epsilon_o} P_e \sin\Theta \frac{e^{-jkR}}{R}$$

$$\qquad\qquad\qquad\qquad\qquad (40)$$

$$H_\phi = -\frac{k^2 c}{4\pi} P_e \sin\Theta \frac{e^{-jkR}}{R}$$

A dipole-type of applicator is shown in Fig. 13, where the radiating element is the protruding central conductor of a coaxial line. The structure is mechanically protected by a teflon bulb, sometimes mounted off-center to modify the radiation pattern. Teflon is transparent for radio waves. The applicator is useful for treating tumors near natural body cavities. A typical frequency of operation is 2450MHz.

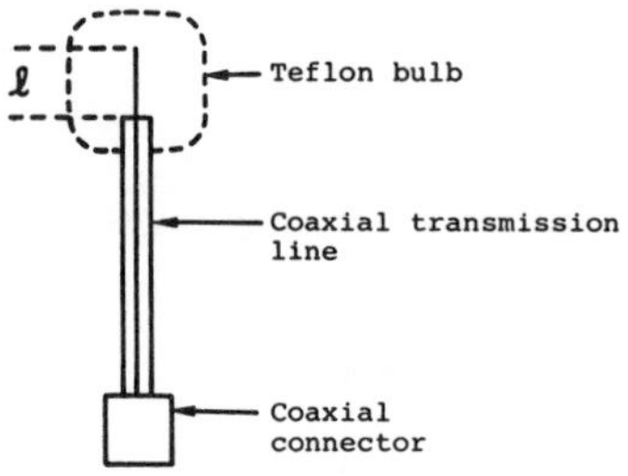

ℓ — Teflon bulb

— Coaxial transmission line

— Coaxial connector

Fig. 13

A second important low-frequency radiator is shown in Fig. 14. It consists of a small current loop, which radiates like a magnetic dipole of moment (Fig. 14)

$$P_m = IS \tag{41}$$

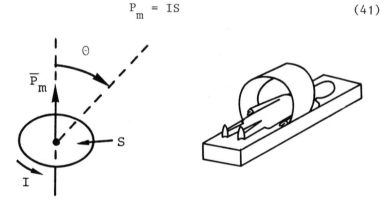

Fig. 14   Fig. 15

The far-fields are now

$$E_\phi = \frac{k^2 R_c}{4\pi} P_m \sin\theta \frac{e^{-jkR}}{R}$$

$$H_\theta = -\frac{k^2}{4\pi} P_m \sin\theta \frac{e^{-jkR}}{R} \tag{42}$$

Another well-known low-frequency applicator, used in whole-body hyperthermia, consists of a single turn of copper sheet (Fig. 15). This loop is an inductance £, which is further tuned out by a series C. The frequency is typically 13.56MHz (λ = 22.1m). The patient is immersed in the near field of the loop.

7. APPLICATORS WITH DIRECTIVE ELEMENTS

As suggested in Fig. 1 the primary fields from $\bar{j}$ are often deflected (and concentrated) by conducting elements V_2. At low frequencies, these elements could be the plates of a capacitor (Fig. 16). At microwave frequencies the target is often fully enclosed in a resonator, to avoid power leakage (Fig. 17). To understand resonator behavior, consider first a low-frequency (R,$\pounds$,C) circuit (Fig. 18a). If we keep the input voltage independent of frequency, and plot the output voltage V_R as a function of ω, we obtain a curve of the type shown in Fig. 18b. Maximum response occurs at an angular frequency ω_o given (for sufficiently small R) by

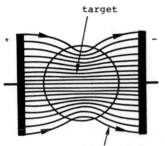

target

lines of force

Fig. 16

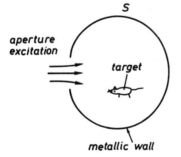

aperture
excitation

target

metallic wall

Fig. 17

$$\omega_{res} = \omega_o = 2\pi\nu_o = \frac{1}{\sqrt{\pounds C}} \quad (43)$$

The sharpness of the peak, which increases as R decreases, is expressed by the quality factor Q, where

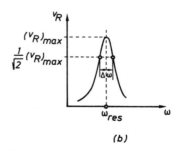

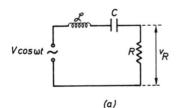

(a)

(b)

Fig. 18

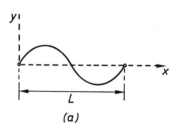

(a)

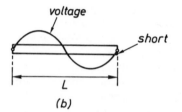

(b)

Fig. 19

$$Q = \frac{\omega_o}{\Delta\omega} = \frac{\nu_o}{\Delta\nu} = \frac{\omega_o \ell}{R} \qquad (44)$$

The interval $\Delta\nu$ is the "band-width", i.e. the frequency difference between the points at which V_R has decreased to $(1/\sqrt{2})$ of its maximum value (the 3dB points). A high quality factor goes with a sharp response and a small bandwidth.

As a next item in our analysis we now consider the flexible string, a one-dimensional structure with distributed constants. Strings are found in numerous musical instruments. They vibrate according to an infinite number of "modes", each of which oscillates independently as an ℓ-C circuit. The oscillating amplitude of mode "n" is

$$y = y_n(x)\cos\omega_n t = A \sin(\frac{n\pi x}{L})\cos(n \frac{\pi c}{L} t) \quad (45)$$

where n is an integer (Fig. 19a). The space part, i.e. $y_n(x)$, is a solution of the differential problem

$$\frac{d^2 y_n}{dx^2} + k_n^2 y_n = 0$$

$$y_n = 0 \quad \text{for } x = 0, \ x = L \qquad (46)$$

The boundary conditions require k_n to be a multiple of $(n\pi/L)$. As the amplitude $y(x,t)$ satisfies the same equation as the voltage on a transmission line, the characteristic vibrations of the string are also relevant for the short-circuited transmission line (Fig. 19b).

The previous considerations show that the three-dimensional resonator of Fig. 17 may be expected to vibrate in a triply infinite number of modes. A detailed analysis (Van Bladel 1964) shows that the electric field of a mode is of the form

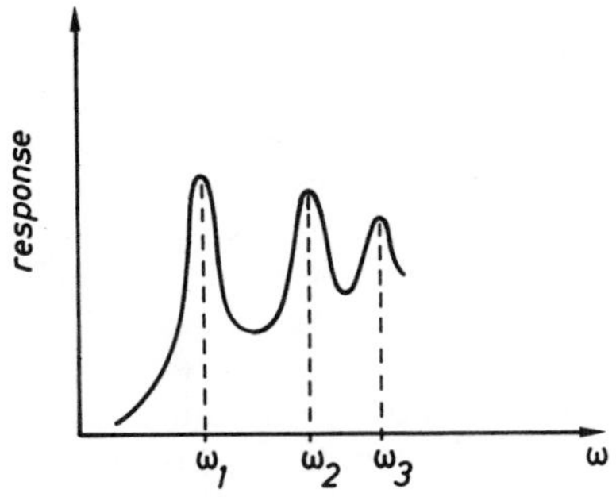

$$\bar{e} = \bar{e}_n(\bar{r})\ \cos\omega_n t \qquad (47)$$

where $\bar{e}_n$ satisfies

$$-\text{curl curl } \bar{e}_n + k_n^2\bar{e}_n = 0$$

$\bar{e}_n$ perpendicular to S

$$(48)$$

The angular frequency ω_n is equal to $(k_n c)$. The response of the cavity as a function of frequency is shown schematically in Fig. 20. We recognize a series of peaks, corresponding to the successive resonant fre-

Fig. 20

quencies of the modes. Around these frequencies the field distribution is practically $\bar{e}_n(\bar{r})$. To ensure that a strong field exists at a given point P, we should therefore select a mode with a strong $\bar{e}_n$ in P, and excite the resonator at the resonant frequency of that mode.

8. WAVEGUIDES

A metallic pipe is capable of carrying an infinite number of waves, of the form (Fig. 21)

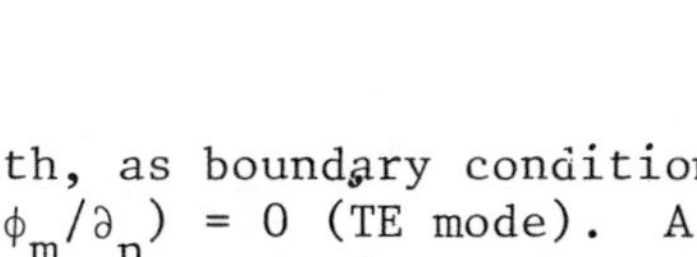

$$\bar{E} = \bar{A}\ e^{-\sqrt{k_n^2-k^2}\,z} \qquad (49)$$

Fig. 21

In this expression $k = \omega\sqrt{\varepsilon\mu}$, and k_n^2 is an eigenvalue of the problem

$$\frac{\partial^2\phi_n}{\partial x^2} + \frac{\partial^2\phi_n}{\partial y^2} + k_n^2\phi_n = 0 \qquad (50)$$

with, as boundary condition on C, either $\phi_n = 0$ (TM mode) or $(\partial\phi_m/\partial_n) = 0$ (TE mode). A look at (49) shows that each mode has a cut-off frequency

$$\nu_c = \frac{c}{2\pi\sqrt{\varepsilon_r\mu_r}}\ k_n \qquad (51)$$

Above this frequency $(k_n^2-k^2)$ is negative, and the wave is propagated. Below this frequency $(k_n^2-k^2)$ is positive, and the mode is attenuated. The frequency scale of Fig. 22, drawn

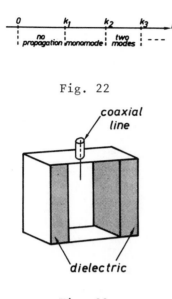

Fig. 22

Fig. 23

with k as a parameter, shows clearly how many modes are propagated. It is seen, from (51), that filling the guide with a dielectric lowers the cut-off frequency or, equivalently, reduces the dimensions of the guide for monomode propagation at a given operating frequency (a desirable feature in most applications).

A classical waveguide applicator is shown in Fig. 23. It is in the form of a parallelepipedic metallic box, open on one side (through which the power escapes towards the biological target), and excited through a short coaxial antenna of the type discussed in Sec. 6. The waveguide is lined with dielectric to reduce its overall dimensions.

By terminating the waveguide with two short-circuiting planes a fully enclosed volume is created (a resonator). A typical modal field distribution is sketched in Fig. 24. Clearly, maximum exposure is obtained by locating the target (a mouse for example) at the center P of the resonator.

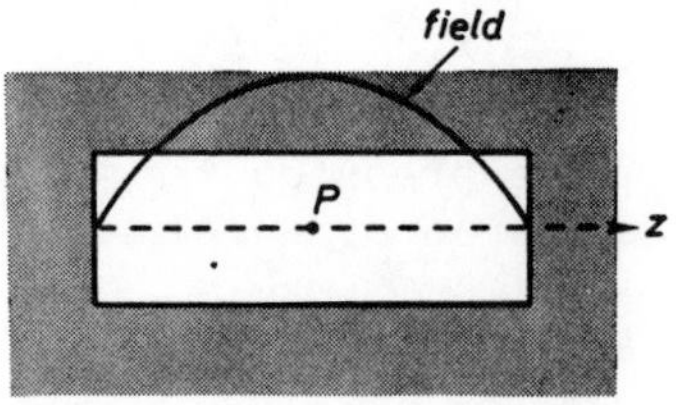

Fig. 24

9. SKIN EFFECT

We now turn to the difficult problem of determining the field distribution in the conducting bio-target V_1 (Fig. 1). Most important here is the limited penetration which the fields can achieve in V_1 at high frequencies. A rough measure of the penetration depth in a good conductor is given by

$$\delta = \sqrt{\frac{2}{\omega \mu \sigma}} \ \text{m} \tag{52}$$

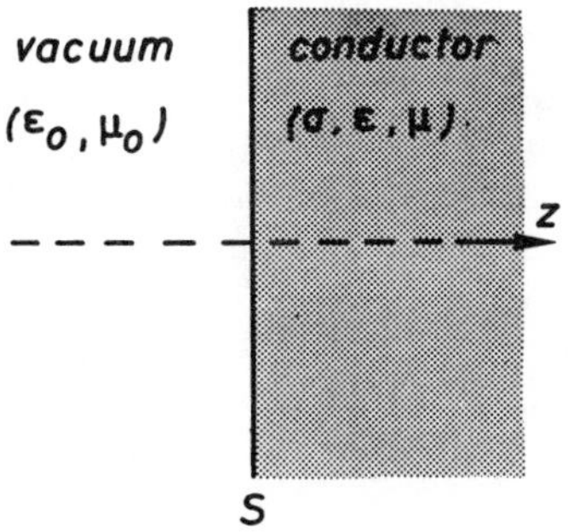

Fig. 25

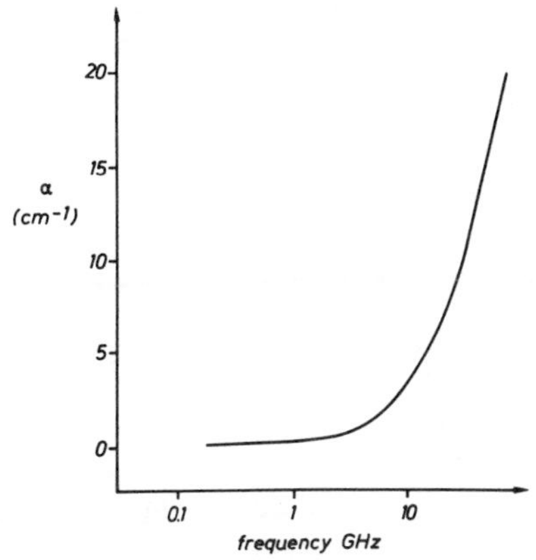

Fig. 26

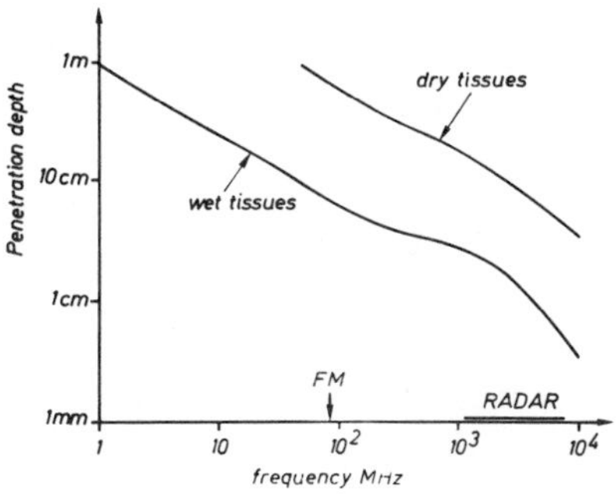

Fig. 27

The phenomenon can be analyzed with particular clarity by considering a plane wave propagating in the z-direction. In vacuum a typical component satisfies

$$\frac{\partial^2 e}{\partial z^2} - \varepsilon_0 \mu_0 \frac{\partial^2 e}{\partial t^2} = 0 \qquad (53)$$

In a conductor, from Maxwell's equations, (53) is replaced by

$$\frac{\partial^2 e}{\partial z^2} - \sigma\mu \frac{\partial e}{\partial t} - \varepsilon\mu \frac{\partial^2 e}{\partial t^2} = 0 \qquad (54)$$

Under time-harmonic conditions :

$$\frac{d^2 E}{dz^2} + \underbrace{(\omega^2 \varepsilon\mu - j\omega\mu\sigma)}_{-(\alpha + j\beta)^2} E = 0 \qquad (55)$$

The general solution of (55) is

$$E = A_1 e^{-\alpha z} e^{-j\beta z} + A_2 e^{\alpha z} e^{j\beta z} \qquad (56)$$

Each term is a wave which decreases exponentially in the direction of propagation. Values of α for water are shown in Fig. 26. The penetration depth (value of z for which the fields decrease to $1/e$ of their value on S) is $(1/\alpha)$. Some typical values of $(1/\alpha)$ are shown in Fig. 27. In a good conductor (i.e. in a medium where $\omega\mu\sigma \gg \omega^2\varepsilon\mu$ or, equivalently, $\omega\varepsilon \ll \sigma$),

$$E = A_1 e^{-\frac{z}{\delta}} e^{-j\frac{z}{\delta}} + A_2 e^{\frac{z}{\delta}} e^{j\frac{z}{\delta}} \qquad (57)$$

where δ is given in (52) Cu, for example, is a very good
conductor up to optical frequencies : its δ is of the order
of 1μm at wavelengths in the cm range. The data appearing
in Fig. 27 underline one of the fundamental problems con-
fronting the bioelectromagneticist. To reach deep regions
of the human body by direct radiation from an outside source,
the frequency must be fairly low, say in the 10-100MHz range.
This requirement conflicts with the rule that an applicator
should be large with respect to λ if its energy is to be
concentrated in a restricted volume (a tumor for example).
In the frequency range indicated λ varies from 30 m to 3 m.
As "large" applicators become enormous in that range,
the latter is mostly used for whole-body hyperthermia. At
slightly higher frequencies focussing arrays become popular,
while in the GHz range the applicators are mostly used for
subcutaneous irradiation.

10. THE TOTAL ELECTROMAGNETIC PROBLEM

Biologists are strongly interested in low-frequency
fields and their effects, particularly at power frequencies
(50 or 60Hz). Of special concern are the strong electric
fields (up to 20kV m^{-1}) which exist under power transmission
lines. At such frequencies Fig. 27 shows that the skin
effect is practically inexistant in humans, hence that
fields and currents permeate the whole body. The general
electromagnetic problem of Fig. 1, so difficult in its
full generality, becomes more tractable at low frequencies.
In that range the fields may be expanded in a series of the
form

$$\bar{E} = \bar{E}_0 + jk\bar{E}_1 + \ldots \tag{58}$$

where $\bar{E}_0$ is the dominant term at low frequencies. It is easy
to show (Van Bladel 1964) that

$$\mathrm{curl}\ \bar{E}_0 = 0$$
$$\mathrm{curl}\ \bar{H}_0 = 0 \tag{59}$$

The low frequency field is therefore irrotational (quasi-
stationary), and can be derived from potentials. We write :

$$\bar{E}_0 = -\mathrm{grad}\ \phi_0$$
$$\bar{H}_0 = -\mathrm{grad}\ \psi_0 \tag{60}$$

The problem sketched in Fig. 1 is now reduced to the solution of a <u>potential</u> problem, the unknowns of which are scalar functions instead of vector functions.

In the more general situation, for arbitrary frequencies, the mathematics become very heavy. Lack of space does not permit any detailed discussion here, hence only a few general comments will be made. It is clear, for example, that the knowledge of the "incident power density" is not sufficient to determine the total field in P (Fig. 1). This field, sum of the incident field and the "target" field, is not simply related to $\bar{E}^i$, $\bar{H}^i$. The total field may, for example, evidence strong variations with respect to frequency, location (hot spots) and polarization. The influence of polarization is illustrated in Fig. 28. In Fig. 28a a thin wire is illuminated by an incident field $\bar{E}^i$ perpendicular to the axis. Induced currents do not develop, as electrons can hardly move transversely. There is little reaction from the wire, hence negligible heat production. In Fig. 28b, $\bar{E}^i$ is parallel with the axis, and strong longitudinal currents can develop. These currents are particularly intense at well-defined <u>resonant frequencies</u>, the lowest of which corresponds to $\ell \approx \lambda/2$. Analog effects can be expected for the human body, as shown in Fig. 29. The lowest resonance frequency for man is about 70MHz, while it is of the order of 1GHz for a small animal. Tests must

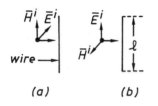

(a)   (b)

Fig. 28

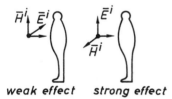

weak effect   strong effect

Fig. 29

therefore mention carefully frequency and direction of linear polarization of the incident wave. Circularly polarised waves are rotation-insensitive, which makes them attractive for certain applications, e.g. rat-exposure systems.

The electromagneticist, confronted with the general numerical problem of Fig. 1, has several methods of solution at his disposal, e.g. finite elements, finite differences, extended boundary conditions and integral equations. To illustrate one of these methods, namely "integral equations",

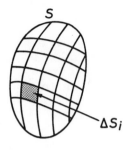

Fig. 30

we consider the simple example of a charged metallic body (Fig. 30). The distribution of the charge density ρ_s on S is the unknown. The charge creates a constant potential on S hence, for $\overline{r}$ on S,

$$\phi(\overline{r}) = \frac{1}{4\pi\epsilon_o} \iint_s \frac{\rho_s(\overline{r}')dS'}{|\overline{r}-\overline{r}'|} = C$$

(61)

Eq. (61) is an integral equation for $\rho_s(\overline{r})$. To solve it numerically we subdivide S into N patches ΔS_i, and choose ρ_s to be constant on each patch. The integral equation now becomes

$$\rho_{s1}\left[\frac{1}{4\pi\epsilon_o} \iint_{\Delta S_1} \frac{dS'}{|\overline{r}-\overline{r}'|}\right] + \ldots + \rho_{sN}\left[\frac{1}{4\pi\epsilon_o} \iint_{\Delta S_N} \frac{dS'}{|\overline{r}-\overline{r}'|}\right] = C$$

(62)

By requiring (62) to be satisfied at N points $\overline{r}$, suitably chosen on S, we obtain N equations with N unknowns, a problem which is amenable to solution on a digital computer. Such a procedure "discretizes" the continuous function $\rho_s(\overline{r})$ through a set of values at N points, with an accuracy which increases with N, i.e. with the fineness of the subdivision.

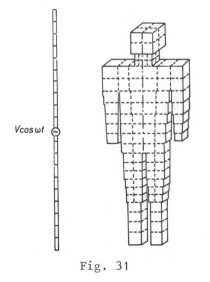

Vcosωt

Fig. 31

In the more general problem of Fig. 1 the unknown is the (complex) current density in the target, for which an integral equation can again be derived. Fig. 31 shows how the numerical solution proceeds by subdividing the target (a human body) into three-dimensional blocks, over which $\overline{J}$ (or $\overline{E}$) is assumed constant. A similar subdivision is performed for the primary source (an antenna), as the exciting voltage Vcosωt is given, but the resulting current distribution I(z) is unknown. The field problem becomes more difficult yet when the media are non-linear, a situation which arises, for example, in the study of cell membranes. Such problems, and the propagation of solitons in these media (A. Scott 1970), are beyond the scope of the present review.

11. REFERENCES

Adair ER (ed)(1983). "Microwaves and Thermoregulation".
   New York : Academic Press.
Nat. Council Rad. Prot. Meas. (1981). "Radiofrequency
   Electromagnetic Fields". Report no. 67, Washington :
   NCRP.
Osepchuk JM (ed)(1983). "Biological Effects of Electromagnetic
   Radiation", New York : IEEE Press.
Presman AS (1970). "Electromagnetic Fields and Life".
   New York : Plenum Press.
Scott A (1970). "Active and Nonlinear Wave Propagation in
   Electronics". New York : Wiley.
Storm FK (ed)(1983). "Hyperthermia in Cancer Therapy".
   Boston : G.K. Hall.
Van Bladel J (1964). "Electromagnetic Fields". New York :
   Mc Graw Hill, p. 191,214,225,297 (to be reprinted, with
   corrections, by the Hemisphere Corp. in april 1985).
Van Bladel J (1984). "Relativity and Engineering". Berlin :
   Springer Verlag, p. 70,108,130.

Electromagnetic Fields and Neurobehavioral Function, pages 23–45
© 1988 Alan R. Liss, Inc.

ELECTROMAGNETIC ORIENTATION: A RELATIVISTIC APPROACH

Ad. J. Kalmijn

Scripps Institution of Oceanography
University of California, San Diego
La Jolla, CA 92093

Through interaction with the earth's magnetic field, tidal and wind-driven ocean currents induce electric fields, which may inform sharks, skates, and rays about their drift with the water. Furthermore, by their swimming movements, the animals induce electric fields, which may provide the physical basis for their magnetic compass sense. Both the ocean-current fields and the fields induced by the animals' movements result from the motion of a conductor, either the water or the fish, through the earth's magnetic field.

To detect the motional-electric fields, elasmobranch fishes would apply their highly sensitive electroreceptors, the ampullae of Lorenzini. According to physical law, however, the animals can measure only the electric fields in the frames of reference in which the sense organs are at rest. But, if the fishes are not moving in the rest frames of their own sense organs, what are the electric fields from which they might infer their drift and magnetic compass headings relative to the earth's frame of reference?

This question assumes that it would be feasible for fishes, when drifting or swimming with constant velocity, to sense their motion electrically by the fields they detect in their receptor frames of reference. However, would not such an idea violate the principle of relativity, as proposed by Galileo in 1632 for mechanical phenomena and extended by Einstein in 1905 to include electromagnetic phenomena as well? The ancestors of modern elasmobranch fishes may have been the first to resolve these fundamental problems.

The theory of electromagnetic orientation has been introduced previously (Kalmijn 1974, 1984). The present article addresses some of the subtle issues that the author has
struggled with for years. The reader will be encouraged to
view the world through the animals' senses, rather than remain an outside observer. The difficulties will be, not so
much in the physics itself, as in its application to animals
moving about in large volumes of seawater, where neither the
fishes nor the water are ideal insulators or conductors.

ELECTRIC AND MAGNETIC FIELD TRANSFORMATIONS

In special relativity, electric and magnetic fields are
measured in different inertial frames of reference, and the
results are related to one another mathematically by transformation formulas. In particular, if in the earth frame of
reference $E_e\perp$ and $B_e\perp$ are the electric and magnetic field
components perpendicular to the velocity $\mathbf{v}$ of a moving animal, then the corresponding components in the animal's frame
of reference are (Panofsky and Phillips 1962)

$$E_a\perp \;=\; \gamma\,(\,E_e\perp \;+\; \mathbf{v}\times B_e\perp\,) \quad \text{and} \tag{1}$$

$$B_a\perp \;=\; \gamma\,(\,B_e\perp \;-\; \frac{1}{c^2}\,\mathbf{v}\times E_e\perp\,), \tag{2}$$

where c is the speed of light and γ denotes $[1-(v/c)^2]^{-1/2}$.
The components $E_e\|$ and $B_e\|$ parallel to the velocity $\mathbf{v}$ re-
main unaltered under transformation from the earth's to the
animal's frame of reference, or

$$E_a\| \;=\; E_e\| \quad \text{and} \tag{3}$$

$$B_a\| \;=\; B_e\|. \tag{4}$$

At speeds much lower than the speed of light, expressions (1) and (2) simplify considerably, as γ tends to unity
and $1/c^2\,\mathbf{v}\times E_e\perp$ becomes negligibly small compared to $B_e\perp$.
Thus, together the perpendicular and parallel field compo-
nents yield to good approximation

$$E_a \;\simeq\; E_e \;+\; \mathbf{v}\times B_e \quad \text{and} \tag{5}$$

$$B_a \;\simeq\; B_e, \tag{6}$$

in which $\mathbf{v} \times \mathbf{B_e} \equiv \mathbf{v} \times \mathbf{B_e}\perp$. If, in the earth's frame, the electric field $\mathbf{E_e}$ is zero, equation (5) reduces further to

$$\mathbf{E_a} \simeq \mathbf{v} \times \mathbf{B_e}. \qquad (7)$$

Hence, an animal moving in the earth's frame of reference with a velocity $\mathbf{v}$, in the presence of a magnetic field $\mathbf{B_e}$, is in its own frame of reference subject to an electric field $\mathbf{E_a}$, which approximately equals the electric field $\mathbf{E_e}$ in the earth's frame, plus the $\mathbf{v} \times \mathbf{B_e}$ induced by the animal's motion (Eq. 5). The magnetic field $\mathbf{B_a}$ in the frame of the moving animal is about the same as the magnetic field $\mathbf{B_e}$ in the frame of the earth (Eq. 6). When $\mathbf{E_e}$ vanishes, $\mathbf{E_a}$ is only due to the animal's motion (Eq. 7, Fig. 1).

The electric and magnetic fields in the earth's frame of reference may also be expressed in terms of the electric field $\mathbf{E_a}$ and the magnetic field $\mathbf{B_a}$ in the animal's frame by

$$\mathbf{E_e} \simeq \mathbf{E_a} - \mathbf{v} \times \mathbf{B_a} \quad \text{and} \qquad (8)$$

$$\mathbf{B_e} \simeq \mathbf{B_a}, \qquad (9)$$

where the minus sign indicates that the earth's frame moves with a velocity $-\mathbf{v}$ with respect to the frame of the animal.

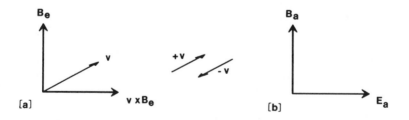

Fig. 1. Electric and magnetic field vectors at position of fish: (a) in earth's frame of reference, in which fish moves with uniform velocity $\mathbf{v}$, and (b) in animal's frame of reference, in which fish is at rest, assuming $\mathbf{E_e} = \mathbf{0}$. The velocity $+\mathbf{v}$ refers to the motion of the animal's frame and equals the fish's velocity $\mathbf{v}$ as observed in the frame of the earth. The velocity $-\mathbf{v}$ refers to the motion of the earth's frame as observed in the frame of the animal.

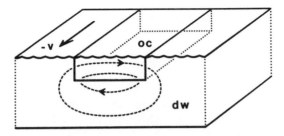

Fig. 2. In the reference frame of an animal drifting with the water, the ocean current (oc) is at rest, while, outside the stream, the whole world is moving with a velocity $-\mathbf{v}$. Indicated is the induced electric current, which gives rise to the ohmic $\rho\mathbf{J}$ field that the drifting animal detects, when in the southern hemisphere. The induced electric current flows across the stream and completes its circuit through deeper water layers (dw) and bottom sediments.

Because, at low velocities, the magnetic fields in the earth's frame and the animal's frame are nearly equal according to equation (6), the subscripts of $\mathbf{B}_e$ and $\mathbf{B}_a$ will be omitted. Nevertheless, the $\mathbf{B}$ in the vector product $\mathbf{v} \times \mathbf{B}$ will still formally refer to the magnetic field in the frame of reference with respect to which the motion takes place.

Approximate equations (5) through (7) express the results of Faraday's (1832) classical researches in motional electricity, and led Einstein in 1905 '... more or less directly to the special theory of relativity ...' (Shankland 1964). For elasmobranch fishes, $\mathbf{v} \times \mathbf{B}$ indeed is '... nothing else but an electric field ...' $\mathbf{E}_a$. The origin of this purely electric field will be further discussed under the heading 'electric versus magnetic field detection.'

Note added in proof: Although purely coincidental in the classical theory, the equivalence of $\mathbf{E}_a$ and $\mathbf{v} \times \mathbf{B}$ is now understood to be a direct consequence of the relativity postulates, as reflected by the above derivation. Actually, Einstein (1905) developed the special theory of relativity, just because he believed that this classical coincidence had a deeper ground. Whereas most relativistic phenomena become apparent only at high speed, the $\mathbf{v} \times \mathbf{B}$ term is a prime example of a low-speed relativistic effect, by decree.

ELECTRIC FIELDS OF OCEAN CURRENTS

In the reference frame of the earth, a tidal or wind-driven ocean current, flowing at a horizontal velocity $\mathbf{v}$, induces, by interaction with the vertical component of the earth's magnetic field $\mathbf{B_V}$, a motional electromotive force per unit length $\mathbf{v} \times \mathbf{B_V}$, normal to $\mathbf{v}$ and $\mathbf{B_V}$, both in the water and in the animals drifting with it (Longuet-Higgins et al. 1954). The relevance of the horizontal component of the earth's magnetic field will be discussed shortly.

In the frame of a fish drifting with the flow of water, the ocean current is at rest (Fig. 2), while, according to equation (7), the world is invaded by a vast electric field

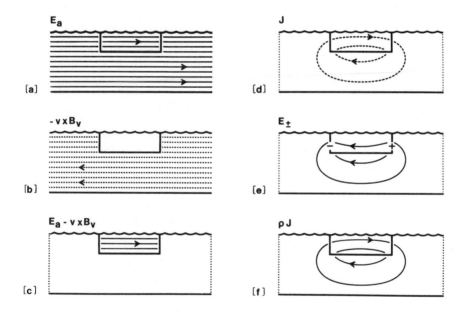

Fig. 3. Motional-electric field of ocean current, observed in reference frame of drifting animal. (a) $\mathbf{E_a}$ field imposed upon fish, assuming $\mathbf{E_e} = \mathbf{0}$, (b) $-\mathbf{v} \times \mathbf{B_V}$ field induced by apparent motion of outside world, (c) vector sum of imposed $\mathbf{E_a}$ field and induced $-\mathbf{v} \times \mathbf{B_V}$ field, (d) current density field $\mathbf{J}$, (e) $\mathbf{E_\pm}$ field of charge accumulations, and (f) ohmic $\rho\mathbf{J}$ field, equal to vector sum of imposed $\mathbf{E_a}$ field, induced $-\mathbf{v} \times \mathbf{B_V}$ field, and $\mathbf{E_\pm}$ field of charge accumulations.

E_a (Fig. 3a). If E_e is assumed to be zero, for the moment, E_a about equals the $v \times B_v$ that the stream induces in the frame of the earth. In the animal's frame, however, the whole world, except the stream, is moving with a velocity $-v$, inducing an electromotive force per unit length $- v \times B_v$ (Fig. 3b), which precisely cancels the electric field E_a in the whole world, but the stream (Fig. 3c).

In other words, in the earth's frame of reference, the charge carriers of the stream are subject to an induced electromotive force per unit length $v \times B_v$, whereas, in the animal's frame, the same charge carriers are subject to a purely electric field E_a. In the earth's frame, the force on the charge carriers is attributed to the flow of water. In the animal's frame, however, the water is at rest, and the force appears to have its cause outside the stream.

If, in the earth's frame, the velocity v and the magnetic field B_v in the vicinity of the drifting animal are considered to be uniform and independent of time, then the electric field E_a, in the animal's frame, is locally uniform as well. Thus, integrated around any measuring loop at rest in the animal's frame of reference, whether completely within the fish or partially through the flowing water, the E_a field as such fails to produce appreciable potential differences across the thin electroreceptive membranes.

However, the E_a field of the stream causes an electric current of density J to flow normal to the drift of the water (Fig. 3d). This current gives rise to accumulations of electrical charges along the boundaries of the stream, where the $E_a - v \times B_v$ field is discontinuous (Fig. 3c). The electric field $E_\pm$ of those charges (Fig. 3e) not only provides the driving force for the current to complete its circuit through deeper water layers and bottom sediments, but also counteracts the E_a field in the stream, thereby yielding a continuous current density J around the circuit.

Along its path, the electric current develops an ohmic field ρJ, with ρ the resistivity of the medium (Fig. 3f). The ρJ provides the force needed to overcome the viscous drag of the charge carriers. The current density J adjusts itself so that the viscous drag just balances the total electrical force. Thus, outside the stream, ρJ equals the $E_\pm$ field of the charge accumulations, driving the external current density J, whereas in the stream, ρJ equals the sum of the E_a field, which drives the current density J, and the $E_\pm$ field of the charge accumulations, tending to diminish J.

Because the local ρJ field depends on the resistivities of the water and the fish, it is far from uniform, unlike the E_a field. Thus, integrated around any measuring loop at rest in the animal's frame of reference, the ρJ can lead to sizeable potential differences across the sensory epithelia, if the fish and, especially, its detection system are sufficiently resistive relative to the seawater medium. It is the strategically distorted ρJ field, not the virtually uniform E_a field, that the drifting animal detects.

But, how does the ρJ field relate to the more informative, yet elusive E_a field? In the stream, ρJ can, in fact, vary from near zero to almost the full E_a. How much ρJ is less than E_a depends on the degree of charge accumulation along the boundaries of the stream, while the charge accumulation itself is determined by the relative resistances of the current path across the stream, by which the charges collect, and of the return path through deeper water and the ocean floor, by which the charges are carried off.

Thus, where the water flows through a highly insulated, rocky channel, such as a fjord, the electric current density J causes substantial charge accumulations at the channel walls, so that the $E_\pm$ field almost completely cancels the E_a field. Consequently, the current density J is negligibly weak in the stream, and the ρJ field, which the drifting animal would have to detect, nearly vanishes.

In the open ocean, however, the electric current tends to flow more freely through deeper water layers and bottom sediments, thereby leading to only small charge accumulations at the boundaries of the stream. Consequently, the often strong, wind-driven surface currents usually lack $E_\pm$ fields of appreciable strength, and, in most of the stream, the ρJ fields closely approach the elusive E_a fields.

Under transformation from the animal's to the earth's frame of reference, ρJ remains virtually the same for the low speeds considered. That is, whether the situation is analyzed in the animal's or the earth's frame of reference, the drifting fish always detects just the ρJ field. Fortunately, ρJ attains its greatest strength in the open ocean, where orientational cues are needed most.

By interaction with the horizontal component of the earth's magnetic field B_h, ocean currents also give rise to vertically directed $v \times B_h$ fields in the earth's frame, and corresponding E_a fields in the animal's frame. The ensuing ρJ fields remain weak, however, as the air-water interface prevents sizeable current densities to develop. Thus, the ρJ fields of wind-driven ocean currents result mainly from interaction with the vertical component of the earth's magnetic field and are predominantly horizontal in direction.

INTERPRETATION OF FIELDS INDUCED BY OCEAN CURRENTS

The question remains whether the drifting animal, by sensing the ohmic ρJ field in its own frame of reference, really can establish the magnitude and direction of its velocity v with respect to the earth's frame of reference. According to the principle of relativity, the animal cannot (Stratton 1941), at least not without further information regarding just that part of the world relative to which it wishes to determine the velocity of its drift.

In the open ocean, the fish may tentatively assume that the ρJ field is exclusively due to the drift of the water, i.e., $E_e = 0$, and that deeper water layers offer suitable, low-resistance return paths, so that little charge accumulation occurs and ρJ nearly attains the full strength of E_a. If correct, the animal could infer the existence of another frame of reference, that of the deeper water, in which the $v \times B_v$ it induces about equals the ρJ it detects.

The drifting fish might further assume that the deeper water layers, forming the main part of the return path, are at rest in the earth's frame of reference. If the animal is correct again, it could, to good approximation, take the reference frame, in which the $v \times B_v$ it induces equals the ρJ it detects, as that of the earth, and identify the velocity v, derived from the ρJ estimate of $v \times B_v$, with that of its drift relative to the bottom. An electrical means of determining B_v will be mentioned in the next section.

By thus inferring its velocity v with respect to the earth's frame of reference, the fish does not violate the principle of relativity, since the interpretation of the ohmic ρJ field in terms of its drift depends entirely on the assumptions that the fish has to make about the ambient electric field E_e in the earth's frame of reference, the relative resistances of the stream and the return path, and the motion of deeper water layers with respect to ground.

If the resistance of the return path is not negligible compared to the resistance across the stream, then the field of the charge accumulations partially cancels the original E_a field, leaving a weaker ρJ for the fish to detect. Thus, to estimate the velocity of its drift correctly, the animal must have information on the degree of field cancelation due to the finite resistance of the return path.

If, in the earth's frame, the ambient electric field E_e differs from zero due to the presence of extraneous fields of various nature (Kalmijn 1974), the fish would, without correction, make a corresponding error in its inferred drift velocity v. If the deeper water layers are not at rest, the inferred velocity would not refer to ground, but rather to the vertically averaged, resistivity-weighted velocity of the water and bottom sediments (Sanford 1971).

In deep-ocean waters, the ρJ fields of strong, wind-driven surface currents may provide the drifting animal with excellent estimates of its ground velocity, if indeed the ambient electric field E_e in the earth's frame of reference and the field $E_\pm$ due to the charge accumulations contribute little to ρJ. When the deeper water layers are moving as well, although with lower velocity, the animal's drift would refer to them rather than to ground.

In coastal waters, the conditions are often less ideal. Yet, the animal can make equally good use of the ρJ field it detects, if it occasionally checks the actual relation between ρJ and its drift v by diving to sufficient depth or, preferably, to the bottom, as sharks have been observed to do (Carey, pers. comm.). Even when the magnitude of the inferred drift is not very accurate, its general direction may still present invaluable orientational cues.

In protected waters, the ρJ fields of nearby ocean currents may be detected even in the absence of any local water flow. By diving to the bottom, the fish could readily identify the ρJ field with the ambient electric field E_e and treat it as such (Kalmijn 1984). Thus, the motional-electric fields of ocean currents offer potentially important orientational cues in those waters as well.

In short, the subtle difficulties of detecting and, especially, of interpreting the oceans' motional–electric fields must not be taken too lightly. Even though the animals receive detectable signals from their drift with the water, they still need, in order to interpret those signals, further knowledge of the physical conditions about which they wish to gather more specific information.

Nevertheless, despite these complexities, the motional-electric fields of ocean currents offer reliable orientational cues for fishes that are familiar with their physical environment, whether by exploration or experience. Marine elasmobranchs indeed have a cunning ability to orient to the electric fields they normally encounter in the oceanic environment, as will be detailed in a later section.

Thus, marine sharks, skates, and rays may have correctly applied the electromagnetic theory long before it was formulated scientifically. Naturally, the fishes need not have any knowledge of the physical principles on which they base their expert behavior, despite the author's objectionable manner of speaking, which often seems to impart great wisdom to the animals that he respects so highly.

ELECTRIC FIELD OF SWIMMING FISH

When, in the earth's frame of reference, a fish swims, on a level course, at a velocity v relative to the water, while the water is at rest, it induces by interaction with the horizontal component of the earth's magnetic field B_h, a motional electromotive force per unit length $v \times B_h$, parallel to its dorsoventral axis (Kalmijn 1974). Interaction with the vertical component of the earth's magnetic field B_v leads to a similar electromotive force along the transverse axis of the animal, as will be detailed presently.

Even though swimming relative to the water, the fish is at rest in its own frame of reference (Fig. 4), in which, by equation (7), it is exposed to a vast electric field E_a (Fig. 5a), where E_a about equals the $v \times B_h$ that the animal induces in the frame of the earth, if E_e may be regarded to vanish. Relative to the fish, however, the whole world is moving with a velocity $-v$, inducing an electromotive force per unit length $- v \times B_h$ (Fig. 5b), which precisely cancels the E_a field everywhere, except in the animal (Fig. 5c).

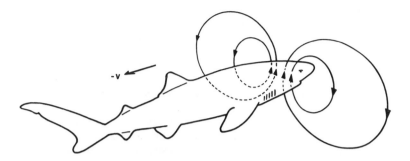

Fig. 4. In the rest frame of a fish heading east, the whole ocean is moving at a velocity −**v**. By interaction with the horizontal magnetic component **B**$_h$, an electric current is induced, which produces the ρ**J** field that the animal detects. The electric current flows dorsoventrally across the body, completing its circuit through the seawater medium.

Thus, in the earth's frame, the charge carriers of the moving fish are subject to an electromotive force per unit length **v** × **B**$_h$. In the frame of the animal, however, the same charge carriers are subject to a purely electric field **E**$_a$, imposed upon the fish. Although of apparent outside origin, the **E**$_a$ field is under control of the swimming fish. Furthermore, the medium relative to which the motion takes place is in direct contact with the animal.

If the fish's velocity **v** and the magnetic field **B**$_h$ are locally uniform and independent of time, the **E**$_a$ field in the vicinity of the animal is uniform as well. Thus, integrated around any measuring loop at rest in the animal's frame of reference, the **E**$_a$ field as such produces only negligible potential differences across the thin electroreceptive membranes. Consequently, the **E**$_a$ field itself escapes detection by the fish. Note that, to measure the **E**$_a$ field directly, the entire path of integration, even if partially outside the fish, must be at rest in the frame of the animal.

However, the **E**$_a$ field causes an electric current of density **J** to flow across the fish (Fig. 5d), giving rise to electrical charge accumulations at the animal's ventral and dorsal surfaces, where the **E**$_a$ − **v** × **B**$_h$ field is discontinuous (Fig. 5c). The electric field **E**$_\pm$ of these charges provides the driving force for the electric current to complete

its loop through the surrounding seawater, while reducing
the current within the body (Fig. 5e), thus establishing a
continuous current density **J** around the circuit.

The electric current develops an ohmic ρ**J** field in the
animal and the seawater medium (Fig. 5f). In the fish, the
ρ**J** field equals the sum of the **E**$_a$ and **E**$_\pm$ fields, whereas in
the water it equals just the **E**$_\pm$ field. Unlike **E**$_a$, the ρ**J**
depends on the resistivities of the animal's tissues and the
outside medium, and is highly non-uniform. Therefore, integrated around the above-mentioned measuring loops, the ρ**J**

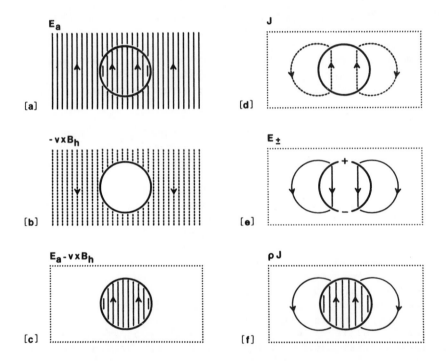

Fig. 5. Motional electric field of swimming fish, observed
in the animal's frame of reference. (a) **E**$_a$ field imposed
upon fish, if in the earth's frame both **E**$_e$ and the velocity
of water are zero, (b) − **v** × **B**$_v$ field induced by the apparent motion of the water, (c) vector sum of imposed **E**$_a$ field
and induced − **v** × **B**$_v$ field, (d) current density field **J**, (e)
E$_\pm$ field of charge accumulations, and (f) ohmic ρ**J** field,
equal to vector sum of imposed **E**$_a$ field, induced − **v** × **B**$_v$
field, and **E**$_\pm$ field of charge accumulations.

field can cause sizeable potential differences, if the fish and, in particular, its sense organs are sufficiently resistive compared to the outside medium. Again, it is not the E_a field, but the ρJ field that the animal detects.

Averaged over the swimming fish, ρJ nearly equals E_a, for the $E_\pm$ field of the charge accumulations, opposing the internal E_a field, remains weak at all times due to the relatively high resistance across the body compared to that of the return path through the seawater medium (Kalmijn 1984). Thus, the electromagnetic orientation mechanism promises to be highly efficient in elasmobranch fishes due to the short-circuiting action of the seawater medium, needed to prevent any charge accumulation from reducing the ρJ field.

The ρJ field hardly changes when transformed from the animal's to the earth's frame of reference. While in the frame of the fish ρJ tends to E_a, in the earth's frame it tends to $v \times B_h$, where E_a and $v \times B_h$ refer to the same field observed in different reference frames. In previous papers, the situation was analyzed in the frame of the earth, with identical results, of course. Biologically, however, the real challenge is to explain the problem of magnetic orientation from the fish's, electrical point of view.

By interacting with the vertical magnetic component B_v, the animal also induces a transversely directed $v \times B_v$. The corresponding E_a field produces again a strong, average ρJ field, as only little charge accumulates, in this instance on the lateral surfaces of the fish. Thus, the ρJ fields resulting from interaction with the horizontal and vertical components of the earth's magnetic field are physically similar, but differ in direction and biological significance.

INTERPRETATION OF FIELDS INDUCED BY SWIMMING FISH

Could the swimming fish, by sensing the direction and strength of the ρJ field in its own receptor frame of reference, really determine its magnetic compass heading in the earth's frame? The animal might, according to the principle of relativity, but only if it has further information about the world relative to which it is moving. Such information, however, is readily available in this case, as the swimming fish not only has direct access to that world, but also can regulate its velocity v with respect to it.

If the animal may assume that E_e is zero and the water is at rest, then it may consider the ρJ it detects to result solely from its swimming motion. As the seawater offers an excellent, low-resistance return path, so that little charge accumulates on the body surfaces, it may furthermore take the internal ρJ, averaged over the height of the body, to approach E_a in strength and direction. Based upon this, the fish may conclude that the ρJ it detects nearly equals the $v \times B_h$ it induces in the earth's frame of reference.

Consequently, by identifying the dorsoventral ρJ in its own frame of reference with the $v \times B_h$ in the frame of the earth, the fish may, when swimming in a level plane at known velocity v, infer the components of the horizontal magnetic field normal to the direction of motion. Moreover, by its swerving mode of swimming, the animal may gather from those components the direction of the resultant horizontal magnetic field B_h and thereby its compass heading (Kalmijn 1984).

To verify whether the ρJ field is solely due to its own motion, the animal could, for example, stop momentarily or seek the compass direction in which the dorsoventral field is weakest, that is, by heading due north or south. If the remaining field is non-zero, then it must be corrected for. Although the fish may not, in fact, follow these particular procedures, they show the feasibility of separating the cues pertaining to its compass heading and to its drift.

Hence, given the velocity of swimming and the low resistivity of the seawater medium, as compared to that of the skin and body tissues, the animal need not infer, but may actually determine the strength and direction of the ambient magnetic field. The fish's normal mode of swimming furthermore suffices to remove any directional ambiguity. Except for the direction of gravity, no additional information is required to comply with the principle of relativity.

The electric fields most relevant to the magnetic compass sense derive from the horizontal component of the magnetic field and are, when the fish maintains a level course, dorsoventral in direction, whereas the fields due to its drift derive mainly from the vertical component of the magnetic field and are predominantly horizontal in direction. The transverse fields resulting from the animal's interaction with the vertical component of the magnetic field are independent of the direction of swimming, whereas the horizontal fields due to its drift change in direction relative to the body axes upon the turning of the fish.

In short, the fields that the animal receives from its own locomotion and from its drift with the water not only tend to act along different body axes, but also are entirely different functions of the fish's swimming movements. That marine stingrays can distinguish between the various types of motional-electric fields has been demonstrated in behavioral tests, as will be reported in a later section.

It must be noted that only the instantaneous, translational velocity of the fish is considered in this article. Certainly, while swerving the fish changes the direction of its velocity from moment to moment, thereby probing, as it were, its physical environment. However, the fields induced by these turning movements as such do not seem to constitute physically adequate stimuli for the electroreceptive system of elasmobranch fishes (Kalmijn 1984).

By sensing the horizontal as well as the vertical component of the earth's magnetic field, the fish could also determine the magnetic inclination and, thereby, the local magnetic latitude (Kalmijn 1974). Besides, the animal needs the strength of the vertical component of the earth's magnetic field B_V, as was pointed out before, in order to interpret the electric fields of its drift with the water. Thus, the electromagnetic orientation mechanism would not only highly versatile, but also largely self-sufficient.

ELECTRIC VERSUS MAGNETIC DETECTION

If elasmobranch fishes use the ampullae of Lorenzini to sense their magnetic compass heading electrically, must this be referred to as electric or magnetic detection? Certainly, the magnetic field in the animal's frame of reference does not differ noticeably from the magnetic field in the earth's frame of reference at the fish's speed of swimming. Nevertheless, the proposed orientation mechanism does not require the electrical charges of the receptor epithelia, on which the stimulus acts, to move in the reference frame of the animal. And, without moving, electrical charges are not affected by the mere presence of a time-independent magnetic field. Thus, from the point of view of the recipient fish, electric detection is the proper term.

If the earth's magnetic field as such is not detected, where do the purely electric fields that the animals orient to originate from? It is learned from the special theory of relativity that electric currents, having zero charge density in the earth's frame of reference, appear negatively charged to an observer moving in the direction of the current, and positively charged to an observer moving in the opposite direction (Resnick 1968). Consequently, a current loop appears negative in the one half and positive in the other (Fig. 6 and 7) to the moving observer thereby creating an electric dipole field (Panofsky and Phillips 1962). The electric fields due to the parts of the current loop that the observer approaches or recedes from perpendicularly are of similar relativistic origin, but do not constitute electrostatic fields (Purcell 1965, footnote at end of section).

According to geophysical theory (Stacey 1969), the main magnetic field of the earth results from electric currents, which can be thought to flow in concentric circles from east

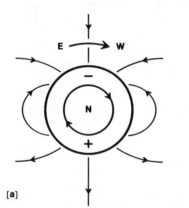 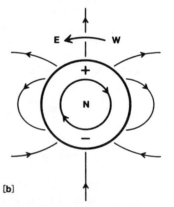

Fig. 6. Earth's sphere viewed from over the north pole. To a fish drifting or swimming along the equator (a) in a westerly and (b) in an easterly direction, the current loops generating the earth's magnetic field appear electrically charged, producing part of the vertical electric field that the animal may infer from the ρJ field it detects. Other relativistic effects not depicted here (see text) decrease the electric field strength at the position of the fish by a factor of two. Note that the strength and direction of the field depends on the animal's compass heading.

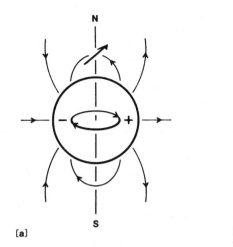
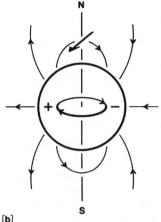

[a]   [b]

Fig. 7. Earth's sphere viewed from a position in the equa-
torial plane. When a fish swims over the north pole in any
direction, as in (a) or (b), the loop currents generating
the earth's magnetic field appear electrically charged, producing part of the horizontal electric field that the fish
may infer from the ρJ field it detects. The relativistic
effects not depicted here (see text) increase the electric
field strength at the position of the fish by a factor of
two. Note that the direction of the field is different when
the fish is either in the northern or southern hemisphere.

to west around the N–S axis of the globe. Consequently, for
a fish swimming or drifting along the equator in westerly
direction, the part of the current loop on the near side
of the earth appears negatively charged, whereas the part of
the current loop on the far side of the earth appears positively charged, producing a global electric dipole field
pointing vertically downwards at the position of the animal
(Fig. 6a). For a fish heading east, however, the global
electric field points vertically upwards at the position of
the animal (Fig. 6b). The nonelectrostatic contribution,
not discussed here, would reduce   the field to half its
strength without changing its direction.

When a fish swims or drifts in polar waters, where feasible, the current loops creating the earth's magnetic field
appear negatively charged on the left and positively charged

on the right with respect to the direction of motion in the northern hemisphere, and positively charged on the left and negatively charged on the right in the southern hemisphere, thereby producing global electric fields that are horizontally directed at the position of the fish (Fig. 7a and b). The nonelectrostatic contribution would double the strength of the field, again without changing its direction. At mid-latitudes, the animal receives electric fields having both vertical and horizontal components.

This leads us to the crucial point of this relativistic digression, namely that the apparent electrical charges and the nonelectrostatic field contributions, in the reference frame of the animal, together constitute exactly the same electric field as that derived from the electric and magnetic field transformations in .n earlier section. Note added in proof: This shows that the familiar relation of equation (7), $E_a \simeq v \times B_e$, although purely empirical in the classical theory (Faraday 1832), indeed is a low-velocity consequence of the relativity postulates (Einstein 1905). As a word of comfort, though, the classical theory is and remains for all practical purposes fully adequate to explain the electromagnetic orientation of sharks, skates, and rays.

If, in special relativity, magnetic fields may be considered to express the relativistic consequences of electric fields, what could be meant with the term magnetic detection? The electrical effects described by the aid of magnetic fields occur only when both the source charges and the test charges are moving in the rest frame of the observer. In the frame of the swimming fish, the source charges, those producing the earth's magnetic field, were moving, but the test charges, those of the receptor cell membranes, did not need to. The equivalent of moving, or rather spinning test charges (Purcell 1965) may be found in the magnetite crystals of various sediment bacteria (Blakemore 1975), causing the organisms to orient by interaction with the magnetic field in their own frames of reference. Thus, for the bacteria, magnetic detection would be the proper term.

----

*) In an earlier version of this paper, to be published by Plenum Press, the nonelectrostatic contributions, having non-zero curl, were loosely described as due to other, relativistically apparent charges, whereas it would be more sensible to relate those to the relativistic radial asymmetry in the electric fields of moving charges.

IMPLEMENTATION OF ORIENTATION MECHANISMS

Elasmobranch fishes are extremely sensitive to electric fields, showing meaningful behavioral responses at voltage gradients as low as 5 nV.cm^{-1} in the frequency range from dc to about 8 Hz (Kalmijn 1966, 1982). The electric sense enables the animals to detect the general bioelectric fields of prey, the motional-electric fields of ocean currents, and the fields that the fishes themselves induce when swimming. Though weak, these fields are well within the dynamic range of the elasmobranchs' electric sense and, consequently, of obvious biological relevance. Various, less-well studied fields remain to be evaluated (Kalmijn 1974).

Bioelectric fields of prey fish and simulations thereof have been presented to sharks, skates, and rays both in the laboratory and at sea (Kalmijn 1971, 1982). When motivated by odor, the predominantly nocturnal predators strike at the electric-field source from distances up to half a meter, in response to dc voltage gradients of 5 nV.cm^{-1} or even less. As a rule, the attacks are remarkable fast, very accurate, and, once initiated, executed without noticeable course corrections (Kalmijn and Weinger 1981). Observations at sea were made at night on bottom-dwelling dogfishes and pelagic blue sharks, off Cape Cod, Massachusetts.

In uniform electric fields, similar to the motionally induced fields of ocean currents, small stingrays were conditioned to seek food by entering an enclosure on the one side, and to avoid punishment by ignoring a similar enclosure on the opposite side of the circular tank, respectively to the left and right relative to the field (Kalmijn 1982). The polarity of the field was selected randomly from trial to trial to exclude the use of alternative cues. The fishes readily learned to orient with respect to dc fields of only 5 nV.cm^{-1}, whereas the fields of ocean currents usually are one to two orders of magnitude stronger (Kalmijn 1974).

To test the stingrays on their ability to direct themselves to the earth's magnetic field, the same circular tank was used, this time provided with Helmholtz coils to control the ambient magnetic field (Kalmijn 1978). By the same behavioral procedure, it was demonstrated that the animals are capable of selecting the enclosure in the magnetic east over the enclosure in the magnetic west in order to earn reward. The strength and inclination of the magnetic fields were those of the California region from where the fish were collected. The animals performed equally well, when strictly horizontal fields were applied (Kalmijn 1984).

Although the latter experiments proved that the stingrays are capable of detecting the direction and polarity of the earth's magnetic field, as expected theoretically, they were not designed to reveal the physical nature of the orientation mechanism. However, that the animals are familiar with the fields they induce themselves follows indirectly from the electric-field experiments, in which the stingrays learned to orient to imposed electric fields up to twenty times weaker than the fields induced by their own locomotion (Kalmijn 1982). Experiments to verify the inferred electromagnetic orientation mechanism are in progress.

The electroreceptors of elasmobranch fishes are the ampullae of Lorenzini (Dijkgraaf and Kalmijn 1963), each featuring a small pore in the skin, giving access to a jelly-filled canal, ending in a blind sensory swelling, the ampulla proper. The canal wall offers high resistance, while the gelatinous core is a good conductor (Murray 1962, Waltman 1966). The ampullae proper are clustered in a few, discrete capsules, allowing the fishes to detect the fields of interest differentially and to suppress undesired, common-mode signals (Kalmijn 1974). The sense organs present extremely high-ohmic input devices, while the skin and body tissues, averaged across the animal, are about a hundred times more resistive than the seawater medium (Kalmijn 1984). Thus, the ampullary system of sharks, skates, and rays seems well-suited for the proposed orientational functions.

The receptor cells in the wall of the ampulla proper are lodged in between supporting cells, together with them forming a simple, single-layered sensory epithelium. The apical membrane of the receptor cell receives the electrical stimulus and passes the excitation on to the basal membrane, from where, by chemical transmission, the signal crosses the synapse to act on the afferent nerve fibers (Bennett and Clusin 1978). When the fish orients to a 5-$nV.cm^{-1}$ threshold field, the apical membranes of the individual receptor cells respond to potential differences of, at most, 50 nV, which is on the same order as the thermal noise of the detection circuit (Kalmijn 1984). These small apical membrane patches thereby exhibit the highest electrical sensitivity presently known in the animal kingdom.

By comparison, the magnetite-based orientation mechanism of magnetic bacteria is extremely simple, without being
less effective. Rather than detecting the magnetic field
and acting accordingly, the bacteria evidently are forced to
swim along the earth's magnetic field lines when separated
from the sediment (Blakemore 1975). The passive nature of
the orientation mechanism has been scrutinized by analyzing
the migration rates of single, living cells as a function of
the ambient magnetic field strength (Kalmijn 1981, Fig. 8).
The role of magnetite in the orientation of higher organisms
remains, however, shrouded in uncertainty.

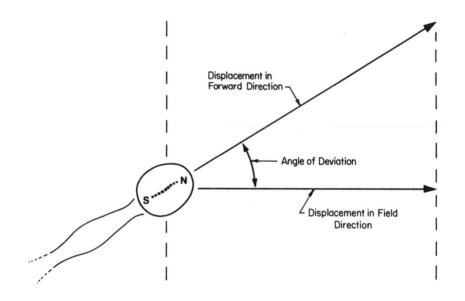

Fig. 8. When separated from the sediments, magnetic bacteria are forced to swim along earth's magnetic field lines,
although they depart randomly from strict alignment due to
thermal agitation (angle of deviation). Indicated are the
string of magnetite grains and the polarity of the northern-
hemisphere bacteria tested on their time of travel over a
1-mm measured distance (between dashed lines, not to scale).
Average cell diameter 1.75 μm. From Kalmijn 1981.

ACKNOWLEDGEMENTS

This paper was presented at the Conference on Electromagnetic Waves and Neurobehavioral Function, Corsendonk,
Belgium, Aug. 1984, and at the International School of Pure
and Applied Biostructure, Erice, Italy, Sept. 1984. The
author thanks Drs. George E. Backus, Alan D. Chave, Charles
S. Cox, Per S. Enger, James R. Enright, Jean H. Filloux,
Mr. Christopher L. Seaman, and the anonymous reviewers for
their constructive comments on the manuscript, without im-
plicating them in any remaining flaws. This research was
conducted under contract with the Office of Naval Research,
Oceanic Biology Program, Drs. Eric O. Hartwig and Bernhard
J. Zahuranec, Program Directors.

REFERENCES

Bennett MVL, Clusin WT (1978). Physiology of the ampulla
of Lorenzini, the electroreceptor of elasmobranchs. In
Hodgson ES, Mathewson RW (eds): "Sensory Biology of
Sharks, Skates, and Rays," Washington DC: Government
Printing Office, pp 483–505.
Blakemore RP (1975). Magnetotactic bacteria. Science 190:
377–379.
Dijkgraaf S, Kalmijn AJ (1963). Untersuchungen ueber die
Funktion der Lorenzinischen Ampullen an Haifischen. Z
Vergl Physiol 47:438–456.
Einstein A (1905). On the electrodynamics of moving bodies.
First published in: Ann Physik 17:891–921. Translated
by Perrett W and Jeffery GB (1952), in: "The Principle of
Relativity," New York: Dover Publications, pp 35–65.
Faraday M (1832). Experimental researches in electricity.
Phil Trans Roy Soc Lond 122(1):125–194.
Galilei G (1632). "Dialogue Concerning the Two Chief
World Systems," translated by Drake S (1967). Berkeley:
University of California Press.
Kalmijn AJ (1966). Electro-perception in sharks and rays.
Nature 212:1232–1233.
Kalmijn AJ (1971). The electric sense of sharks and rays.
J Exp Biol 55:371–383.
Kalmijn AJ (1974). The detection of electric fields from
inanimate and animate sources other than electric organs.
In Fessard A (ed): "Handbook of Sensory Physiology," Vol
III/3, Berlin, Heidelberg, New York: Springer Verlag,
pp 147–200.

Kalmijn AJ (1978). Electric and magnetic sensory world of sharks, skates, and rays. In Hodgson ES, Mathewson RF (eds): "Sensory Biology of Sharks, Skates, and Rays," Washington DC: Government Printing Office, pp 507–528.

Kalmijn, AJ (1978). Experimental evidence of geomagnetic orientation in elasmobranch fishes. In Schmidt-Koenig K, Keeton WT (eds): "Animal Migration, Navigation, and Homing," Berlin, Heidelberg, New York: Springer Verlag, pp 347–353.

Kalmijn AJ (1981). Biophysics of geomagnetic field detection. IEEE Trans Magnetics 17:1113–1124.

Kalmijn AJ (1982). Electric and magnetic field detection in elasmobranch fishes. Science 218:916–918.

Kalmijn AJ (1984). Theory of electromagnetic orientation: a further analysis. In Bolis L, Keynes RD, Maddrell SHP (eds): "Comparative Physiology of Sensory Systems," Cambridge: Cambridge University Press, pp 525–560. Together with present paper announced in Kalmijn (1981) under the title of "A relativistic approach to animal orientation."

Kalmijn AJ, Weinger MB (1981). An electrical simulator of moving prey for the study of feeding strategies in sharks, skates and rays. Ann Biomed Eng 9:363–367.

Longuet-Higgins MS, Stern ME, Stommel H (1954). The electrical field induced by ocean currents and waves, with applications to the method of towed electrodes. Papers Phys Oceanog Meteorol 13:1–37.

Murray RW (1962). The response of the ampullae of Lorenzini of elasmobranchs to electrical stimulation. J Exp Biol 39:119–128.

Panofsky WKH, Phillips (1962). "Classical Electricity and Magnetism." Reading, Massachusetts: Addison-Wesley.

Purcell EM (1965). "Electricity and Magnetism." Berkeley Physics Course, Vol 2, New York, London: McGraw-Hill.

Resnick R (1968). "Introduction to Special Relativity," and texts listed herewith. New York, London, Sydney: Wiley.

Sanford TB (1971). Motionally induced electric and magnetic fields in the sea. J Geophys Res 76:3476–3492.

Shankland RS (1964). Michelson-Morley experiment. For quote of Einstein's statement, Am J Phys 32:16–35.

Stacey FD (1969). "Physics of the Earth." New York, Sydney, Toronto: Wiley.

Stratton JA (1941). "Electromagnetic Theory." New York, London: McGraw-Hill.

Waltman B (1966). Electrical properties and fine structure of the ampullary canals of Lorenzini. Acta Physiol Scand 66, Suppl 264, pp. 1–60.

Electromagnetic Fields and Neurobehavioral Function, pages 47–61
© 1988 Alan R. Liss, Inc.

THE MAGNETIC DETECTION SYSTEM OF THE PIGEON:INVOLVEMENT OF PINEAL AND RETINAL PHOTORECEPTORS AND THE VESTIBULAR SYSTEM.

Peter Semm

University Frankfurt
Dept.of Zoology
Frankfurt, FRG

In the last 20 years, a number of studies have been conducted to determine if exposure to natural and/or earth-strength artificial magnetic fields can give rise to measurable behavioral and physiological effects (for review see Ossenkopp and Barbeito, 1978). From such studies many lines of evidence have resulted which indicate that a variety of organisms are clearly affected by geomagnetic cues.
From this body of experimental work it seems important to note that most behavioral responses fall into two categories: either they involve magnetic compass orientation, or imply some form of physiological sensitivity to weak fluctuations in natural magnetic intensity, i.e. the extraction of time or map information from changing background geomagnetic activity.

THE MAGNETIC COMPASS

The magnetic compass is much simpler than any mechanisms involving celestial information, as the sun and the stars change their position with time and geographical latitude.

These temporal and spatial variations must be taken into account, since seeing the sun or the stars alone does not provide the basis of a direction finding mechanism. Whereas the astronomical systems are established by learning processes, the ability to perceive the magnetic field provides animals with a reference system at birth (Wiltschko, 1983).

Before the magnetic compass was found in birds, the sun compass and the star compass had already been described, and thus the magnetic compass was at first considered a second order mechanism, used only when the use of the sun or the stars was prevented by adverse weather conditions.However, additional findings soon indicated that the magnetic compass played a much more important role in bird orientation, and suggested that it might represent the fundamental compass of the bird´s directional reference system, by which the other factors used for directional orientation can be calibrated.

To act as a basic directional reference system for birds is not the only function of the magnetic compass. Several findings suggest (for review see Wiltschko, 1983), that magnetic directional information gathered ´ en route ´ is used to determine where home lies, implying that magnetic information is used not only during active flying but also during passive displacement.

Young pigeons are apparently able to register that they are transported, for example, magnetically south and they reverse this direction and fly north to come home, whereas older and more experienced birds normally employ different strategies. In these experienced animals, any effect of treatment during transportation is minimal, and we must assume that they switch to site - specific information as soon as they become familiar with it. The ideas about the nature of such ´ map factors ´ are unfortunately still very vague, but some observations suggest that the magnetic field is somehow involved.

SENSITIVITY TO SMALL MAGNETIC FLUCTUATIONS

There is another effect of the earth´s magnetic field on the orientation of birds which is entirely different from its use as a compass. Southern (1972) working with Ring - billed Gulls has obtained data that suggest a sensitivity to magnetic fluctuations of less than 50 gamma (the natural magnetic field ranges between 0.25 and 0.6 Gauss = 10^5 gamma = 10^{-6} nTesla). Because the daily heating and cooling of the atmosphere displaces the jet stream north and south, a more or less regular circadian variation of the intensity of the magnetic field is observed on the ground. After solar flares an enormous number of extra ions appear in the jet streams, causing irregular changes in the magnetic field (less than 100 gamma). These magnetic storms have roughly dose-dependent effects on birds , indicating that the magnetic sensitivity of pigeons is in the range of 10 - 30 nTesla. Since even a 1.000 nTesla storm could not rotate a compass needle 2 degrees, and since these effects on pigeons and gulls are observed when the sun is clearly visible, the phenomenon is discussed as being possibly related to the map sense (for review see Wiltschko, 1983). On the other hand, these findings make it probable that the nearly circadian rhythmicity in magnetic field intensity could be used as a time cue, an idea which is discussed later in relation to the findings of magnetic sensitivity in the pineal gland.

THE MAGNETIC SENSORY SYSTEM IN THE BRAIN

A final problem for the magnetic compass and the magnetic map system is how the central nervous system could measure direction and small intensity changes. Whether or not the recently

discovered single domains of magnetite in birds
(for review see Baker,1982) have anything to
do with pigeon magnetic orientation is unclear
yet. In the opinion of the author, the
involvement of magnetite crystals require a
sense organ, which must be equipped with sensory
hairs in order to monitor movements of the
material within the magnetic field. However,
experimental support for this assumption is
still lacking.
There is clear evidence from behavioral studies
(Wiltschko and Wiltschko, 1972) that in contrast
to a technical compass, the bird's magnetic
compass functions as an "inclination compass" in
that the birds apparently pay no attention to
field polarity but read north as that direction
where the magnetic and gravity vectors form the
most acute angle. This implies the simultaneous
sensing of the direction of both gravity and the
magnetic field, suggesting that the two
detection processes may be integrally locked
together. Leask (1977) proposed that magnetic
field detection in birds takes place in the
retina as an adjunct to the normal processes of
vision. According to this hypothesis magnetic
information would therefore initially be
available in the visual system. These
theoretical assumptions have received
experimental support in young unexperienced
pigeons transported in total darkness (
Wiltschko and Wiltschko,1981), in the visual
system of the pigeon (Semm et al., 1984;) and
in the retinae of quails, humans (
Cremer-Bartels et al., 1983; 1984), turtles (
Rayburn, 1982) and frogs (Lövsund et al.,
1981).
In order for magnetic and gravity cues to be
integrated, the vestibular system is likely to
receive the magnetic message via the known
visual-vestibular projections (for review see
Emmerton,1982).
Thus, the effects of magnetic stimulation on
electrical activity in the vestibular nuclei and
the vestibulo-cerebellum and the nucleus of the

basal optic root (nBOR) which has a projection to the vestibular system, were investigated (Semm et al,1984)

In order to assess the possible integration of magnetic information in known neuronal pathways, a comparison of the responses of cells to their normal physiological stimuli with those to magnetic stimulation was made.

MATERIALS and METHODS

Experiments were performed, in dim light, during daytime on anaesthetized pigeons (Columba livia).The anaesthetised pigeon was mounted in a stereotaxic frame and the brain exposed by boring a hole in the skull to accommodate the recording electrode. The eyes were protected against corneal drying by contact lenses with artificial pupils. A glass micropipette was mounted on a micromanipulator attached to the frame and stereotaxically (Karten and Hodos, 1967) inserted into the nBOR, the lateral or superior vestibular nuclei or that part of the vestibulo-cerebellum (paraflocculus and folia IXc,d), which receives an input from the nBOR (Brecha et al.,1980). Individual, spontaneously active units were located by advancing the micropipette in nm steps using a motorized nanostepper, the motor of which was switched off during recording times and magnetic stimulation. Recorded signals were amplified and further elaborated using conventinal electrophysiological techniques.

Three pairs of Helmholtz-coils (1.0 m in diameter) were used to produce alterations in the horizontal and vertical components of the natural magnetic field, with one of the horizontal coils placed exactly in north - south orientation and the second placed in east - west orientation. The stereotaxic frame in which the pigeon was held, was placed on a plastic tilt-table at the centre of the coils with the animal´s head pointing to the magnetic north-pole. In this area in the center of the coils, the artificial magnetic field is homogeneous.

The artificial magnetic field was controlled by the computer which was interfaced to a power supply with three outputs. The coil system was steered to invert the horizontal and/or vertical component in a gradual manner, with the same inclination and intensity as in the natural field . Inversion of the horizontal component took the needle of a compass from magnetic north via east to south , i.e. a clockwise half-circle in our system; inversion of the vertical component moved the needle of a perpendicular oriented inclinatorium from pointing to the center of the earth until it indicated the opposite direction. The natural magnetic field (field strength in the experimental room = 0.42 Gauss) and the artificial changes were continously monitored by a Gaussmeter . The intensity of the natural magnetic field within the coil system was measured just before experimentation and the value manually entered into the computer to provide a basis for the generation of the intensity level of the artificial fields.

Just prior to magnetic stimulation, units in the nBOR were identified and tested by applying white light stimuli provided by a narrow beam tungsten lamp (30W). In order to assess the movement and direction selectivity, the beam was directed onto the eye through a slit which could be moved either horizontally or vertically. During magnetic stimulation, no light stimuli were applied.

In the vestibular nuclei, cells were tested by tilting the whole animal out of the horizontal plane by 10 to 45 degrees, depending on the sensitivy of a given cell to the grade of tilting. The same was done in the vestibulo-cerebellum.

Single unit electrical activity was recorded extracellularly in the lateral and superior vestibular nuclei, the vestibulo-cerebellum and the nucleus of the basal optic root (nBOR) under earth-strength magnetic stimulation. Units in the vestibular system responded with either inhibition or excitation to the magnetic stimuli only if the animal was moved out of the horizontal plane. No responses to the artificial magnetic field were observed when enucleation was performed contralateral to the recording site or when magnetic stimuli were applied in total darkness.

Most of the units in the nBOR responded to slow direction changes in the magnetic field with a gradual augmentation of activity. The responses were generally weak but nevertheless statistically significant and seemed to be direction selective, i.e.different cells responded to a different distinct direction change of the magnetic field.

The results indicate, that information provided by magnetic cues in the earth's strength range may be conveyed from the visual to the vestibular system via a projection from the nBOR and then related to active movements of the animal.

Although we were of course not able to test all cells in the nBOR, the results of the present study reveal that all direction selective units investigated so far and the majority of cells exhibiting an axis specifity respond to direction changes of the magnetic field,whereas the movement sensitive cells do not appear to respond. Interestingly, it is these direction selective cells which project to the vestibulo-cerebellum. Surprisingly, most of the cells which were directionally sensitive to light also showed a clearcut directional selectivity to the magnetic stimulus, i.e. most of them responded to only a distinct part of the total range involved in the complete inversion of one magnetic vector. Whether or not there is a relationship between a given visual directional preference and the magnetic directional selectivity, remains to be elucidated.

In contrast to the effects in the nBOR, the majority cells in the vestibular nuclei and in the vestibulo-cerebellum responded with either a sustained excitation or sustained inhibition to the gradual inversion of one magnetic vector. This phenomenon may be caused by a convergence of the output of the nBOR cells onto vestibular neurons, and thus represent more or less the whole direction change of the magnetic field.

However, the magnetic responsiveness of the vestibular influenced neurons investigated so far is dependent on the following two prerequisites:(1.) The photoreceptors of the eyes must be intact and activated by light and (2.) the vestibular system must be activated by displacement just prior to the magnetic stimulation.

The first point is demonstrated by the fact that unilateral enucleation causes an insensitivity to magnetic stimulation in the vestibular system contralateral to the operated side and that total darkness abolished the magnetic responsivess of these cells. This suggests that magnetic field detection may initially take place in the eyes. Leask (1977) postulated on a theoretical basis that magnetic field detection takes place in the retina,as an adjunct to the normal process of vision. Specifically,he proposed an optical/radio frequency double resonance process involving the lowest excited molecular triplet state of the rhodopsin,which provides for anisotropy which in turn is essential if such detection is to be of directional use. It was pointed out by Leask, that the response in the visual system is much weaker than other directional cues and is difficult to detect experimentally.

Moreover, the intrinsic sensitivity of the pigeon pineal gland to both light (Semm and Demaine,1983) and magnetic (Semm, 1983) stimulation fits nicely into this concept. In the present study, the possibility that the independent pineal magnetic detection system and pineal related brain mechanisms (Ossenkopp and Ossenkopp,1983; Ossenkopp et al.,1983; Kavaliers et al., 1984) influenced responses in the vestibular system was excluded by the observation that the effects of MF stimulation were unaltered in pinealectomized pigeons.

The second point is demonstrated by our findings that, in the absence of displacement, the spontaneous electrical activity of vestibular neurons is not affected by changes of the magnetic field, indicating that under natural conditions, changes in the gravity and magnetic inclination vectors relative to the animal are implicated in the integration of magnetic information. These observations therefore may provide a neural basis for the "inclination compass" system used by birds for orientation, in which the angle between gravity and the dip of magnetic field lines is assessed, rather than the technically used polarity of the field (Wiltschko and Wiltschko, 1972). The integration of magnetically biased information with that derived from the detection of the position of the animal relative to gravity would possibly allow for an output to the motor system which would enable orientation movements to be fully compensated for any change in the angle between the two vectors.

THE AVIAN PINEAL GLAND AS AN INDEPENDENT MAGNETIC SENSOR.

We have recorded the effects of alterations in the earth's magnetic field on the electrical activity of pineal cells in anaesthetised pigeons under three conditions:(a) in intact birds; (b) after bilateral section of the optic nerves and (c) following section of the pineal stalk and the administration of the beta-adrenergic blocker, propranolol. We report here that responses to magnetic stimulation still occur in treated birds although the magnitude is reduced. This demonstration of the magnetic sensitivity in denervated glands implies that pineal photoreceptors are sufficiently organized to detect magnetic fields as well as light, and is in line with the concept that photoreceptors are inherently capable of magnetic field detection.

Responses to magnetic stimulation were of a general nature in that the average firing rate of responding units was either elevated or lowered to an extent well outside the range of spontaneous fluctuations in basal activity for the whole of the time for which the natural magnetic field was altered. The responses did not appear to reflect any of the obvious characteristics of the stimulus e.g the direction or extent of the field change or the rate of change.
Thus the hypothesis originally put forward by Leask, that magnetic detection may be a property of retinal photoreceptors, can be supported. However, in birds, photoreceptors also occur in the pineal gland (Semm and Demaine, 1983). The persistence of magnetic sensitiivity in the pineal of blinded pigeons implies that pineal photoreceptors are sufficiently organized to detect magnetic fields as well as light. Since there are as yet no reports of responses to earth's strength magnetic field stimulation originating in structures which do not have a photoreceptive capacity, our results suggest that the Leask hypothesis should be extended to include pineal photoreceptors.
Although we and other authors have tested the role of the pineal gland in magnetic compass navigation (Maffei et al.,1982) and magnetic orientation during times of migratory restlessness in handraised young unexperienced birds (Semm et al.,1984), the pineal magnetic detection system is much more likely to be involved in neuroendocrine responses to geomagnetic disturbances (Ossenkopp et al.,1983; Kavaliers et al.,1983). Since pineal melatonin synthesis is influenced by changes in

the natural magnetic field (Welker et al.,1983), the hormonal output of the gland may be subject to the dual inputs of light and magnetism.

Finally, I would like to present a scheme summarizing the findings of magnetic reactions in the CNS of birds (see Schema 1):
Two magnetic detection systems have to be distinguished:

1. The neural magnetic compass system and the so called photoneuroendocrine "vegetative" magnetic system.
In both systems, magnetic detection takes place in photoreceptors and magneticinformation is transformed in an hormonal and/or neural output.
The magnetic compass system appears to involve magnetic and vestibular information, which is locked together integratively and at least transduced to the motor system. The question remaines, how in both the visual and the vestibular system magnetic information is differentiated from the intrinsic activity of these sensory channels.
The photoneuroendocrine "vegetative" magnetic system appears to respond to natural and artificial fluctuations in the natural magnetic environment by lowering the synthesis of melatonin and thereby influencing circadian rhytmicity. In case of the mammalian pineal, which has no functioning photoreceptors, the retinal influence via the suprachiasmatic nucleus (SCN), the paraventricular nucleus (PVN)and the sympathetic innervation from the superior cervical ganglia (SCG) is essential for magnetic effects on melatonin secretion. Target organs of melatonin are subsequently also responding to these magnetic stimuli. Moreover, the pineal is some how involved in the time compensation of the sun compass, thus causing a magnetic influence on this second compass system. Whether there exists in addition a pinealofugal neural magnetic output, remains to be elucidated. Furthermore, the melatonin formation in the retina also responds to magnetic stimulation both in vivo and in vitro.

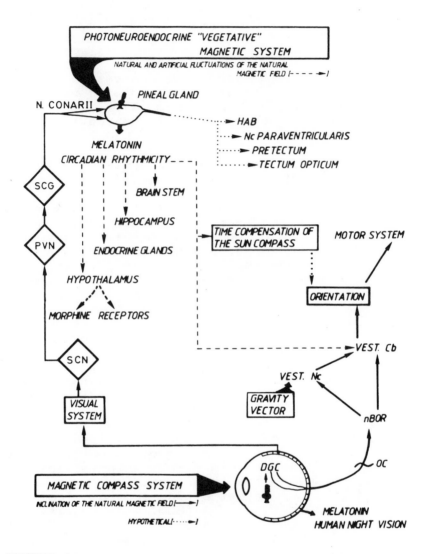

SCHEMA 1

(Abbreviations: DGC=displaced retinal ganglion cells; OC=optic chiasma; VEST.Nc=vestibular nulcei+ Vest.Cb=vestibulo-cerebellum)

CONCLUSION

As a consequence of these observations, it may be speculated that MF detection could take place in all animal and human photoreceptors. However, we dont know whether all animals make use of the available magnetic information in the visual system and whether they have the ability of integratively locking together vestibular and magnetic cues. It may well be that there exist different adaptations in different species and that during evolution some animals, as migratory birds and homing pigeons, have developed a special magnetic system.

REFERENCES

Baker RR (1984). Signal magnetite and direction finding. Phys Technol 15:30

Brecha N, Karten HJ, Hunt SP (1980). Projections of the nucleus of the basal optic root in the pigeon: an autoradiographic and horseradish peroxidase study. J Comp Neurol 189:615

Cremer-Bartels G, Krause K, Küchle HJ (1983). Influence of low magnetic field strength variations on retina and pineal glands of quail and humans. Graefe's Arch Clin Exp Ophthalmol 220:248

Cremer-Bartels G, Krause K, Mitoskas G, Brodersen D (1984) Magnetic field of the earth as additional Zeitgeber for endogenous rhythms? Naturwissenschaften 71:567

Emmerton J (1982). Functional morphology of the visual system. In Abs M (ed): "Physiology and behavior of the pigeon," Academic press,London, p 221

Karten HJ, Hodos W (1967). A stereotaxic atlas of the brain of the pigeon (columba livia). John Hopkins Press,Baltimore

Kavaliers M, Ossenkopp K-P, Hirst M (1984). Magnetic fields abolish the enhanced nocturnal analgesic response to morphine in mice. Physiol Behav 32:261

Leask MJM (1977). A physikochemical mechanism for magnetic field detection by migratory birds and homing pigeons. Nature 267:144

Lövsund P,Nilsson SEG, Oberg PA (1981). Influence on frog retina of alternating magnetic fields with special reference to ganglion cell activity. Med Biol Eng Comput 19:679

Maffei L, Meschini E, Papi F (1983). Pineal body and magnetic sensitivity: homing in pinealectomized pigeons under overcast skies. Z Tierpsychol 62:151-156.

Ossenkopp K-P, Barbeito R (1978). Bird orientation and the geomagnetic field. Neurosci Biobehav Rev 2:255

Ossenkopp K-P, Ossenkopp MD (1983). Geophysical variables and behavior:XI. Open field behaviors in young rats exposed to ELF rotating magnetic field. Psychol Rep 52:343

Ossenkopp K-P, Kavaliers M, Hirst M (1983). Reduced nocturnal morphine analgesia in mice following a geomagnetic disturbance. Neurosci Lett 40:321

Rayburn MS (1983). The effects of direct-current magnetic fields on turtle retinas in vitro. Science 220:713

Semm P (1983). Neurobiological investigations on the magnetic sensitivity of the pineal gland in rodents and pigeons. J Comp Biochem Physiol 76:683

Semm P, Demaine C (1983). Electrical responses to direct and indirect photic stimulation of the pineal gland of the pigeon. J Neural Transm. 58:281

Semm P, Nohr D, Demaine C, Wiltschko W (1984). Neural basis of the magnetic compass: interactions of visual,magnetic and vestibular inputs in the pigeon´s brain. J Comp Physiol 155:283

Semm P, Beck W, Wiltschko W (1984). Migratory orientation of hand-raised Pied Flycatchers (Ficedula hypoleuca) after pinealectomy. Proceedings of the German Zoological Society (in press)

Southern WE (1972). Influence of disturbances in the earth´s magnetic field on Ring-billed gull orientation. Condor 74:102

Welker HA, Semm P, Willig RP, Commentz JC, Wiltschko W, Vollrath L (1983). Effects of an artificial magnetic field on serotonin N-acetyltransferase activity and melatonin content of the rat pineal gland. Exp Brain Res 50:426

Wiltschko W (1983). Compasses used by birds. J Comp Biochem Physiol 76:709

Wiltschko W, Wiltschko R (1972). Magnetic compass of European robins. Science 176:627

Wiltschko W, Wiltschko R (1982). Disorientation of unexperienced young pigeons after transportation in total darkness. Nature 291:433

Electromagnetic Fields and Neurobehavioral Function, pages 63–80
© 1988 Alan R. Liss, Inc.

HUMAN MAGNETORECEPTION FOR NAVIGATION

R. Robin Baker, B.Sc., Ph.D.

Reader in Zoology
University of Manchester
M13 9PL, U.K.

There is a widespread misconception that only long-distance migrants, such as some birds, need to be able to navigate and that only such animals would thus benefit from a magnetic sense. In fact, navigational ability is essential to any animal with a home base to which the animal returns after occasional exploratory forays into surrounding unfamiliar terrain (Baker 1981). As all mammals, including Man, and perhaps even all vertebrates, seem to organize their movements in this way (Baker 1978), a magnetic sense would be expected to be widespread, if not universal, amongst such animals (Baker 1985a). Even so, no animal is expected to navigate solely by reference to the earth's magnetic field. Magnetoreception is just one element in an integrated navigational armory that involves all the available senses and uses a wide range of environmental information (Keeton 1972).

At Manchester University, the location and physiology of the magnetoreceptor and the role of magnetoreception in navigation are being studied for three species of mammal: the woodmouse (*Apodemus sylvaticus*), horse (*Equus caballus*) and Man (*Homo sapiens*). For all three, we have evidence of a role for magnetoreception in navigation (Mather and Baker 1981; Baker 1985a; Baker 1986a). This paper is a brief summary of such evidence for Man with an emphasis on implications for the nature and location of the human magnetoreceptor. At the same time, the data presented show that applied dc magnetic fields, little stronger than that of the Earth, can have a significant influence on the behavior of a whole organism.

EXPERIMENTS ON NAVIGATION AND COMPASS ORIENTATION

We have used three major types of experiment in our studies of human orientation and navigation. All three types produce data for the level of ability to recognise compass directions (i.e. north, south, east, west, etc.) and one, the so-called 'chair' experiment, tests only this ability. The other two types, which we term 'bus' and 'walkabout', experiments, test in addition the ability of humans to navigate; to judge the direction of home from a site being visited for the first time. As such, these latter two experiments are similar to those carried out on other animals, such as homing pigeons.

'Chair' Experiments

In chair experiments a blindfolded, ear-muffed subject sits on a rotating chair. The chair is turned to disorient the subject and is then stopped, whereupon the subject estimates the compass direction in which he or she is facing. The chair is then turned again and a second estimate made. Currently, one test-run involves 9 such estimates. Details of experimental protocol such as turning procedure, computer generation of sequences of directions to be estimated, double-blind organization, and of blindfolds, ear-muffs and test-rooms are given elsewhere (Baker 1984b; Baker 1986a). Variants of the protocol used at Manchester have been tried at Tulsa (Zusne and Allen 1981) and Caltech (Kirschvink et al. 1985). At Keele University, U.K., Dr. Mary Campion (personal communication) has repeated the Tulsa protocol.

'Bus' Experiments

In bus experiments, groups of blindfolded subjects are displaced by van or bus along tortuous routes, usually tens of kilometers long. At one or several sites during the journey, the bus stops. While still blindfolded the subjects estimate the direction of the starting point of the journey (i.e. 'home'). This is done by: 1) pointing or drawing an arrow towards home: and/or 2) describing the compass direction of home relative to the test site. Details of the experimental protocol at Manchester are given elsewhere (Baker 1980; Baker 1981; Baker 1985b; Baker 1986a;

for a critical discussion of techniques see Adler and Pelkie 1985; Baker 1985c). Bus experiments using essentially the Manchester protocol have been repeated at Princeton (Gould 1980; Gould and Able 1981), Albany (Gould and Able 1981; Able and Gergits 1985; Judge 1985) and Cornell (Adler and Pelkie 1985).

In some experiments at Manchester, after being displaced while blindfolded, subjects were allowed to remove their blindfold before pointing (Baker 1981). This last protocol is the most similar to conventional navigation experiments on homing pigeons in that birds are allowed to see their surroundings while 'estimating' home direction.

'Walkabout' Experiments

In walkabout experiments groups of subjects without blindfolds are led through unfamiliar woodland by experienced guides. Journeys are usually 3-5 km long leading to a test site about 1 km or so from the starting point of the journey. Subjects first draw an arrow pointing toward 'home' (i.e. the starting point of the journey) and then estimate the compass direction of the arrow they have drawn. Details are given elsewhere (Baker 1985a; Baker 1986a).

Statistics

Data generated by experiments on orientation and navigation are usually analyzed by an esoteric branch of statistics known as circular statistics. The tests used in this paper are all described by Batschelet (1981). Briefly, estimates are treated as vectors and subjected to a form of vector analysis. A mean vector is calculated which has both direction ($a°$) and length (r). Most often, estimates of direction are expressed relative to some predicted direction (e.g. 'home' direction; true compass direction) as an error, clockwise errors having a positive sign, counter-clockwise errors negative. Thus, the mean direction ($a°$) of a set of estimates is usually presented as a mean error ($e°$) relative to the predicted direction ($0°$). The length (r) of the mean vector takes a value between limits of 0.0, when estimates are completely uniform, and 1.0, when estimates show complete agreement. As long as the scatter of estimates is

not too great, 95% confidence limits to the mean vector may
be calculated. The often-called 'homeward component' (h) of
the mean vector (i.e. the component in the direction 0°)
takes a value between limits of +1.0 when all estimates are
0° in error, and -1.0, when all estimates are 180° in error.
The probability that a given homeward component is greater
than 0.0 by chance is determined by the Rayleigh V-test. A
set of estimates is considered to show significant homeward
orientation when the V-test yields significance AND the 95%
confidence interval of the mean vector includes the
predicted ('home') direction (Aneshansley and Larkin 1981).

There has been some discussion (Adler and Pelkie 1985,
Baker 1985b; Baker 1985c; Dayton 1985) of how to analyze
the results of bus experiments when more than one test site
are used during a single journey. General agreement seems
to have been reached (but see Gould 1985) that in such cases
second order analysis should be used. First, a mean error
is calculated for each subject. Individual means are then
subjected to higher order analysis to calculate the mean for
the group. In this paper, data from bus experiments (and
data from chair experiments) are analyzed in this way.
However, the most recent suggestion (Adler and Pelkie 1985;
Baker 1985c; Baker 1986a) is that future bus experiments
should have only one test site per journey and that only
data for the first test site on previous journeys should be
used. The problem of second order analysis does not arise
for data from walkabout experiments, all recent journeys
have used only one test site.

When testing data for significance in this paper I have
adopted the convention of giving exact probabilities and
distinguishing between 'significant' and 'non-significant'
values by expressing the former (i.e. $< 5.0 \times 10^{-2}$) in
exponential form.

Alteration of the Ambient Magnetic Field

As in experiments on other animals, a role for
magnetoreception in human orientation and navigation may be
studied by comparing the performance of 'experimentals'
(subjects exposed to an altered ambient magnetic field) with
'controls' (subjects exposed to an unaltered ambient field).
If magnetoreception is involved, experimental manipulation
of the magnetic field should influence the strength of

homeward orientation. Experiments at Manchester have used both electromagnetic helmets and bar magnets to alter the ambient field. Elsewhere, at Princeton (Gould 1980; Gould and Able 1981) and Cornell (Adler and Pelkie 1985), only magnets have been used.

The electromagnetic helmets used at Manchester are made of PVC with lateral copper coils (details in Baker 1981). Current is provided by a 9v battery on the subject's lap. A dc field is generated that is horizontal at the helmet's centre and has an intensity about three times that of the horizontal component of the geomagnetic field (about 0.18 G in Manchester). Away from the centre of the helmet the field is complex (Baker 1981). Controls wear identical but inactive helmets disconnected from the battery by a false connection.

Bar magnets used at Manchester measure 77 x 15 x 6 mm and have a pole strength of about 20 mT (Baker 1985b; Baker 1986a). Controls wear brass bars of the same dimensions. All bars are sealed inside opaque cotton or brown-paper envelopes. Other precautions taken to ensure that neither subjects nor experimenters know which subjects are controls and which are experimentals are described by Baker (1985b).

Differences in the strength of homeward orientation are tested for significance by Wallraff's modification of the Mann-Whitney U-test (Batschelet 1981, pp 126-7).

ABILITY AT COMPASS ORIENTATION AND NAVIGATION

Compass Orientation

Levels of ability to recognise compass direction as measured in chair, bus and walkabout experiments are summarized in Table 1.

The Manchester experiments show humans to have a weak but significant ability to perceive and name compass directions, even when blindfolded. Not surprisingly, compass orientation is stronger when subjects can see and the sun is shining ($h = 0.299$) than when they are blind-folded ($h = 0.10$ to 0.18; table 1). A surprise is that, although significant, h is as low as 0.299 when the sun is shining. Under such conditions, a homeward component of 0.9 or even more might reasonably have been expected. This weakness of performance emphasizes the inexperience of the test subjects (mainly University Biology students, 19-21 y old), to most of whom the recognition of compass direction will never have been important in their everyday lives.

In experiments at Tulsa (Zusne and Allen 1981), blindfolded people were disoriented by first leading them along a twisting path. They were then seated in a chair and turned before being asked to estimate the direction of north. The authors found no evidence of compass orientation (h = 0.0, approximately) but sample size was only 25. Campion (personal communication) repeated Zusne and Allen's experiment on students at Keele University. Sample size was 153 and compass orientation was significant (Table 1) with a homeward component of 0.116.

Table 1. Level of compass orientation in walkabout, bus and chair experiments

	n	e $\pm$ CI	r	h	P (V-test)
SIGHTED					
Walkabout (under sun)					
Manchester	130	$-22\pm22°$	0.323	0.299	8.7×10^{-7}
BLINDFOLDED					
Bus					
Manchester	354	$4\pm32°$	0.107	0.107	2.2×10^{-3}
Cornell	86	$21\pm51°$	0.191	0.179	9.7×10^{-3}
Chair					
Manchester	875	$-7\pm11°$	0.175	0.174	3.3×10^{-14}
Keele	153	$-11\pm70°$	0.118	0.116	2.1×10^{-2}
Tulsa	25	?	?	app 0.000	0.500

Data from: Adler and Pelkie 1985; Baker 1985b; Baker 1986a; Campion (personal communication)

Adler and Pelkie (1985) give data for compass orientation by blindfolded subjects (their Table 1; 'hypothesis E') on five bus journeys at Cornell University. Orientation was significant (Table 1) with a homeward component of 0.179.

It is clear from these experiments that the level of ability of inexperienced subjects to perceive and name compass directions is relatively weak. In the introductory section on the statistics used in these studies it was pointed out that the statistic 'h' (the homeward component) varies between limits of +1 (all estimates 0° in error) to -1 (all estimates 180° in error), with guesswork producing h = 0. Observed values when blindfolded range from 0.0 (at Tulsa) to 0.179 (at Cornell) or, when sighted and with the sun shining, to 0.299 (at Manchester). The near-astronomic significance value of h = 0.174 for blindfolded subjects in chair experiments at Manchester owes more to the sample size of 875 than to the strength of the phenomenon. Equally, the lack of significance at Tulsa may owe more to the small sample size of 25 than to the absence of an ability observed independently at Manchester, Keele and Cornell. A homeward component of 0.0 when n = 25 will not be significantly different from h = 0.116, n = 153 (at Keele) or from h = 0.179, n = 86 (at Cornell) and may not even be different from h = 0.174, n = 875 (at Manchester). Unfortunately, the form in which the Tulsa data were published do not allow the necessary statistical tests to be applied.

Navigation

Table 2 summarizes the results of 20 walkabout and 49 (31 British; 18 American) bus experiments in which control subjects exposed to the unaltered geomagnetic field estimated home direction. All series show that humans do have an ability to estimate the direction of home from a novel site, both by pointing and by judging compass direction. Moreover, the ability is significant when subjects are blindfolded as well as when they can see.

Data from bus experiments in which subjects were displaced while blindfolded but then allowed to remove the blindfold before pointing towards home are directly comparable to data for homing pigeons. The level of homeward orientation shown by these inexperienced humans (h = 0.205) compares favourably with the level (h = 0.15 to 0.25) shown by inexperienced homing pigeons over similar distances in Germany (Foa et al 1982).

Table 2. Navigational performance in unaltered magnetic fields in bus and walkabout experiments in Britain and the United States

	n	e $\pm$ CI	r	h	P (V-test)
COMPASS ESTIMATES OF HOME DIRECTION					
Walkabout (day & night)					
Manchester	222	$-50\pm39°$	0.157	0.101	1.7×10^{-2}
Bus					
blindfolded					
Britain	414	$18\pm14°$	0.256	0.243	3.7×10^{-13}
U.S.A.	226	$-4\pm38°$	0.156	0.156	4.9×10^{-4}
POINTING TO HOME					
Walkabout (day & night)					
Manchester	238	$10\pm13°$	0.369	0.364	5.2×10^{-16}
Bus					
blindfolded					
Britain	372	$2\pm15°$	0.245	0.245	3.4×10^{-12}
U.S.A.	202	$-29\pm71°$	0.104	0.091	3.4×10^{-2}
blindfold removed					
Britain	166	$13\pm32°$	0.210	0.205	9.7×10^{-5}

British data from: Baker 1985b; Baker 1986a.
US data compiled from: Able and Gergits 1985; Adler and Pelkie 1985; Dayton 1985; Judge 1985. See Baker 1985c.

The navigational performances in Table 2 do not, and are not intended to, reflect level of ability to navigate by magnetoreception. In walkabout experiments in particular, subjects were free to use and integrate information from all mechanisms in their navigational armory. In bus experiments, visual mechanisms are impaired by blindfolds but rotational, acoustic, olfactory, and (non-visual) topographic information are still available. Adler and Pelkie (1985) tried to remove acoustic and olfactory information during bus experiments at Cornell but failed to observe any apparent deterioration in navigational performance (see also Baker 1985c).

The only way to evaluate any contribution of magneto-reception to the performances shown in Table 2 is to influence the subjects' ability to detect the geomagnetic field. As long as tests are suitably controlled, such evaluation is as possible for sighted subjects on walkabout experiments as for blindfolded subjects on bus and chair experiments. The available data are summarized in the next section.

THE INFLUENCE OF MAGNETS

Magnets on the back of the head have little, if any, influence on compass orientation (Baker 1984b; Baker 1985b) or navigation (Baker 1980; Baker 1981; Baker 1985a). However, magnets on the forehead (Gould and Able 1981; Adler and Pelkie 1985) or between the ear and the eye (Baker 1984a; Baker 1984b; Baker 1985a) have a significant influence on both orientation and navigation (Baker 1985c). Magnets behind the ear have an intermediate effect (Baker 1985a).

Three American bus journeys, two at Princeton (Gould 1980; Gould and Able 1981) and one at Cornell (Adler and Pelkie 1985) have involved some subjects wearing magnets. Sample size in each experiment was small (15-20 with magnets) but the combined data for the three experiments show a significant difference in strength of homeward orientation ($N_{1,2}$ = 48,53; z = -2.276; P(2-tailed) = 2.3×10^{-2}; Wallraff's test) between subjects wearing magnets (N = 53; e = -38+30; r = 0.38; h = 0.299; P = 1.1×10^{-3}; V-test) and control subjects wearing magnetically inert bars (N = 48; e = -88+54; r =0.24; h = 0.008; P = 0.47; V-test) (Baker 1985c).

Even when, as on walkabout experiments, inexperienced subjects can see and are free to use any environmental cue they wish, they are influenced in their compass orientation (Table 3) and navigation (Table 4) by exposure to an artificial magnetic field through the front half of their head. In homing pigeons, the influence of magnets on navigation decreases as the birds gain in experience (Keeton 1972; Wiltschko and Wiltschko 1982). We may anticipate that the same is true for humans but none of our experiments have yet used experienced navigators as subjects.

Table 3. The influence of exposure to an artificial magnetic field on compass orientation during 20 walkabout experiments, 1980-1984

	n	e ± CI	r	h	P (V-test)
COMPASS ORIENTATION					
Controls	222	−25+26°	0.225	0.204	9.4×10^{-6}
Experimentals	360	−46+42°	0.092	0.064	4.3×10^{-2}

Comparison of strength of homeward orientation:
z = 2.293; P(2-tailed) = 2.2×10^{-2}; Wallraff's test

    Magnets do not have to be worn throughout an experiment to influence orientation and navigation. Subjects who have worn magnets on the head for only 10-15 minutes continue to be influenced in their ability to orientate in the normal geomagnetic field for some time after the magnet has been removed. This influence of 'pre-treatment' was first demonstrated in chair experiments (Baker 1984a; Baker 1984b) but has since also been shown in walkabout experiments (Baker 1985a and Table 4). The 'after-effect' persists for at least 1.5 hours in walkabout experiments and preliminary chair experiments suggest that orientation may not return to its pre-exposure level for 10-15 hours. However, more extensive tests are needed before a 'decay curve' can be plotted.

Table 4. The influence of a 15 minute 'pre-exposure' to bar magnets on navigation during 11 walkabout experiments, 1983-1984

	n	e ± CI	r	h	P (V-test)
NAVIGATION					
Pointing to start					
Brass	146	9+24°	0.289	0.286	5.8×10^{-7}
Magnets	211	0+13°	0.419	0.419	1.6×10^{-18}

Comparison of strength of homeward orientation:
z = −2.097; P(2-tailed) = 3.6×10^{-2}; Wallraff's test

It is not hard to imagine ways in which artificial magnetic fields may DISRUPT compass orientation (Table 3). It is less easy to see how such fields can IMPROVE navigational performance (Table 4; see also Gould 1980; Walcott 1982; Baker 1984a; Baker 1985a; Adler and Pelkie 1985; Baker 1985c; Baker 1986a). The fact that they do, and continue to do so even after the applied field is removed, must give a strong clue as to the nature of the receptor by which the Earth's magnetic field is sensed.

THE SEARCH FOR THE MAGNETORECEPTOR

The Sinal Magnetite Hypothesis

A wide range of animals is now known to be able to detect the geomagnetic field (Kirschvink et al. 1985). For none of these animals, however, has the magnetic sense organ on which this ability is based been identified.

There are many suggestions (reviewed by Baker 1984b) as to the most likely form of the magnetoreceptor but the current favourite is what may be termed 'the magnetite hypothesis'. This idea derives from observations by Lowenstam (1962) and Blakemore (1975) and postulates the existence in specialized tissue of large numbers of single-domain particles of the iron oxide, magnetite (see reviews by Kirschvink and Gould 1981; Kirschvink et al. 1985). Nerves would connect this specialized tissue to the central nervous system. It is suggested that, as the tissue is moved within the geomagnetic field, physical, electrical or magnetic events around the magnetite will trigger the firing of nerves which thus deliver directional information to the brain. The popularity of this hypothesis has led to an intensive search for magnetite in animal tissue (collected papers in Kirschvink et al. 1985).

Magnetometric examination of various tissues from the heads of five human corpses within two days of death found no magnetic remanence in any soft tissue (e.g. brain, dura, pineal) (Baker et al. 1983). Only the bones that form the walls of the sphenoid and ethmoid sinuses showed a level of magnetic remanence that was significantly greater than background. Histological examination of these bones for deposits of ferric iron, using the Prussian Blue reaction, revealed a dense layer of positive-staining material about 5µ beneath the surface (Baker and Mather 1982; Baker et al. 1983). Similar magnetic remanence and apparent deposits of ferric iron have been reported from the ethmoid sinus region of a variety of other vertebrates (Kirschvink et al. 1985), including woodmice (Mather and Baker 1981; Baker and Mather 1982). In some species, the ferric deposits are confirmed to be or to contain magnetite. Such reports have led to speculation that sinal magnetite may be the basis of direction finding in vertebrates (Baker 1984a; Walker et al. 1984).

The Case Against Magnetite

The presence of magnetite in specific tissue is proving to be notoriously inconsistent. For example, magnetite in the dura of the first few homing pigeons examined (Walcott et al. 1979) was not present in the next 80 (Walcott and Walcott 1982); nor could magnetite at this site be found by other authors (Presti and Pettigrew 1980) though it was reported from the neck muscles. Presti and Pettigrew found greater magnetic remanence in the heads of long-distance migrants among birds than among residents. However, Ueda et al. (1982) found no significant magnetic remanence in either. Histological studies of the pigeon head (Walcott and Walcott 1982) found little consistency in the location of deposits of ferric iron. Kuterbach et al. (1982) were unable to demonstrate magnetite among ferric deposits in the abdomen of honey bees where magnetic remanence had previously been reported (Gould et al. 1978).

The apparent ferric deposits that were such a conspicuous feature of the sinus bones of human corpses, were not evident in ethmoid sinus bones removed from a living person (Baker, Kennaugh and Canty, unpublished). Proton probe analysis of unstained sinus bones from human corpses also failed to find a layer of ferric iron (Baker 1985b) as did electron microscopy of the analagous ethmoturbinal bones of woodmice (Jorgenson, in Mather 1985).

Bees without single-domain magnetite nevertheless appear to show magnetic sensitivity (Gould et al. 1980). Salmon fry, although able to orient to the ambient magnetic field, showed no significant magnetic remanence (Ueda et al. 1982). Cave salamanders, which are sensitive to magnetic fields (Phillips and Adler 1978), showed no consistent ferric deposits other than at the base of the teeth (Walcott and Walcott 1982).

An inability to find magnetite in a particular animal may, of course, mean only that the material is present in quantities too small to detect. Such small amounts may nevertheless be sufficient for magnetoreception (Kirschvink 1982). Even so, the continuing absence of a demonstrable link between magnetite and magnetoreception, magnetite's erratic occurrence and distribution in animal tissue and its possible absence in animals capable of magnetoreception, all suggest that the current excitement surrounding the magnetite hypothesis may be premature.

Other Hypotheses

Non-magnetite hypotheses of magnetoreception are reviewed by Baker (1984b). The only suggestion for which there is any support from experimental data for land vertebrates is that postulated by Leask (1977). Leask hypothesized that magnetoreception might take place in the eye, in the molecules of the retina, as a by-product of the normal visual process. Specifically, his suggestion is for an optical or radio frequency double-resonance process involving the lowest excited triplet state of a particular molecule (rhodopsin being the favoured candidate). These triplet states have a magnetic moment and their energy variations with the magnetic field are anisotropic, depending on field magnitude as well as on field direction.

Support for Leask's hypothesis has come from two recent discoveries with homing pigeons. First, inexperienced young birds are as disoriented on release when transported in total darkness as they are when transported in a disrupted magnetic field (Wiltschko and Wiltschko 1981). Secondly, there is single unit electrical activity in the nucleus of the basal optic root under earth-strength magnetic stimulation that does not occur when magnetic stimuli are applied in total darkness (Semm et al. 1984).

In this context, it may be relevant that Judge (1985) found no evidence of non-visual navigational ability in bus experiments on blind and partially blind people. Although sample size was very small (N = 9), the results could imply a role for the eyes in magnetoreception. Against this is the apparent ability of normally sighted subjects to detect the magnetic field when blindfolded. Whether this is taken to be evidence against Leask's model depends on two factors: 1) how much light energy is needed to drive a retinal magnetoreceptor? and 2) how much light reaches the retina through the blindfolds used? Neither question has yet been answered.

The Human Magnetoreceptor

The studies of orientation and navigation summarized in this paper highlight two specific features of the human magnetoreceptor: 1) exposure to a 20 mT bar magnet for 15 minutes continues to influence magnetoreception for at least 1.5 h after the magnet has been removed; and 2) the magnetic sense can be improved, as well as disrupted, by applied magnetic fields. Any model of the magnetoreceptor has to accommodate both of these characteristics.

A case has been made, both for pigeons (Walcott 1982) and Man (Baker 1984a), that such characteristics are consistent with a magnetoreceptor based on magnetite. The models developed, however, would require a fairly specific relationship between the viscosity of the medium in which the particles are embedded, the effects of thermal agitation, and the torque imposed on the magnetite particles by both geomagnetic and applied fields.

A molecular system of the type suggested by Leask (1977) at first seems even less able to account for such a persistent after-effect, reactions at molecular and sub-molecular levels usually having much shorter time bases. However, Adey (this volume) reports an influence of magnetic fields on the distribution of calcium ions that persists for several hours after removal of the applied field. Perhaps molecular phenomena such as resonance and triplet states may yet be found to show a similarly persistent response.

Currently, the sphenoid/ethmoid sinus region on the one hand and the eye on the other are the only contenders for the site of human magnetoreception. Neither is a clear front-runner and it may yet be a few years before we can point at any specific tissue and say with confidence that "this is the human magnetoreceptor".

ACKNOWLEDGEMENTS

I thank: Dr. Mary Campion, University of Keele, for use of her chair data on students; Gai Murphy, University of Manchester, for use of her chair data on schoolchildren; and Sandra Hardman for preparing the camera-ready manuscript. Research on magnetoreception at Manchester University is supported by SERC research grant GR/B74337.

REFERENCES

Able KP, Gergits WF (1985). Human navigation: attempts to replicate Baker's displacement experiment. In Kirschvink JL, Jones DS, McFadden BJ (eds): "Magnetite Biomineralization and Magnetoreception in Organisms: A new Magnetism," New York: Plenum.

Adler K, Pelkie CR (1985). Human homing orientation: critique and alternative hypotheses. In Kirschvink JL, Jones DS, MacFadden BJ (eds): "Magnetite Biomineralization and Magnetoreception in Organisms: A new Magnetism," New York: Plenum.

Adey R (this volume).

Aneshansley DJ, Larkin TS (1981). V-test is not a statistical test of "homeward" direction. Nature, London 293:239.

Baker RR (1978). "The Evolutionary Ecology of Animal Migration." London: Hodder and Stoughton.

Baker RR (1980). Goal orientation by blindfolded humans after long-distance displacement: possible involvement of a magnetic sense. Science 210:555.

Baker RR (1981). "Human Navigation and the Sixth Sense." London: Hodder and Stoughton.

Baker RR (1984a). Sinal magnetite and direction finding. Physics in Technology 15:30.

Baker RR (1984b). "Bird Navigation: Solution of a Mystery?" London: Hodder and Stoughton.

Baker RR (1985a). Exploration and navigation: the foundation of vertebrate migration. In Rankin MA (ed): "Migration: Mechanisms and Adaptive Significance," Port Aransas Marine Laboratory.

Baker RR (1985b). Magnetoreception by man and other primates. In Kirschvink JL, Jones DS, MacFadden BJ (eds): "Magnetite Biomineralization and Magnetoreception in Organisms: A new Magnetism," New York: Plenum.

Baker RR (1985c) Human navigation:a summary of American data and interpretations. In Kirschvink JL, Jones DS, MacFadden BJ (eds): "Magnetite Biomineralization and Magnetoreception in Organisms: a new Magnetism," New York: Plenum.

Baker RR (1986a). "Human Navigation and Magnetoreception" Manchester: University Press.

Baker RR, Mather JG, Kennaugh JH (1983). Magnetic bones in human sinuses. Nature, London 301:78.

Batschelet E (1981). "Circular Statistics in Biology." London: Academic Press.

Blakemore RP (1975), Magnetotactic bacteria. Science 190:377.

Dayton T (1985). A comment on Baker's methodology and statistics. In Kirschvink JL, Jones DS, MacFadden BJ (eds): "Magnetite Biomineralization and Magnetoreception in Organisms: A new Magnetism," New York: Plenum.

Foa A, Wallraff HG, Ioale P, Benvenuti S (1982) Comparative investigations of pigeon homing in Germany and Italy. In Papi F, Wallraff HG (eds): "Avian Navigation," Heidelberg: Springer, p 232.

Gould JL (1980). Homing in on the home front. Psychology Today 14:62.

Gould JL (1985). Absence of human homing ability as measured by displacement experiments. In Kirschvink JL, Jones DS, MacFadden BJ (eds): "Magnetite Biomineralization and Magnetoreception in Organisms: A new Magnetism," New York: Plenum.

Gould JL, Able KP (1981). Human homing: an elusive phenomenon. Science 212:1061.

Gould JL, Kirschvink JL, Deffeyes KS (1978). Bees have magnetic remanence. Science 201:1026.

Gould JL, Kirschvink JL, Deffeyes KS, Brines ML (1980). Orientation of demagnetized bees. Journal of experimental Biology 86:1.

Judge TK (1985) A study of the homeward orientation of visually handicapped humans. In Kirschvink JL, Jones DS, MacFadden BJ (eds): "Magnetite Biomineralization and Magnetoreception in Organisms: A new Magnetism," New York: Plenum.

Keeton WT (1972). Effects of magnets on pigeon homing. In Galler SR, Schmidt-Koenig K, Jacobs GJ, Belleville RE (eds): "Animal Orientation and Navigation," Washington DC: NASA SP 262 US Govt Print Office, p 579.

Kirschvink JL (1982). Birds, bees and magnetism. A new look at the old problem of magnetoreception. Trends in Neuroscience 5:160.

Kirschvink JL, Gould JL (1981). Biogenic magnetite as a basis for magnetic field sensitivity in animals. BioSystems 13:181.

Kirschvink JL, Jones DS, MacFadden BJ (eds) (1985). "Magnetite Biomineralization and Magnetoreception in Organisms: A new Magnetism." New York: Plenum.

Kirschvink JL, Peterson KA, Chwe M, Filmer P, Roder B (1985). An attempt to replicate the spinning chair experiment. In Kirschvink JL, Jones DS, MacFadden BJ (eds): "Magnetite Biomineralization and Magnetoreception in Organisms: A new Magnetism," New York: Plenum.

Kuterbach DA, Walcott B, Reeder RJ, Frankel RB (1982). Iron-containing cells in the honey bee (*Apis mellifera*). Science 218:695.

Leask MJM (1977). A physico-chemical mechanism for magnetic field detection by migratory birds and homing pigeons. Nature, London 267:144.

Lowenstam HA (1962). Magnetite in denticle capping in recent chitons (Polyplacophora). Geological Society of America bulletin 73:435.

Mather JG (1985) Magnetoreception by rodents. In Kirschvink JL, Jones DS, MacFadden BJ (eds): "Magnetite Biomineralization and Magnetoreception in Organisms: A new Magnetism," New York: Plenum.

Mather JG, Baker RR (1981). Magnetic sense of direction in woodmice for route-based navigation. Nature, London 291:152.

Phillips JB, Adler K (1978). Directional and discriminatory responses of salamanders to weak magnetic fields. In Schmidt-Koenig K, Keeton WT (eds): "Animal Migration, Navigation and Homing," Heidelberg: Springer, p. 325.

Presti D, Pettigrew JD (1980). Ferromagnetic coupling to muscle receptors as a basis for geomagnetic field sensitivity in animals. Nature, London 285:99.

Semm P, Nohr D, Demaine C, Wiltschko W (1984). Neural basis of the magnetic compass: interactions of visual, magnetic and vestibular inputs in the pigeon's brain. Journal of Comparative Physiology A 155:1.

Ueda K, Kusunoki M, Kato M, Kakizawa R, Nakamura T, Yaskawa K, Koyama M, Maeda Y (1982). Magnetic remanences in migratory birds. Journal Yamashina Institute of Ornithology 14:166.

Walcott B, Walcott C (1982). A search for magnetic field receptors in animals. In Papi F, Wallraff HG (eds): "Avian Navigation," Heidelberg: Springer, p 338.

Walcott C (1982). Is there evidence for a magnetic map in homing pigeons? In Papi F, Wallraff HG (eds): "Avian Navigation," Heidelberg: Springer, p 99.

Walcott C, Gould JL, Kirschvink JL (1979). Pigeons have magnets. Science 205:1027.

Walker MM, Kirschvink JL, Chang S-BR, Dizon AE (1984). A candidate magnetic sense organ in the yellowfin tuna, *Thunnus albacares*. Science 224:751.

Wiltschko W (1978). Further analysis of the magnetic compass of migratory birds. In Schmidt-Koenig K, Keeton WT (eds): "Animal Migration, Navigation and Homing," Heidelberg: Springer, p 50.

Witschko W, Wiltschko R (1972). Magnetic compass of European robins. Science 176:62.

Wiltschko W, Wiltschko R (1981). Disorientation of inexperienced young pigeons after transportation in total darkness. Nature, London 291:433.

Wiltschko W, Wiltschko R (1982). The role of outward-journey information in the orientation of homing pigeons. In Papi F, Wallraff HG (eds): "Avian Navigation," Heidelberg: Springer, p 239.

Zusne L, Allen B (1981). Magnetic sense in humans? Perceptual and Motor Skills 52:910.

Electromagnetic Fields and Neurobehavioral Function, pages 81–106
© 1988 Alan R. Liss, Inc.

THE CELLULAR MICROENVIRONMENT AND SIGNALING THROUGH CELL
MEMBRANES

W. Ross Adey, M.D.

Departments of Physiology and Surgery
Loma Linda University School of Medicine
Loma Linda, California 92357   USA

INTRODUCTION

In its earliest forms, life on earth may have existed
in the absence of cells, simply as a "soup" of unconstrained
biomolecules at the surface of primitive oceans. It is a
reasonable assumption that the first living organisms
existed as single cells floating or swimming in these
primordial seas. Concepts of a cell emphasize the role of a
bounding membrane surrounding an organized interior that
participates in the chemistry of processes essential for all
terrestrial life; as for example, in metabolism,
respiration, reproduction and responses to environmental
stimuli.

This enclosing membrane is the organism's window on the
world around it. For unicellular organisms that swim freely
through large fluid volumes, the cell membrane is both a
sensor and an effector. As a sensor, it detects altered
chemistry in the surrounding fluid. It provides a pathway
for inward signals generated on its surface by a wide
variety of stimulating ions and molecules, including
hormones, antibodies and neurotransmitters; and as discussed
below, these most elemental signals crossing the membrane
are susceptible to manipulation by a wide variety of natural
or imposed electromagnetic fields that may also pervade the
pericellular fluid. As effectors, cell membranes may induce
cell movement by such devices as flagellae or pseudopodia;
or secrete substances synthesized internally, including
hormones, antibodies and structural proteins such as
collagen. These effector functions are also sensitive to
manipulation by intrinsic and imposed electromagnetic fields.

This situation is sharply changed in cellular
aggregates that form the tissues of higher animals. No
longer moving freely in a virtually limitless ocean, cells
are separated by narrow fluid channels that take on a
special importance in signaling from cell to cell. These
channels act as windows on the electrochemical world
surrounding each cell. Hormones, antibodies and
neurotransmitter molecules move along them to reach binding
sites on cell membrane receptors. These tiny fluid
"gutters", typically not more than 150 Å wide, are also
preferred pathways for intrinsic and environmental
electromagnetic fields in tissue, since they offer a much
lower electrical impedance than cell membranes. They are
also the channels through which all cellular nutrients must
pass and products of cellular metabolism are removed.

Intercellular spaces (ICS) are not simple saline filled
channels. Numerous stranded protein molecules protrude into
these spaces, sensing chemical and electrical signals in
surrounding fluid. These strands are external terminals of
helical proteins that pass through the lipid bilayer (plasma
membrane), as discussed below. On the membrane surface,
they also form specialized receptor sites for hormones and
antibodies and for neurotransmitters at synapses. They
offer an anatomical substrate for the first detection of
weak electrochemical oscillations in pericellular fluid,
including field potentials arising in activity of adjoining
neurons or as tissue components of environmental fields.

Research in molecular biology has increasingly
emphasized communication between cells that occurs more or
less directly due to their mutual proximity, as in the liver
or pancreas, or even between moving cells in blood.
However, for brain tissue, concepts of direct communication
between neurons have gained slower acceptance. They
obviously usurp key tenets of the Waldeyer neuronal doctrine
which has served for more than a century in development of
all connectionist brain models; in other words, the flux of
signals in brain tissue should exclusively follow nerve
fiber paths from neuron to neuron in a network organization,
proposed by Sherrington (1947) in his "enchanted loom" that
grew out of Waldeyer's concepts and the elegant histological
studies of Ramon y Cajal (1911). Field potentials have
traditionally held no place in these schemes, and the
oscillations of the EEG have been considered only as "the
noise of the brain's motor".

2.   Evolving Models of Cerebral Tissue Organization.

There has been a strong trend away from cerebral models that consider fiber connections as the only basis for information handling that must include transaction, storage and retrieval. A broad spectrum of anatomical, physiological and behavioral data now supports the view that there is an intrinsic communication system in cerebral tissue that permits these neurons to "whisper together" (Young, 1951).

The traditional concept of CNS function that emphasizes all-or-none spike discharges (an equilibrium process) as the sole means of intercellular communication has been challenged. Recent research that has provided new data through the use of electromagnetic fields gives support to the concept that incremental changes in potential in single neurons significantly affect adjoining neurons through their intimately intertwined dendritic trees, and through weaker pericellular components of these dendritic potentials. These data clearly imply new models of field-tissue interactions through nonequilibrium processes. In this chapter, I will relate these field interactions to appropriate cellular and molecular substrates with the expectation that this will provide an experimentally grounded, testable theory to guide future research.

Numerous dendro-dendritic contacts, arranged as gap junctions or chemical synapses, allow direct interaction between adjoining neurons (Shepherd, 1974). A unique aspect of electrical activity of cerebral dendrites is the occurrence of large slow wave trains with amplitudes of 10-20 mV in intracellular records (Fujita et al., 1964; Creutzfeldt et al., 1966) and closely related to the genesis of the EEG in the surrounding extracellular fluid (Elul, 1967,1972). The EEG has an electric gradient of the order of 100 mV/cm across the dimensions of a single cell. Its amplitude of about 50 uV at these dimensions is about one two hundredth of intracellular dendritic waves from which it is derived. Power spectra of dendritic waves and the EEG from the same tissue domain closely resemble one another.

Imposed electromagnetic fields that mimic frequencies of EEG rhythms are associated with behavioral modifications, including aspects of conditional behavior, at tissue field levels far lower than the membrane potential, and even far weaker than the EEG. A 10 Hz square wave field at 2.5 V/m modulates circadian periodicities in man and birds (Wever, 1968,1977). Sinusoidal 7 and 10 Hz electric fields at 10 to 50 V/m alter subjective estimates of the passage of time in monkeys. Calculated tissue field levels in these experiments were around 10^{-7} V/cm (Gavalas et al., 1970; Gavalas-Medici and Day-Magdaleno, 1976). A 16 Hz sinusoidal magnetic field producing 10 uV/cm in rat body tissues lowered body core temperature by $0.12^{\circ}C$ ($p < 0.05$), but was without effect at 7 or 30 Hz (Smith, 1984).

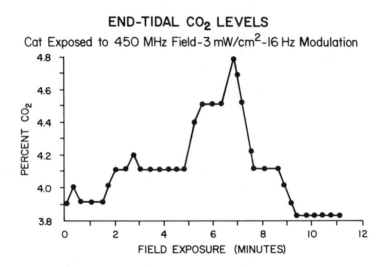

END-TIDAL CO_2 LEVELS

Cat Exposed to 450 MHz Field-3 mW/cm^2-16 Hz Modulation

Fig. 1. Transient increase in end-tidal CO_2 at onset of exposure of unanesthetized cat to a 3 mW/cm^2 450 MHz field, 16 Hz sinusoidal modulation. (From Adey, Bawin and Lawrence, 1982).

Increased carbon dioxide excretion followed initiation of exposure of unanesthetized cats to a 16 Hz sinusoidally modulated 450 MHz field and correlated with increased cerebral calcium efflux (Adey, et al., 1982), (Fig. 1) but hypoventilation-induced hypercapnea did not increase calcium efflux. Conditioned EEG rhythms in cats are modified by 147 MHz 0.8 mW/cm^2 field sinusoidally modulated at the same frequencies as the EEG (Bawin et al., 1973).

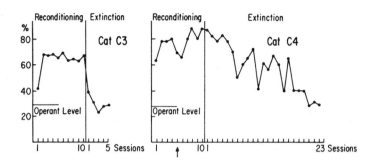

Fig. 2. Comparison of performance of two cats trained to produce a "burst" of EEG waves in response to a light flash. Cat C3 was overtrained and extinguished on a 14 Hz rhythm in the nucleus centrum medianum. No field was imposed. Cat C4 was similarly manipulated on a 4.5 Hz hippocampal rhythm but was also exposed to a 147 MHz 1.0 mW/cm^2 field, sinusoidally modulated at 4.5 Hz. Arrow marks first day of field exposure. Data are normalized over the total number of CS presentations within a session. Irradiated animals differed markedly from the control group in rate of performance, accuracy (in terms of frequency bandwidth) of the reinforced patterns and resistance to extinction (minimum of 50 vs. 10 days). (From Bawin, Gavalas-Medici and Adey, 1973).

Physiological experiments with imposed fields have added impressive data on the sensitivity of cerebral tissue to fields orders of magnitude weaker than the membrane potential. In the awake cat, cortical stimulation with a pulse train at the same intensity as the EEG gradient (200/sec, 1.0 msec, 50–100 mV/cm) increased efflux of calcium and of the neurotransmitter GABA by almost 20 percent (Kaczmarek and Adey, 1974). In the awake cat, cyclic increments in calcium efflux with a periodicity of about 20 min occurred during and following exposure to a 450 MHz microwave field sinusoidally modulated at 16 Hz and producing a tissue gradient of 330 mV/cm (Adey et al., 1982). Other data on sensitivity of cultured nerve cells to weak pulsed magnetic fields are discussed below (Dixey and Rein, 1982).

Cerebral tissue slice preparations have produced growing evidence on the capacity for propagation of wave phenomena in the absence of synaptic transmission.

Following chemical synaptic blockade in the hippocampal
slice with lowered calcium and raised manganese levels,
paroxysmal wave discharges occur with electric stimulation
(Jefferys and Haas, 1982; Taylor and Dudek, 1984; Bawin et
al., 1984). This propagation is attributed to the
extracellular electric field causing a passive current flow
across inactive cell membranes, exciting and synchronizing
populations of neurons.

3.   Cerebral Electrical Impedance and the Extracellular
     Space.

From a quite different perspective, "electrical
impedance changes accompanying physiological responses may
arise in perineuronal fluid with a substantial
macromolecular content and calcium ions may modulate
perineuronal conductivity" (Adey, 1966). Since cell
membranes exhibit typical resistances in the range
1,000-1,000,000 ohm.cm^2, and since the specific resistance
of extracellular fluid is of the order of 50 ohm.cm^{-1}, most
measuring current flows along membrane surfaces.
Macromolecular strands derived from intramembranous proteins
lie in the ECS and may modulate conductance as a function of
cerebral tissue state; thus, there are impedance
"transients" accompanying alerting, orienting and visual
discriminative responses (Adey et al., 1966) (Fig. 3). They
exhibit differential characteristics in different brain
regions. Long lasting but reversible impedance changes
occur with anesthetic and psychotropic drugs. We have shown
that this impedance relates to extracellular calcium levels
(Nicholson, 1965).

4.   The Physiological Dilemma in Observed Tissue
     Sensitivities to Weak Imposed Electromagnetic Fields.

Ever since the turn of the century, excitability of
nerve membranes has been addressed on the basis of
equilibrium phenomena, with emphasis on massive
perturbations in transmembrane ionic states associated with
depolarization of the membrane potential. These concepts
have been elegantly expressed in models for the squid axon
(Hodgkin and Huxley, 1952) and for the spinal motoneuron
(Eccles, 1953).

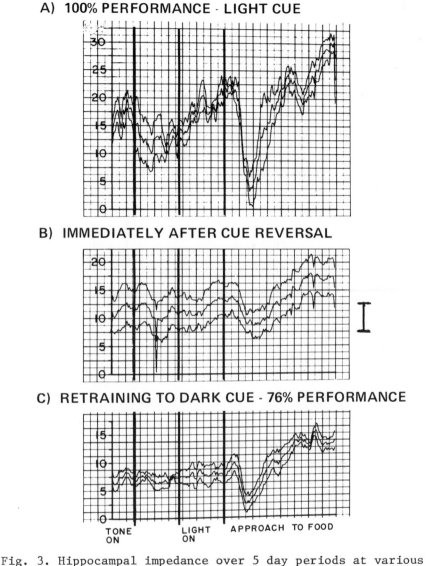

A) 100% PERFORMANCE - LIGHT CUE

B) IMMEDIATELY AFTER CUE REVERSAL

C) RETRAINING TO DARK CUE - 76% PERFORMANCE

TONE
ON

LIGHT
ON

APPROACH TO FOOD

Fig. 3. Hippocampal impedance over 5 day periods at various levels of training, with successive presentations of alerting, orienting and discriminative stimuli. In each graph, middle trace shows mean. Upper and lower traces show one standard deviation. Variability was low at 100 percent performance (A), increased substantially after cue reversal (B), but decreased again after retraining (C). Calibration, 50 pf. (From Adey, Kado, McIlwain and Walter, 1966).

These models define lower limits for theshold
transmembrane currents inducing depolarization of the
membrane potential that exists across the lipid bilayer.
For example, the typical membrane potential of 70 mV exists
across 40 Å, equivalent to an electric gradient of 10^5 V/cm.
Threshold current levels to depolarize this gradient are
about 1.0 mA/cm^2 through the membrane. Current densities in
pericellular fluid to achieve this threshold will be 2 or 3
orders of magnitude higher, due to the disparity in
conductances between EC fluid and cell membranes. Clearly,
it would appear unlikely that extracellular electric
gradients of the order of the EEG (10^{-1} V/cm) or the far
weaker gradients induced by many environmental fields would
have physiological significance.

How is this amplification achieved? Weak pericellular
fields at least six orders of magnitude less than the
membrane potential exercise major control over intracellular
metabolic and messenger enzyme systems. The sequence of
steps from membrane surface to cell interior is consistent
with nonlinear, nonequilibrium processes. The following
synthesis of experimental data has considered the role of
both cooperative (dissipative) and dispersive processes in
modeling ionic and molecular behavior in cell membrane
transductive coupling (Adey, 1981a and b, 1983, 1984).

5.   Cell Membrane Substrates of Weak Electrochemical
Sensitivities

Experimental findings are consistent with the "fluid
mosaic" model of cell membranes (Singer and Nicolson, 1972).
External protrusions of intramembranous helical protein
particles (IMPs) "floating" in the lipid bilayer have amino
sugar (sialic acid) polyanionic terminals. They form a huge
negatively charged sheet that attracts hydrogen and calcium
ions in a "counterion" layer (Fig. 4).

Internal strands of IMPs may have further connections
with elements of the cytoskeleton, including microtubules
(Edelman, 1976). Thus, this series of pathways would
provide relatively direct communication from receptor sites
on the cell surface to intracellular organelles, including
the nucleus. Altered cytoskeletal elements have been
reported in cerebellar Purkinje neurons of rabbits exposed
to 50 Hz power line fields (14 kV/m, expected tissue

FLUID MOSAIC CELL MEMBRANE MODEL
(after Singer & Nicolson, 1972)

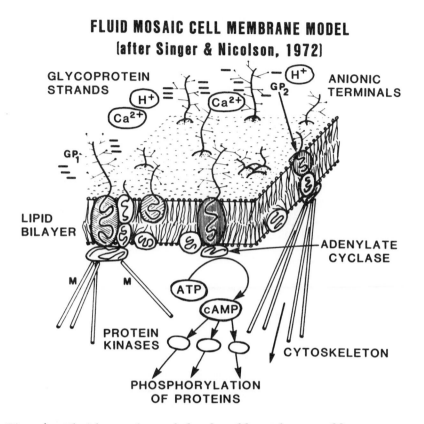

Fig. 4. Fluid mosaic model of cell membrane offers a
structural basis for tissue interactions with EM fields.
Intramembranous protein particles (IMPs) in the lipid
bilayer have protruding external glycoprotein strands,
negatively charged on their amino sugar terminals. They
form receptor sites for antibodies, hormones and
neurotransmitters. They attract calcium ions. Stimulating
molecules and EM fields alter surface calcium binding in the
first step of transmembrane signal coupling. In the second
stage, transmembrane signals pass along IMPs which act as
coupling proteins to the interior. The third stage
modulates intracellular enzyme activity, including adenylate
cyclase and protein kinase messenger enzymes. (Modified
from Singer and Nicolson, 1972).

components of the order of 1 mV/cm), and similar but less
severe changes in hippocampus, cerebral cortex and thalamic
nuclei (Hansson, 1981).

Stranded glycoproteins also form an intercellular
matrix in developing tissues essential for migration of
major cell masses in the embryo. A pulsed 100 Hz, 1.2 μT
magnetic field (about 1 percent of the intensity of the
earth's magnetic field) inhibited embryogenesis in
experiments where a major reduction in extracellular
glycoproteins was a key finding (Delgado et al., 1982). The
neural tube failed to close. Elegant studies by Edelman and
his colleagues (1984) have identified morphogenetic genes
responsible for production of glycoproteins on the surface
of nerve cells (nCAMs). They are necessary for cell
adhesion and migration in regional brain development and in
subsequent maturation. Delgado's findings are consistent
with EM field modulation of this essential morphogenetic
system.

6. A Three Stage Model of Cell Membrane Transductive
    Coupling of Electromagnetic Fields and Humoral
    Stimuli.

We have briefly considered anatomical and physiological
evidence pointing to the cell membrane as a prime site of
interaction with EM fields in tissue. Although the picture
remains incomplete in important aspects, the collected data
from recent research is consistent with a sequence of steps
that couple signals from oscillating fields and from humoral
stimuli from the cell surface to the interior. We have used
EM fields to manipulate humoral events at cell membranes,
including responses to hormones and antibodies associated
with enzymatic activity within cells, and in other
instances, field effects on cellular secretions, such as
insulin and collagen.

As predicted a decade ago, EM fields that either
oscillate at low frequencies or are radiofrequency fields
amplitude-modulated at low frequencies have proved powerful
tools in understanding intimate qualities of communication
between cells (Adey, 1975). Their use has allowed
determination of the sequence of key steps in transmembrane
coupling. It has also permitted relatively precise
examination of aspects of energetics in the coupling

sequence. Manipulation of neurohumoral, endocrine and immune processes has disclosed highly nonlinear, nonequilibrium mechanisms in cell membrane sensitivities to extracellular electrochemical oscillations. Finally, examination of these membrane electrochemical sensitivities in widely differing cell types suggests that this may be a general biological property; and that further search may determine its occurrence in varying degree in many tissues.

There is a minimal sequence of three steps in transductive coupling (Adey, 1984a and b) and each is calcium-dependent: (a) cell surface glycoproteins sense the first weak electrochemical events associated with binding of neurohumoral molecules, hormones and antibodies; (b) transmembrane portions of IMPs signal these surface events to the cell interior; (c) internally, there is coupling of this signal to intracellular enzyme systems and to the cytoskeleton (and thus to the nucleus and other organelles).

6a.   Stage 1: Cooperative Modification of Calcium Binding in "Amplification" of Initial Signal.

Initial cell surface events appear to involve modulation of calcium binding to the numerous negative charges on the surface glycoprotein sheet. This step is presumed to occur along the plane of the membrane surface. A longitudinal spread would be consistent with spreading calcium-dependent enzymatic activation from a single membrane molecular locus proposed by Nishizuka (1984) and discussed below.

In brain tissue, two distinct and contrasting patterns of calcium efflux occur in response to differing types of imposed fields. RF fields at intensities around 1.0 mW/cm^2 and with sinusoidal amplitude-modulation from 3 to 35 Hz produced a "tuning curve" of increased calcium efflux, with a maximum increase at 16 Hz and smaller increments at higher and lower frequencies (Bawin, Kaczmarek and Adey, 1975). Unmodulated fields had no effect. Essential aspects of these studies in isolated cerebral tissue have been confirmed in awake cats at tissue field gradients around 0.1 V/cm (Adey, Bawin and Lawrence, 1982). Far weaker sinusoidal electric fields in the same low frequency range (calculated levels in isolated cerebral tissue six orders of magnitude lower) also produced a "tuning curve" of modified

calcium efflux, essentially as a mirror image of that from
the stronger RF fields, with a decrease rather than an
increase (Bawin and Adey, 1976). These responses are
"windowed" with respect to field frequency and also to field
intensity (Bawin, Sheppard and Adey, 1978; Blackman et al.,
1979). This is the strongest single line of evidence about
the essential nonlinearity of these effects.

As a finer focus on the structural and functional basis
of this field-sensitive calcium efflux in brain tissue, we
have examined this relationship in synaptosome fractions
(Lin-Liu and Adey, 1982). Cerebral synaptosomes, typically
0.7 µm in diameter, retain the synaptic junction and
adjoining postsynaptic membrane. They have characteristics
typical of brain chemical synapses. Calcium efflux was
studied in synaptosomes preloaded with $^{45}Ca^{2+}$, using a
continuous perfusion technique in a calcium-free
physiological solution. This minimized Ca-Ca exchange
between intra- and extracellular compartments. A 450 MHz
0.5 mW/cm^2 field (measured gradient in air, 43 V/m) and
sinusoidally modulated at 16 Hz increased the rate constant
of the efflux by 38 percent (Fig. 5). Unmodulated and 60
Hz-modulated fields were without effect. This field-induced
change was distinguishable from $CaCl_2$-stimulated efflux,
which is most probably derived from intracellular sites.
Thus, these tiny elements of cerebral nerve fiber terminals
also exhibited a frequency-selective calcium efflux to field
exposure. The data support a model of field interaction
with calcium at cell membrane surface sites.

We have proposed the following model for these highly
cooperative interactions (Adey, 1981b). From intracellular
sources, anionic charge sites on terminals of protruding
glycoprotein strands are raised to energy levels
substantially above ground state, forming "patches" or
domains with coherent states between neighboring charge
sites. Weak triggers at the boundaries of these coherent
domains, such as oscillating EM fields or proton tunneling,
may initiate a domino effect, with release of much more
energy than in the initial triggering events. Modulation of
membrane surface calcium binding is thus an "amplifying"
step in the transductive sequence, and is sensitive to
imposed EM fields.

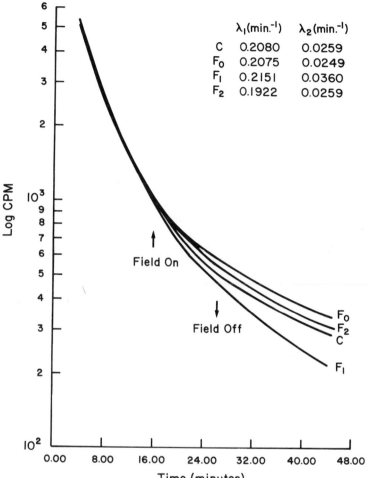

Fig. 5. Computer fitting of composite calcium efflux data from rat cerebral synaptosomes, each obtained by averaging at every time point all experimental data, which were first normalized for a $^{45}Ca^{2+}$ efflux of 2000 cpm at time 10 minutes. Rate constants computed for the 4 composites are shown at upper right: (C) control; (Fo) unmodulated 450 MHz field; (F1) same field with 16 Hz modulation; (F2) same field with 60 Hz modulation. (From Lin–Liu and Adey, 1982).

6b.   Stage 2:   Signaling Along Proteinaceous Molecules
      Spanning the Plasma Membrane.

The "avalanche" effect of weak fields on calcium
binding to cell membrane surfaces appears to be one of the
first steps in membrane signal processing. Are there
measurable field effects on calcium-dependent cell membrane
functions, as for example, in the direct action of one cell
membrane on another; or in the cell's internal responses to
hormones and antibodies; or in the secretion of hormones or
in the synthesis of cement substances or supporting tissue?
The questions have all been answered affirmatively in
studies of this second step in transmembrane signal
coupling. Aspects of energetics of signals passing both
inward and outward across the cell membrane have been
evaluated with imposed EM fields.

Imposed fields modify release of noradrenalin from
cultured pheochromocytoma cells (Dixey and Rein, 1982). A
500 Hz pulsed magnetic field with an 8 g peak intensity that
induced only 0.1 mV/cm in the pericellular fluid sharply
increased noradrenalin release. The response depended on
calcium levels and on the calcium/magnesium ratio in the
bathing fluid. Accepted models based on equilibrium
considerations, such as the Hodgkin-Huxley model, do not
account for these sensitivities to fields far weaker than
the membrane potential (10^5 V/cm).

Secretion of insulin from cultured pancreatic islets
stimulated by glucose was reduced by 35 percent in the
presence of a low frequency pulsed magnetic field that
induced a current density of about 1.0 uA/cm^2 (Jolley et
al., 1983). Formation of collagen is the first step in
deposition of new bone. This is inhibited by the peptide
parathyroid hormone (PTH) which binds to receptor
glycoproteins on the cell surface. A 72 Hz pulsed magnetic
field at the same intensity as in the insulin experiments
blocked this inhibitory action of PTH at receptor sites;
leading to the conclusion that this field action is on
coupling proteins carrying signals across the cell membrane
(Luben et al., 1982).

Direct membrane-to-membrane interactions have been
assayed in studies of the cytolytic capacity of allogeneic T
lymphocytes targeted against human lymphoma cells (Lyle et
al., 1983). Cytolysis was reduced more than 20 percent in

vitro with a 450 MHz field (peak energy 1.5 mW/cm^2) and
sinusoidally amplitude-modulated at 60 Hz (Fig. 6). This
sensitivity followed a "window" with respect to modulation
frequency over the range 3-100 Hz. Maximum effects occurred
at 60 Hz and declined at higher and lower frequencies.
Unmodulated fields caused no change. Also, this altered
lymphocyte membrane status persisted after termination of
field exposure, with discernible changes for as long as 12
hours. These fields thus modify some forms of direct
cell-to-cell communication that depends on the precise
pattern of cell surface antigen-antibody mosaic.

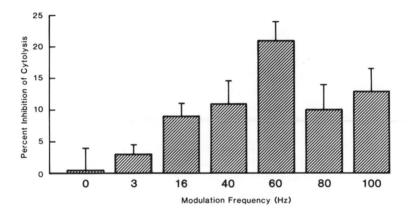

Fig. 6. Inhibition of cytotoxicity of allogeneic
T-lymphocytes targeted against human lymphoma cells as
modulation frequency was varied between 0 and 100 Hz. (From
Lyle et al., 1983).

6c. Stage 3: Signal Coupling from Cell Membranes to
      Intracellular Systems.

The third step couples signals from cell membranes to
intracellular systems. There is good evidence that
transmembrane signaling occurs along intramembranous helical
proteins (IMPs). Their stranded inner ends may interact
directly with enzyme molecules lying close to the membrane,
as in the case of adenylate cyclase. However, within the
cell, a tertiary communication system distributes these
signals more widely. Although the full extent of this
system is not known, it clearly involves the great messenger
system of the protein kinase enzymes, and it probably also
involves the tiny tubules and filaments of the cytoskeleton.

In bone cells and cultured embryonic bones, binding of parathyroid hormone (PTH) to cell surface receptors activates membrane-bound adenylate cyclase, initiating conversion of ATP to cAMP, releasing metabolic energy and activating some protein kinases. This sequence is inhibited by a 70 Hz pulsed magnetic field (20-30 g peak intensity) (Luben et al., 1982). Activation of adenylate cyclase bound to the inside of the membrane is inhibited, even though PTH is still bound to surface receptors, and the bone cells resume synthesis of collagen. The field appears to "jam" signals that would otherwise pass across the membrane to the cell interior and activate adenylate cyclase.

Sinusoidal 10 Hz electric fields capacitively coupled to cultured embryonic chick and mouse bones (estimated culture fluid gradient 10^{-7} V/cm) increase bone formation. A 30 minute daily exposure was more effective than continuous exposure. Indices of bone formation included increased release of a glycoprotein skeletal growth factor (SGF), increased cell proliferation, increased collagen formation, and increased mitogenic response to SGF. Fields at 1 and 50 Hz had no effect and 100 Hz fields decreased bone formation to 51 percent of controls ($p < .001$) (Fitzsimmons et al., 1984).

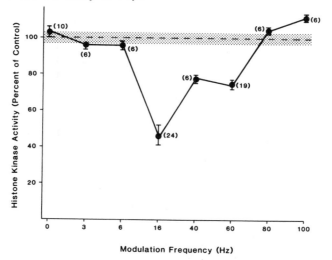

Fig. 7. Activity of cAMP-independent protein kinase in human lymphocytes is sharply reduced by a 450 MHz field (1.0 mW/cm^2 peak envelope power) amplitude modulated at frequencies between 16 and 60 Hz, but not at higher or lower frequencies, nor with unmodulated fields. (From Byus et al., 1984).

Protein kinase enzymes act as intracellular messengers by phosphorylating other proteins. Some kinase enzymes are activated following production of cyclic adenosine monophosphate (cAMP) from adenosine triphosphate (ATP) by action of membrane-bound adenylate cyclase. These are the AMP-dependent kinases. AMP-independent kinases are activated by messages from the cell membrane that do not follow the cAMP pathway. AMP-independent kinase activity in cultured human lymphocytes is sharply reduced by a 450 MHz field (peak intensity 1.0 mW/cm^2) when sinusoidally modulated at frequencies between 16 and 60 Hz, but not at higher or lower frequencies (Fig. 7), nor with unmodulated fields. This reduction occurred only in the first 15 to 30 minutes after onset of exposure (Byus et al., 1984). Thus, in addition to windows in frequency and amplitude discussed above, there is a "window in time" for field action (Fig. 8). It is a matter of conjecture whether such major but transient responses would be associated with a significant immune insult in the intact subject; and whether their transient nature may imply that repeated intermittent exposures may each have their separate effects.

7. Biophysical Perspectives on Future Research in Nonlinear Electrodynamics of Cell Membranes.

These experimental data emphasize the need for new models of field-tissue interactions. They should consider those data which clearly imply nonequilibrium interactions and should relate them to appropriate cellular and molecular substrates; with the expectation that they would fill needed predictive capabilities in future research.

The quest for predictive models of transmembrane signaling current research focuses on mechanisms underlying sensitivities at low field frequencies in both ionic and molecular interactions; on the windowed character of many of these responses; on the precise nature of membrane surface macromolecular changes arising in joint interactions with calcium ions and imposed fields; and on resonant interactions of millimetric and other microwave fields with biological macromolecules, including DNA.

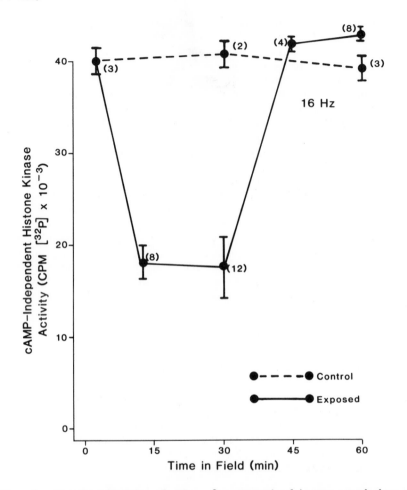

Fig. 8. In the fields of Fig. 3, protein kinase activity was reduced only 15 to 30 minutes after onset of field exposure, thus establishing a "window in time" for field action. (From Byus et al., 1984).

No known mechanisms explain ELF bioeffects on the basis of direct interactions with component dipoles of molecular systems oscillating at these low frequencies. Therefore, a structural and functional basis must reside in properties of molecular systems; as, for example, in phase transition models proposed by Frohlich (1975) and Grodsky (1976); or possibly in a coherent motion of ions bound at the membrane surface in the counterion layer (Polk, 1984).

Mon Jan 06 1997

The item below is now available for pickup at designated location.

Ohio State University
OSU Main Library

Jerome Library
CALL NO: RC350.N48R31990
AUTHOR: Rattay, Frank
Electrical nerve stimulation : theo
BARCODE: A113098197750
REC NO: i19898381
PICKUP AT: My Office

ROBERT DAVID WELLS
PHYSICS
2011 SMITH LAB
174 W EIGHTEENTH AVE
CAMPUS

AM

Mon Jan 06 1997

PAGING SLIP - The item/s listed below has been requested. Go to
the stacks and pull it.

Ogg Science Library
Math/Science Bldg, Room 308
BGSU
Bowling Green, Ohio 43403

Science Stacks
CALL NO: RC350.N48R31990
AUTHOR: Rattay, Frank
Electrical nerve stimulation : theo
BARCODE: A113098197 50
REC NO: i19898381
PICKUP AT: My Office

ROBERT DAVID WELLS
PHYSICS
2011 SMITH LAB
174 W EIGHTEENTH AVE
CAMPUS
INSTITUTION: Ohio State University
PATRON TYPE: ohlnk faculty

We have considered modulation of calcium binding in the plane of the membrane surface by highly cooperative processes. There is now striking evidence for a simultaneous calcium-dependent enzyme activation that spreads over the whole cell membrane surface from a single molecular locus. Studies of the calcium-dependent membrane enzyme phosphatidyl serine kinase (kinase C) have shown it to be both an enzyme and a receptor. It occurs in higher concentrations in brain cell membranes than elsewhere. It is also a focus of interest in cancer research, since it is a receptor for powerful cancer promoting substances, the phorbol esters. Its role in brain cells may be linked to regulation of transmembrane calcium currents, since phorbol esters act in this way in Aplysia ganglion cells (DeRiemer et al., 1984). Nishizuka and his colleagues (1984) have shown that one molecule of diacylglycerol, produced in the course of excitation by the breakdown of one molecule of inositol phospholipid in the membrane, can activate every molecule of kinase C in the presence of calcium. These findings clearly offer a new avenue for studies of EM field bioeffects, and as Nishizuka points out, "these findings provide an entirely new concept of receptor function."

Development of highly stable signal sources in the millimetric and far-infrared regions has led to testing of theoretical models of resonant interactions with helical proteins and DNA (Illinger, 1981; Kohli et al., 1981; Mei et al., 1981). At 11 GHz, energy absorption by DNA fragments is about 400 times higher than in the surrounding aqueous medium, with evidence for a chain length dependence in the absorption (Edwards et al., 1983). At still higher frequencies around 42 GHz, Grundler et al. (1983) have shown increased and decreased growth of yeast cells with a periodicity around 8 MHz as a function of field frequency. Related experiments at the same field frequency have correlated this effect with nonlinear vibrational energy exchanges between hydrogen atoms in amide groups that form the spines of helical proteins and DNA (Genzel et al., 1983). All these experiments were conducted with athermal levels of field exposure.

Do these highly nonlinear vibrational energy exchanges in helical proteins play a role in signal transmission across cell membranes? We have considered the possibility that this may involve the passage of solitary waves, or solitons, down the length of the long spirals of the helical protein molecules spanning the membrane (Lawrence and Adey,

1982). These solitons may be considered as traveling
"packets" of a vibrational state, forming quasiparticles
that pass along the triple spines of the protein molecule.
These concepts suggest a fundamentally new aspect to the
organization of matter at molecular and atomic levels, and
there is an intense search to detect solitons in biological
and physical systems. Atoms in solitons are not necessarily
randomly located, as classic statistical mechanics of matter
has postulated, and in this "clustering" or graininess,
first perceptions indicate some unique properties of these
quasiparticles.

There is strong but inconclusive evidence for the
occurrence of solitons in biomolecules. The triple parallel
spines of helical proteins and DNA are formed of amide
groups with the repeating atomic sequence -C-O-H-N. Davydov
(1979) has modeled energy exchanges in this system in the
formation of "packets" of vibrating elements. Vibrational
energy of the hydrogen atom is exchanged nonlinearly with
exciton states in the amide group and vice versa. When this
nonlinear exchange reaches a threshold energy level and
involves a sufficient number of elements, the packet behaves
as a quasiparticle and moves as an entity along the linear
macromolecule as a soliton. They may be detected by Raman
scattering that occurs when they encounter anisotropies in
the molecular chain as they propagate. Raman scattering
with millimeter microwave exposure was first reported in
bacterial cultures by Webb (1975). Scott (1981) modeled
vibrational modes in the Davydov soliton and calculated
Raman scattering numbers for amide spine sequences,
producing an excellent fit with Webb's data. Toboada and
Mrotek (1984) have examined human nasal and mouse adrenal
cancer cells for solitons induced by 514 nm laser light,
reporting that anti-Stokes Raman spectra support the
existence of two fundamental solitons predicted by Scott.

The precise nature of this second step in transductive
cell membrane coupling awaits future research, which will
doubtless determine the precise mechanisms of the striking
and beautiful nonlinearities within and between cells
revealed by these manipulations with weak electromagnetic
fields. There may well be a series of these nonlinear
interatomic processes, of which solitons would be but one
manifestation.

SUMMARY

The structural and functional aspects of communication between cells have been reviewed, with emphasis on the cell membrane in detection and transductive coupling of oscillating electromagnetic fields in the pericellular environment. Imposed fields are powerful and highly specific tools in manipulation of the sequence of events in membrane transductive coupling. They have revealed nonlinear and nonequilibrium aspects of these interactions. In cerebral tissue, extracellular fields orders of magnitude weaker than the membrane potential can modulate cell firing patterns, entrain EEG rhythms, alter neurotransmitter release and modulate behavioral states. These sensitivities have also been widely detected in non-neural tissues. It is therefore proposed that an intrinsic communication system between cells based on these weak electromagnetic influences may be a general biological property. A three-step model of transductive coupling is presented. First, a highly cooperative modification of calcium binding occurs in the plane of the membrane surface following a focal event at a receptor site. This "amplifying" stage releases substantially more energy than in the initial events. Cerebral extracellular conductance changes accompanying physiological responses may arise in perineuronal fluid with a substantial macromolecular content and calcium ions may modulate perineuronal conductivity. In the second stage, coupling occurs along transmembrane helical proteins and may be mediated by solitons. The third stage couples transmembrane signals to the cytoskeleton and to intracellular enzyme systems, including membrane-bound adenylate cyclase and the protein kinase system of intracellular messengers. Activation of these intracellular systems is calcium-dependent.

ACKNOWLEDGEMENTS

Our studies have been generously supported by the US Department of Energy, the US Environmental Protection Agency, the Southern California Edison Company, the USFDA Bureau of Radiological Health, and the US Veterans Administration.

REFERENCES

Adey WR (1966). Intrinsic organization of cerebral tissue
  in alerting, orienting and discriminative responses. In
  Quarton GC, Melnechuk T, Schmitt FO, (eds): "The
  Neurosciences. First Study Program," New York:
  Rockefeller University, p 615.
Adey WR (1975). Effects of electromagnetic radiation on the
  nervous system. Ann NY Acad Sci 247:15.
Adey WR (1981a). Tissue interactions with electromagnetic
  fields. Physiol Rev 61:435.
Adey WR (1981b). Ionic nonequilibrium phenomena in tissue
  interactions with electromagnetic fields. In Illinger KH
  (ed): "Biological Effects of Nonionizing Radiation,"
  Washington DC: American Physiological Society, p. 271.
Adey WR (1983). Molecular aspects of cell membranes as
  substrates for interactions with electromagnetic fields.
  In Basar E, Flohr H, Haken H, Mandell AJ (eds):
  "Synergetics of the Brain," Berlin: Springer, p 201.
Adey WR (1984a). Biological models of electromagnetic field
  interactions with tissues: a review and synthesis of
  recent findings. In Anderson L (ed): "Interaction of
  Biological Systems with Static and ELF Electric and
  Magnetic Fields," Washington DC: Department of Energy.
Adey WR (1984b). Nonlinear, nonequilibrium aspects of
  electromagnetic field interactions at cell membranes. In
  Adey WR, Lawrence AF (eds): "Nonlinear Electrodynamics of
  Biological Systems," New York: Plenum, p 3.
Adey WR, Bawin SM, Lawrence AF (1982). Effects of weak
  amplitude-modulated microwave fields on calcium efflux
  from awake cat cerebral cortex. Bioelectromagnetics
  3:295.
Adey WR, Kado RT, McIlwain JT, Walter DO (1966). The role
  of neuronal elements in regional cerebral impedance
  changes in alerting, orienting and discriminative
  responses. Exptl Neurol 15:490.
Adey WR, Lawrence AF (eds) (1984). "Nonlinear
  Electrodynamics of Biological Systems," New York: Plenum,
  608 pp.
Bawin SM, Adey WR (1976). Sensitivity of calcium binding in
  cerebral tissue to weak environmental electric fields
  oscillating at low frequency. Proc Nat Acad Sci USA
  73:1999.
Bawin SM, Gavalas-Medici R, Adey WR (1973). Effects of
  modulated very high frequency fields on specific brain
  rhythms in cats. Brain Res 58:365.

Bawin SM, Kaczmarek LK, Adey WR (1975): Effects of modulated VHF fields on the central nervous system. Ann NY Acad Sci 247:74.

Bawin SM, Sheppard AR, Adey WR (1978). Possible mechanisms of weak electromagnetic field coupling in brain tissue. Bioelectrochem Bioenergetics 5:67.

Bawin SM, Sheppard AR, Mahoney MD, Adey WR (1984). Influences of sinusoidal electric fields on excitability in the rat hippocampal slice. Brain Res 323:227.

Blackman CF, Elder JA, Weil CM, Benane SG, Eichinger DC, House DE (1979). Induction of calcium ion efflux from brain tissue by radio frequency radiation; effects of modulation frequency and field strength. Radio Sci 14:93.

Byus CV, Lundak RL, Fletcher RM, Adey WR (1984). Altered protein kinase activity following exposure of cultured human lymphocytes to modulated microwave fields. Bioelectromagnetics 5:341.

Cajal R (1911). Histologie du Systeme Nerveux. A. Maloine, Paris.

Creutzfeldt OD, Watanabe S, Lux HD (1966). Relations between EG phenomena and potentials of single cortical cells. II. Spontaneous and convulsoid activity. Electroenphalogr Clin Neurophysiol 20:19.

Davydov AS (1979). Solitons in physical systems. Physica Scripta 20:387.

Delgado JMR, Leal J, Monteagudo JL, Gracia MG (1982). Embryological changes induced by weak, extremely low frequency electromagnetic fields. J Anat (Longdon) 134:533.

DeRiemer SA, Albert KA, Strong JA, Greengard P, Kaczmarek LK (1984). Electrophysiological effects of phorbol ester and protein kinase C on the bag cell neurons of Aplysia. Proc Soc Neurosci 14th Annual Meeting, p 867 (abstract).

Dixey R, Rein G (1982). H-noradrenaline release potentiated in a clonal cell line by low-intensity pulsed magnetic fields. Nature 296:253.

Eccles JC (1953). "The Neurophysiological Basis of Mind," Oxford: University Press.

Edelman GM (1976). Surface modulation in recognition and cell growth. Science 192:218.

Edelman GM (1984). Cell-adhesion molecules: a molecular basis for animal form. Scientific American 250(4):118.

Edwards GS, Davis CC, Saffer JD, Swicord MS (1984). Resonant absorption of microwave energy by DNA. Proc Bioelectromangetics Soc, 6th Annual Meeting, Atlanta GA, p 33 (abstract).

Elul R (1967). Statistical mechanisms in generation of the EEG. In Fogel LJ, George FW (eds): "Progress in Biomedical Engineering," Washington DC: Spartan, p 131.

Elul R (1972). The genesis of the EEG. Internat Rev Neurobiol 15:227.

Fitzsimmons R, Farley J, Adey R, Baylink D (1984). Bone formation is increased after short term exposure to very low amplitude electric fields in vitro. J Cell Biol 99:422a (abstract).

Frohlich H (1975). Evidence for Bose condensation-like excitation of coherent modes in biological systems. Phys Lett 51A:21.

Fujita Y, Sato T (1964). Intracellular records from hippocampal pyramidal cells in rabbit during theta rhythm activity. J Neurophysiol 27:1012.

Gavalas RJ, Walter DO, Hamer J, Adey WR (1970). Effects of low-level, low-frequency electric fields on EEG and behavior in Macaca nemestrina. Brain Res 18:491.

Gavalas-Medici R, Day-Magdaleno SR (1976). Extremely low frequency, weak electric fields affect schedule-controlled behavior of monkeys. Nature 261:256.

Genzel L, Kremer F, Poglitsch A, Bechtold G (1983). Relaxation processes on a picosecond time scale in hemoglobin and poly-1-alanine observed by mm-wave-spectroscopy. Biopolymers 22:1715.

Grodsky IT (1976). Neuronal membrane: a physical synthesis. Math Biosci 28:191.

Grundler W, Keilmann F, Putterlik V, Santo L, Strube D, Zimmermann I (1983). Nonthermal resonant action of millimeter microwaves on yeast growth. In Frohlich H, Kremer F (eds): "Coherent Excitations in Biological Systems," Heidelberg: Springer, p 25.

Hansson H-A (1981). Lamellar bodies of Purkinje nerve cells experimentally induced by electric field. Brain Res 203:47.

Hodgkin AL, Huxley AF (1952). A quantitative description of membrane current and its application to conduction and excitation in nerve. J Physiol (London) 117:500.

Illinger KH (1981). Electromagnetic-field interaction with biological systems in the microwave and far-infrared region. In Illinger KH (ed): "Biological Effects of Nonionizing Radiation," Washington DC: American Chemical Society, Symposium Series No. 157, p 1.

Jefferys JGR, Haas HL (1982). Synchronized bursting of CA1 hippocampal pyramidal cells in the absence of synaptic transmission. Nature 300:448.

Jolley WB, Hinshaw, DB, Knierim K (1983). Magnetic field effects on calcium efflux and insulin secretion in isolated rabbit islets of Langerhans. Bioelectromagnetics 4:103.

Kaczmarek LK, Adey WR (1974). Weak electric gradients change ionic and transmitter fluxes in cortex. Brain Res 66:537.

Kohli M, Mei WN, Van Zandt LL, Prohofsky EW (1981). Calculated microwave absorption by double-helical DNA. In Illinger KH (ed): "Biological Effects of Nonionizing Radiation," Washington DC: American Chemical Society, Symposium Series No. 157, p 101.

Lawrence AF, Adey WR (1982). Nonlinear wave mechanisms in interactions between excitable tissue and electromagnetic fields. Neurol Res 4:115.

Luben RA, Cain CD, Chen MC-Y, Rosen DM, Adey WR (1982). Effects of electromagnetic stimuli on bone and bone cells in vitro: inhibition of responses to parathyroid hormone by low-energy low-frequency fields. Proc Nat Acad Sci USA 79:4180.

Lyle DB, Schechter P, Adey WR, Lundak RL (1983). Suppression of T-lymphocyte cytotoxicity following exposure to sinusoidally amplitude-modulated fields. Bioelectromagnetics 4:281.

Mei WN, Kohli M, Van Zandt LL, Prohofsky EW (1981). Long-range forces in DNA. In Illinger KH (ed): "Biological Effects of Nonionizing Radiation," Washington DC: American Chemical Society, Symposium Series No. 157, p 95.

Nicholson PW (1965). Specific impedance of cerebral white matter. Exper Neurol 13:386.

Nishizuka Y (1984). The role of protein kinase C in cell surface transduction and tumor promotion. Nature 308:693.

Polk C (1984). Time varying magnetic fields and DNA synthesis: magnitude of forces due to magnetic fields on surface-bound counterions. Proc Bioelectromagnetics Soc, 6th Annual Meeting, Atlanta GA, p 77 (abstract).

Scott AC (1981). The laser-Raman spectrum of a Davydov soliton. Phys Letters 86A:60.

Shepherd GM (1974). "The Synaptic Organization of the Brain," Oxford: University Press.

Sherrington C (1947). The Integrative Action of the Nervous System. University Press, Cambridge, 433 pp.

Singer SJ, Nicolson GL (1972). The fluid mosaic model of cell membrane. Science 175:720.

Smith RF (1984). Core temperature as a behavioral indicant of the rat's reaction to low frequency magnetic fields. Ph.D. Thesis, Department of Psychology, University of Kansas.

Taboada J, Mrotek J (1984). Evidence for Davydov solitons in the anti-Stokes Raman spectra of living HEP-2 cells and Y-1 cancer cells. Bull Amer Phys Soc 28:30 (abstract).

Taylor CP, Dudek FE (1984). Excitation of hippocampal pyramidal cells by an electrical field effect. J Neurophysiol 52:126.

Webb SJ (1975). Genetic continuity and metabolic regulation as seen by the effects of various microwave and black light frequencies on these phenomena. Ann NY Acad Sci 247:327.

Wever R (1968). Einfluss schwacher elektro-magnetischer Felder auf die circadiane Periodik des Menschen. Naturwissenschaften 55:29.

Wever R (1977). Effects of low-level low-frequency fields on human circadian rhythms. Neurosci Res Program Bull 15:39.

Young JZ (1951). "Doubt and Certainty in Science," New York: Oxford University Press.

Electromagnetic Fields and Neurobehavioral Function, pages 107–117
© 1988 Alan R. Liss, Inc.

STIMULATION OF BRAIN TISSUE IN VITRO BY EXTREMELY LOW
FREQUENCY, LOW INTENSITY, SINUSOIDAL ELECTROMAGNETIC FIELDS

Carl F. Blackman

Health Effects Research Laboratory (MD-74)
U.S. Environmental Protection Agency
Research Triangle Park, NC 27711 USA

INTRODUCTION

Extremely low frequency (ELF) and sub-ELF electromagnetic signals (1-300 Hz) have been shown by many investigators to affect biological systems. Extremely low frequency
fields have been reported to cause alterations in reaction
time of human beings (Konig and Ankermuller 1960, Hamer
1968, Konig 1971) and of monkeys (Gavalas et al. 1970,
Gavalas-Medici and Day-Magdaleno 1976), and alterations in
circadian activity of human beings (Wever 1973). Friedman
et al. (1967) observed that magnetic fields modulated at
ELF also change human reaction times. One research group
investigated the biochemical basis responsible for these
effects by examining changes in physiologically-significant
neurochemicals. Non-linear releases of calcium ions and of
a neurotransmitter, gamma amino butyric acid (GABA), were
characterized in surgically-exposed cerebral cortex of cats.
The non-linear release of either substance was found to occur
both in response to increasing calcium ion concentrations
in the surrounding solution, and in response to low intensity
200-Hz electric currents applied directly to the surface of
the cerebral cortex (Kaczmarek and Adey 1973, 1974). Subsequently, to increase the penetration of ELF signals into
the brain tissue, intact cats were exposed to 147-MHz
carrier-wave radiation, amplitude modulated at sub-ELF. In
an operant paradigm, the exposed cats exhibited changes in
their electroencephalogram (EEG) during the training period
and the extinction period (Bawin et al. 1973).

The observed EEG and behavioral changes caused by exposure to electromagnetic fields may have been due to stimulation of the central nervous system (CNS) receptors directly or indirectly through an initial stimulation of peripheral receptors. To distinguish between these two possible interaction sites, brain tissues were extracted from 1- to 7-day-old chickens, labeled with radioactive calcium-ions, subjected to radiofrequency (RF) fields, amplitude modulated between 0.5 and 35 Hz, and assayed for alterations in calcium-ions flux. As described above, changes in calcium ion association with the brain tissue had already been correlated with neurotransmitter (GABA) release (Kaczmarek and Adey 1974). The results indicated a change in calcium-ion flux due to exposure to a single intensity of the 147-MHz carrier waves, when amplitude modulated at frequencies between 6 and 20 Hz (Bawin et al. 1975). Subsequently, these results were corroborated (Blackman et al. 1979) but only for a narrow range of intensity values using modulated 147-MHz carrier-waves. In further work, the narrow range of intensities that could produce the response (Blackman et al. 1980a, Joines et al. 1981) was confirmed and extended to demonstrate at least two effective intensity regions, separated by regions of no effect, for 147-MHz and 50-MHz carrier waves, amplitude modulated at 16 Hz (Blackman et al. 1980b). The effective intensities for the two carrier frequencies were consistent only when compared through a relationship that utilized the dielectric constant of the tissues at each carrier frequency (Blackman et al. 1981; Joines and Blackman 1980). This unusual intensity-dependent response has not yet been confirmed by others with the chicken brain-tissue preparation. Sheppard et al. (1979) showed that modulated 450-MHz carrier waves could cause enhanced calcium-ion flux over one sparsely-delineated intensity range that was consistent with the effective intensities observed for the other carrier frequencies. No attempt was made to develop a high-resolution dose-response curve. Because both Bawin and Blackman had reported that unmodulated RF carrier waves would not induce changes in calcium-ion flux from the brain tissue, attention focused on the role played by the ELF and sub-ELF signals.

The initial report of changes in calcium-ion flux from brain tissue in vitro exposed to 16-Hz electric fields was reported by Bawin and Adey (1976), who showed 10 and 56 volts peak-to-peak per meter (V/m) to be effective while 5 and 100 V/m were not. We reported a detailed dose response for 16-Hz electromagnetic fields that indicated two effective intensity regions, between 5 to 7.5 and 35 to 50 V/m, separated by

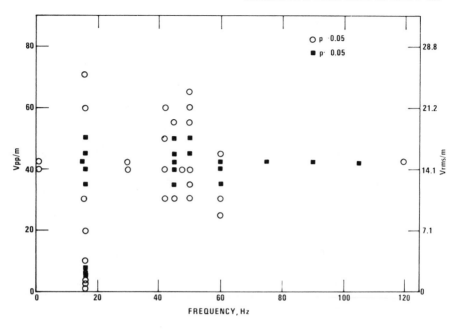

Fig. 1. Summary of frequency and intensity combinations of
ELF electromagnetic fields that have been tested for ability
to cause calcium-ion efflux enhancement from brain tissue in
vitro. Exposure to those combinations of frequency and intensity that produce statistically significant enhancements of
efflux when compared to sham (zero intensity) treatments are
indicated by the darkened squares. Conversely, those exposure
combinations that produce no significant enhancements when
compared to sham treatments are denoted by open circles. Data
from Blackman et al. (1985a).

regions that were ineffective (Blackman et al. 1982). This
work was extended to include specific combinations of frequency and intensity from 1 to 120 Hz (Blackman et al. 1985a).
There appear to be specific frequency and intensity combinations that are effective in altering calcium flux, inter-
spersed with combinations that are not (Figure 1). The major
disagreement between the reports of Bawin and Blackman is the
direction of the change in calcium-ion flux induced by the
ELF fields. Bawin reported decreased flux from the brain
tissue whereas Blackman reported enhanced flux. It was pos-

sible that the difference in direction of flux was due to an oscillating magnetic component present in our experiments but absent in Bawin's experiments (Blackman et al. 1982).

ROLE OF THE MAGNETIC COMPONENT

Blackman et al. (1985b) reduced the oscillating magnetic component of the 16-Hz signal to essentially zero, and observed no field-induced alterations in calcium flux from the brain tissue in vitro at electric field intensities of 6, 10, or 40 V/m. Thus, the oscillating magnetic component must be present in the exposure chamber to alter the calcium flux under the exposure conditions that were examined.

In addition, we demonstrated the importance of the local geomagnetic field (LGF). Specifically, the density of the LGF is directly related to the frequencies of the oscillating (AC) electromagnetic field that cause enhanced flux of calcium ions from the chick brain tissue. The effective frequency was directly proportional to the density of the LGF times an index, $2n + 1$, where $n = 0$ or 1. A 40 V/m electromagnetic field at 15 Hz was effective in causing enhanced flux of calcium ions when the density of the LGF was 38 microtesla (μT), but not when it was reduced to 19 μT; similarly, a 30-Hz field that was ineffective at 38 μT was effective at ±25.3 μT and at ±76 μT. In all the previous work published by Blackman and co-workers the density of the LGF was 38 μT.

Although we showed that the AC magnetic component must be present for a 16-Hz, 40-V/m electromagnetic field to cause enhanced efflux, its precise role is uncertain (Blackman et al. 1985b). Because the orientation of the LGF was always perpendicular to the plane formed by the electric and magnetic AC vectors, there is insufficient information to distinguish between a cyclotron resonance-like mechanism and a magnetic resonance-like mechanism. In the former case, the electric component of the AC signal must be perpendicular to the LGF for maximum coupling; in the latter case, it is the magnetic component that must be perpendicular. Of course, the actual mechanism operating at the transduction sites may be so complicated that simple manipulations of the field orientations cannot resolve this issue. While the influence of the LGF is an additional factor complicating any theoretical analysis of the calcium-ion efflux phenomenon, it may provide an essential clue to the underlying mechanism of action. Further, different densities of the LGF in various laboratories may be one reason that otherwise identical experiments with ELF electromagnetic signals would not produce the same results. Other possibilities for non-replication are cited below.

ESSENTIAL STEPS IN A MECHANISM OF ACTION

The field-induced calcium-ion flux phenomenon can be conceptualized as a multistep process. First, there is the transduction step that converts the minute amount of energy in the electromagnetic field into an initial chemical change in the biological system.

Second, this small initial change must be amplified by some process in order to produce a larger change that can be detected and measured. A relatively direct approach is to assume that the initial chemical change acts as a seed to trigger some cooperative phenomenon in the biological system.

Third, there will be secondary reactions that result from the cooperative phenomenon that result in changes both inside and outside the cell. These changes may be observed in biochemical events or processes associated with the cell membrane and with biochemical pathways within the cell.

This multistep process may occur within the same molecular species and be experimentally inseparable. In the other extreme, it may occur between different molecular species that are chemically coupled and distinguishable under appropriate conditions.

CURRENT STATUS

The research reports describing the biological influence of ELF electromagnetic fields can be evaluated from the perspective developed above. The calcium-ion flux phenomenon has been sufficiently well studied to serve as an example. First, the electromagnetic signal must have the appropriate values of frequency and intensity to satisfy the characteristics of the transduction apparatus. The frequency-specific pattern of response observed with ELF sinusoidal electromagnetic fields can be interpreted as resulting from at least two different primary interaction sites: non-excitable tissue, e.g. lymphocytes, appear to respond to a broad frequency range extending from 16 Hz through 100 Hz (Lyle et al. 1983) whereas excitable tissue (brain hemispheres) appears to respond to a similar broad band of frequencies that includes 60 and 90 Hz and also to a narrower bandwidth of electromagnetic signals at odd multiples of 15-Hz (Blackman et al. 1985a). It is possible that either of these two patterns could be modified by various conditions such as age, prior treatment, physiological or biochemical state, and species. Although it is too early to make definitive conclusions, it is reasonable to suspect that the intensity and alignment of the local geomagnetic field may play a critical role in determining the frequencies that can cause changes in the transducing entity involved in the calcium-ion flux phenomenon observed with brain tissue in vitro. It is currently unclear whether and how the observed intensity specificity is involved in this transduction process.

Second, the minor chemical change caused by the field is unlikely to be responsible for the biological and biochemical changes observed without some amplification process, because the amount of energy contained in the electromagnetic field is minute and because the transduction process is probably not 100% efficient. Thus, amplification will only occur if the transducing entity is coupled to the amplification process. Such an amplification phenomenon could be a cooperative transition in a membrane complex between two coexisting states of a molecular system. This general idea has been advanced for many years by Adey and his associates (Adey 1975, Bawin et al. 1975, Adey 1981). One such biochemical system could be two phases of the lipid or lipid-protein domains in the same membrane. The cooperative nature of a transition could lead to an increase in or rearrangement of one of the phase states compared to the other. Similarly, biopolymers such as DNA or RNA that can undergo cooperative transitions without the intervention of a membrane are also possible sites for the amplification process [see report of effects on DNA transcription (Goodman et al. 1983)]. This model would predict that chemical or physical conditions that alter cooperative or phase transitions could be affected by the radiation-induced process, provided the system is energetically-poised in its non-linear response region. Thus any experimental data that results from this amplification step may exhibit large variances and even deviations from an idealized mean if all the conditions required for amplification are not constant and identical within or between experiments. We have observed both of these outcomes (Blackman et al. 1979, 1980a, 1982). Alternatively, failure to detect biological or biochemical change upon exposure to effective combinations of frequency and intensity, both AC and DC, may be due to conditions that poise the amplification process outside the boundaries of its non-linear response region.

Third, the amplification process may cause subsequent changes both inside and outside the cell, thus leading to an initially confusing and perhaps conflicting spectrum of biological and biochemical changes that do not fit any pattern observed after chemical stimulation. For example, the alteration of calcium-ion flux outside the cell as has been reported by Bawin and by Blackman, and intracellular change in protein kinase activity has been observed by Byus et al. (1984).

The experimental results involving changes in calcium-ion flux from chick brain tissue have been replicated within one laboratory and corroborated by an independent laboratory. Thus they should be accepted as a phenomenon caused by low-intensity electromagnetic fields. Singular reports have noted field-induced changes in calcium-ion flux from synaptosomes prepared from rat cerebri (Lin-Liu and Adey 1982), from neuroblastoma cells of human origin (Dutta 1984), and from the cortex of awake, immobilized cats (Adey et al. 1982).

It is too early in the descriptive stages of this phenomenon to develop strong positions vis-a-vis each change that has been reported in any given system; for example, contrast the more conservative approach taken in reviews by Greengard et al. (1982) and Postow and Swicord (1985) with the more aggressive review by Myers and Ross (1981). Sometimes lost in the review process is the premise that experimental results are free to deviate from current theory, while it is the requirement of theory to be consistent with all the relevant experimental results.

CONCLUSION

Many reports of effects of RF fields, amplitude modulated at extremely low frequencies, have not been independently corroborated. The major exception is calcium-ion flux from chick brain tissue in vitro at intensity levels far below those that cause heating. When this exception is considered in conjunction with the results of biochemical studies in synaptosome preparations and human neuroblastoma cells in culture, and EEGs in animals, the evidence indicates that CNS tissues from several species, including human beings, can be affected by low-intensity RF fields sinusoidally amplitude modulated at specific extremely low frequencies or by those extremely low frequencies directly. Although a single agent caused these diverse observations, they may result from a single or from multiple causal mechanisms. Nevertheless, the occurrence of multiple effective-intensity ranges and the influence of the local geomagnetic field are factors that underscore the unusual nature of these findings.

In addition to the CNS-related changes, RF fields amplitude-modulated at ELF have been reported to alter an immune response (Lyle et al. 1983) and a pancreatic tissue function (Albert et al. 1980). These reports with diverse biological systems are not obviously connected except for the physical agent causing the change. The critical parameter common to all the experiments discussed here is the specificity of the ELF electromagnetic signal. Most studies do not report dose response curves and action spectra, viz. magnitude of the response as a function of frequency. More detailed parametric manipulation of these factors, with appropriate allowances for the local geomagnetic field vector, would permit comparisons and correlations between widely differing biological endpoints to assist in focusing on potential common, underlying mechanism(s) of action. Unfortunately, this viewpoint is currently not appreciated by researchers who narrowly focus on the biological or biochemical ramifications in their own specialized systems, in the search for the underlying mechanisms and physiological significance. By adopting this approach, they may be missing an opportunity to join the individual efforts and to identify the common critical parameters. Perhaps the discovery of the influence of the local geomagnetic field will provide a unifying guide for future research.

It is essential that the underlying mechanism of action be established so that the consequences of exposure to ELF electromagnetic signals can be fully determined. Knowledge of the mechanism will facilitate the assessments of potential hazard and therapeutic value. The accomplishment of this goal in the most expeditious manner will require the concerted efforts of experts in many different disciplines.

ACKNOWLEDGMENT

The author acknowledges the helpful discussions and constructive criticisms received from colleagues during the course of these studies. Particularly useful were comments made during manuscript preparation by Drs. Miller, Elder, Berman, and Kawanishi. Mrs. Sawaya is also thanked for her resiliency and good nature during the typing and reformatting processes.

DISCLAIMER

Mention of trade names or commercial products does not constitute endorsement or recommendation for use.

REFERENCES

Adey WR (1975). Introduction: effects of electromagnetic radiation on the nervous system. Ann NY Acad Sci 247:15-20.
Adey WR (1981). Tissue interaction with nonionizing electromagnetic fields. Physiol Rev 61:435-514.
Adey WR, Bawin SM, Lawrence AF (1982). Effects of weak amplitude-modulated microwave fields on calcium efflux from awake cat cerebral cortex. Bioelectromagnetics 3:295-307.
Albert E, Blackman C, Slaby F (1980). Calcium dependent secretory protein release and calcium efflux during RF irradiation of rat pancreatic tissue slices, in Berteaud AJ and Servantie B (eds): Ondes Electromagnetiques et Biologie, Paris, France, pp. 325-329.
Bawin SM, Gavalas-Medici RJ, Adey WR (1973). Effects of modulated very high frequency fields on specific brain rhythms in cats. Brain Res 58:365-384.
Bawin SM, Kaczmarek LK, Adey WR (1975). Effects of modulated VHF fields on the central nervous system. Ann N Y Acad Sci 247:74-81.
Bawin SM, Adey WR (1976). Sensitivity of calcium binding in cerebral tissue to weak environmental electric fields oscillating at low frequency. Proc Natl Acad Sci USA 73:1999-2003.
Blackman CF, Elder JA, Weil CM, Benane SG, Eichinger DC, House DE (1979). Induction of calcium-ion efflux from brain tissue by radio-frequency radiation: Effects of modulation frequency and field strength. Radio Sci 14(6S):93-98.
Blackman CF, Benane SG, Elder JA, House DE, Lampe JA, Faulk JM

(1980a). Induction of calcium-ion efflux from brain tissue by radio-frequency radiation: Effect of sample number and modulation frequency on the power-density window. Bioelectromagnetics 1:35-43.

Blackman CF, Benane SG, Joines WT, Hollis MA, House DE (1980b). Calcium-ion efflux from brain tissue: Power-density versus internal field-intensity dependencies at 50 MHz RF radiation. Bioelectromagnetics 1:277-283.

Blackman CF, Joines WT, Elder JA (1981). Calcium ion efflux induction in brain tissue by radiofrequency radiation. In: Biological Effects of Nonionizing Radiation, Illinger KH, (ed): ACS Symposium Series 157:299-314.

Blackman CF, Benane SG, Kinney LS, Joines WT, House DE (1982). Effects of ELF fields on calcium-ion efflux from brain tissue in vitro. Radiat Res 92:510-520.

Blackman CF, Benane SG, House DE, Joines WT (1985a). Effects of ELF (1-120 Hz) and modulated (50 Hz) RF fields on the efflux of calcium ions from brain tissue, in vitro. Bioelectromagnetics 6(1):1-11.

Blackman CF, Benane SG, House DE, Rabinowitz JR, Joines WT (1985b). A role for the magnetic field in the radiation-induced efflux of calcium ions from brain tissue in vitro. Bioelectromagnetics 6 (4):327-337.

Byus, CV, Lundak RL, Fletcher RM, Adey WR (1984). Alterations in protein kinase activity following exposure of cultured human lymphocytes to modulated microwave fields. Bioelectromagnetics 5:341-351.

Dutta SK, Subramoniam A, Ghosh B, Parshad R (1984). Microwave radiation-induced calcium efflux from human neuroblastoma cells in culture. Bioelectromagnetics 5:71-78.

Friedman H, Becker RO, Bachman CH (1967). Effect of magnetic fields on reaction time performance. Nature 213:949-950.

Gavalas RJ, Walter DO, Hamer J, Adey WR (1970). Effect of low-level, low-frequency electric fields on EEG and behavior in Macaca Nemestrina. Brain Res 18:491-501.

Gavalas-Medici R, Day-Magdaleno SR (1976). Extremely low frequency weak electric fields affect schedule-controlled behavior of monkeys. Nature 261:256-258.

Goodman R, Bassett CAL, Henderson AS (1983). Pulsing electromagnetic fields induce cellular transcription. Science 220:1283-1285.

Greengard P, Douglas WW, Nairn AC, Nestler EJ, Ritchie JM (1982). Effects of electromagnetic radiation on calcium in the Brain, USAF School of Aerospace Medicine, Report Number SAM-TR-82-15, 113 pp.

Hamer J (1968). Effects of low level, low frequency electric fields on human reaction time. Commun Behav Biol 2(5) Part A:217-222.

Joines WT, Blackman CF (1980). Power density, field intensity, and carrier frequency determinants of RF-energy-induced calcium ion efflux from brain tissue. Bioelectro-magnetics 1:271-275.

Joines WT, Blackman CF, Hollis MA (1981). Broadening of the RF power-density window for calcium-ion efflux from brain tissue. IEEE Trans Biomed Eng BME-28:568-573.

Kaczmarek LK, Adey WR (1973). The efflux of $^{45}Ca^{2+}$ and $[^3H]\gamma$-aminobutyric acid from cat cerebral cortex. Brain Res 63:331-342.

Kaczmarek LK, Adey WR (1974). Weak electric gradients change ionic and transmitter fluxes in cortex. Brain Res 66:537-540.

Konig H, Ankermuller F (1960). Über den einfluss besonders niederfrequenter elektrischer vorgange in der atmosphare auf den menschen. Naturwissenschaften 21:486-490.

Konig H (1971). Biological effects of extremely low frequency electrical phenomena in the atmosphere. J Interdiscipl Cycle Res 2:317-323.

Lin-Liu S, Adey WR (1982). Low frequency amplitude modulated microwave fields change calcium efflux rates from synapto-somes. Bioelectromagnetics 3:309-322.

Lyle DB, Schechter P, Adey WR, Lundak RL (1983). Suppression of T-lymphocyte cytotoxicity following exposure to sinusoi-dally amplitude modulated fields. Bioelectromagnetics 4:281-292.

Myers RD, Ross DH (1981). Radiation and brain calcium: A review and critique. Neurosc and Biobehav Rev 5:503-543.

Postow E, Swicord ML (1985). Modulated fields and "window" effects, in: Polk C, Postow E (eds): CRC Handbook of Biological Effects of Electromagnetic fields, CRC Press, Boca Raton, FL.

Sheppard AR, Bawin SM, Adey WR (1979). Models of long-range order in cerebral macromolecules: effect of sub-ELF and of modulated VHF and UHF fields, Radio Sci 14(6S):141-145.

Wever R (1973). Human circadian rhythms under the influence of weak electric fields and the different aspects of these studies. Int J Biometeor 17:227-232.

about 1 - 2^0 C) during 1 h per day during three days resulted in no obvious initial changes in behaviour. Minimal acute dam- age could be demonstrated. However, after two to four months and later on both structural, immunohistochemical and biochemical changes could be documented.

Radar technicians accidently and/or occupationally exposed to microwaves showed psychoneurological signs of affection as well as changes in cerebrospinal fluid protein pattern. No related changes have been noticed among matched controls.

Exposure of nervous tissue to electromagnetic fields ranging from power frequency to microwaves may thus exert a wide range of effects, mostly by mechanisms we know little about.

BACKGROUND

The increasing exposure of humans to electromagnetic fields of a wide spectrum of frequencies and intensities has rised the question of risks for affection of humans ultimately resulting in damage (Cf. Sheppard and Eisenbud 1977,Lerner 1980). The nervous system has been paid special attention as it under normal conditions is using electromagnetic fields of low intensity generated within itself (Cf Shepherd 1979. Adey 1981). It is, how-ever, still a question of debate to what extent the electromagnetic fields may induce damage and possible mechanisms (Sheppard and Eisenbud 1977,Becker and Marino 1982, Adey 1981, 1984).

We have during the last years studied effects of electromagnetic exposure on the nervous system with special attention paid to power frequencies and to micro-waves. Our results will be summarized, as will also some ongoing clinical studies on possible brain damage in humans accidently and/or occupationally exposed to micro-waves.

Effects of Experimental Exposure to Power Frequency Electromagnetic Fields

Animals have in several different experimental systems been exposed to electromagnetic fields of power frequency (50 or 60 Hz). The initial studies were performed on rabbits kept outdoors in a substation under a live 400 kV line or under a disconnector (Hansson 1981a, b). The electric field was about 14 kV/m and the magnetic field 12 - 60 mG, depending on the actual current. The animals were exposed during 23 to 24 hours per day from conception and then postnatally for one to eight weeks more. Even longer exposure times were used in some series. In parallel to these outdoor exposures other animals (albino and lop eared rabbits, rats and mice) have been exposed in a laboratory system to 10 or 14 kV/m (Hansson 1984). Precautions were taken to minimize the risk of spark discharges and corona effects. In parallel, other animals were kept in Farady's cages or outside measurable electric fields. At predecided times the exposed and the corresponding control animals were anaesthetized and fixed by transcardial perfusion with buffered formaldehyde or glutaraldehyde. After dissection, various parts of the nervous system were identified and isolated. Specimens were prepared for light and electron microscopic examination. In parallel, tissue pieces were processed for demonstration of neuron specific enolase and markers for neurolemmal glycoproteins, the neuroglial marker proteins S-100 and gliofibrillary acidic protein (GFA), neurofilaments and microtubules using immunohistochemical methods at light and electronmicroscopic levels (Hansson 1984). Unfixed tissue pieces were used for biochemical and immunochemical analysis of soluble brain proteins as well as the neuroglial cell markers S-100 and GFA.

Light and electronmicroscopic examination of brains from exposed rabbits revealed variable loss of Nissl bodies in large nerve cells in the cerebellum, hippocampus, superior colliculus and in some thalamic regions (Hansson 1981a, b), as compared to animals either kept in Farady's cages or outside measurable electric field. The diminuation of the Nissl bodies was due to rebuilding of parts of the granular endoplasmic reticulum into lamellar bodies (Figs 1,2). Concomitantly, there was loss of

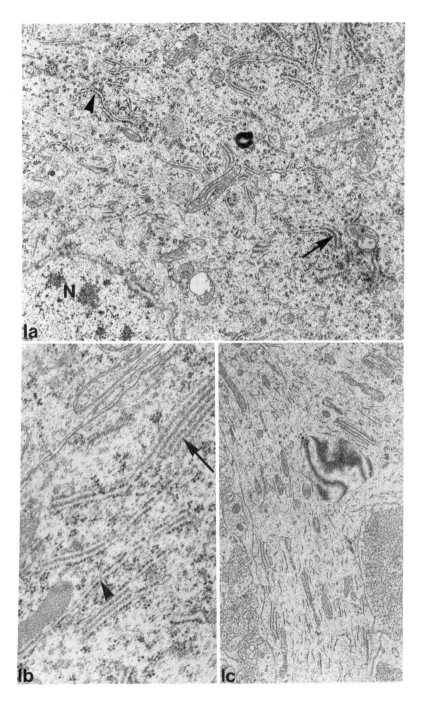

microtubules as compared to the controls. The residuing microtubules appeared to a large extent twisted and even branched, a structural pattern not observed in the controls. To a variable extent alterations of filaments as well as increase of fuzzy material in the neuronal cytoplasm could be observed. Other cell organelles appeared to be without obvious changes. Quantitative morphometric studies are in preparation to enable further evaluation of the significans of the observed changes. Lamellar bodies were observered not only in the cell bodies of large cerebellar nerve cells but also in the postsynaptic terminals of Purkinje nerve cells, which normally do not have such structural components (Palay and Chan-Palay 1974, Shepherd 1979). The most extensive changes were observed in large nerve cells in rabbits exposed to 14 kV/m from conception up to the age of 6-8 weeks outdoors in a substation under a 400 kV line. The magnetic field under a live line was mainly rotatory and varied according to the load . However, in contrast, rabbits similarly exposed indoors in a laboratory to electric fields showed much less prominent changes in their large nerve cells. In none of these animals all Purkinje nerve cells contained lamellar bodies as regularly observed in those exposed outdoors. The same was true for both rats and mice exposed similarly indoors to 10 or 14 kV/m either from conception or birth up to the age of 4-8 weeks. It must thus be concluded that the outdoor exposure system induced more prominent effects on nerve cells as compared to what could be seen after indoor exposure. Albert (1984) recently reported that about every third Purkinje nerve cell contained lamellar bodies in four out of ten rats long term exposed to 100 kV/m for 18 h/day. However, the animals were allowed to recover for 17 to 27 days after the last exposure, which according to my experience may have influenced the results(Hansson 1984). No lamellar bodies were observed in any of the controls. Similar structures were also seen in the hippocampal

---

Fig. 1 Electron micrographs of Purkinje nerve cells in cerebellar vermis from rabbits exposed for 7-8 weeks postnatally to 14 kV/m outdoors in a substation. Figs. 1a & b demonstrate lamellar bodies (arrows) in continuity with granular endoplasmic reticulum (arrow head). The nerve cell nucleus marked by N. Fig. 1c shows an obliquely sectioned lamellar body in a large dendrite.

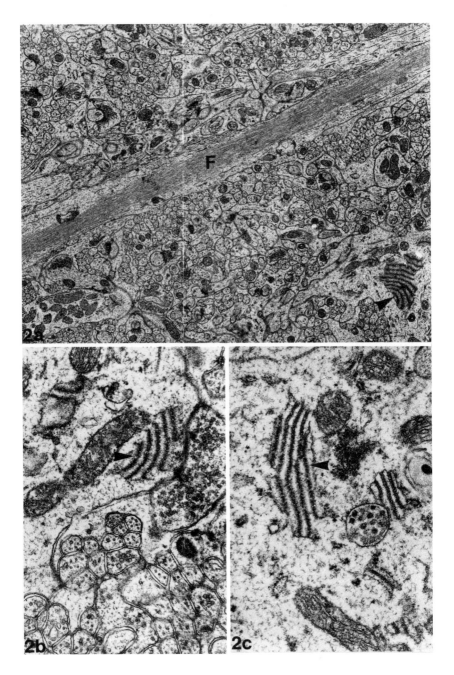

pyramidal nerve cells. Portet et al (1984) failed to detect lamellar bodies in nerve cells in rabbits exposed to 50 kV/m in a laboratory 18 hours per day from birth up to the age of six weeks. A possible explanation for the discrepancies may be the differences in exposure conditions. Blackman et al (1984) recently reported that the efflux of calcium ions from chicken brain tissue exposed to electric fields are significantly influenced by the magnitude of the magnetic field, indicating synergistic interaction between the electric and magnetic fields under certain conditions. During the outdoor exposure the relative intensities of the electric and magnetic fields differed from those at indoor exposures.

The importance of the disappearance of Nissl bodies and appearance of lamellar bodies is due to the fact that the granular endoplasmic reticulum is the main center for protein and lipid syntheses, detoxication and other key activities in cells. Further studies are necessary to elucidate possible importance of formation of lamellar bodies and imduction of cytoskeletal changes as well as reasons for the discrepancies in appearance of lamellar bodies in nerve cells in animals exposed to electromagnetic fields under various conditions.

Significant changes in the structure and function of nerve cells are likely to cause reactive changes in adjacent supporting neuroglial cells (Palay and Chan-Palay 1974, Shepherd 1979). Therefore, analyses were performed with regard to the distribution, structure and chemical characteristics of the neuroglial cells. We have mainly concentrated our studies on the cerebellum as the Bergmann radial glial cells are very regularly arranged parallel to the large Purkinje nerve cells. Due to their structural characteristics it is possible to recognize even discrete structural ,immunohistochemical and immunochemical changes (Hansson 1984). The glial proteins S-100 and GFA were visualized using immunohistochemical

---

Fig. 2 Electron micrographs of specimens treated as in Fig. 1. Fig. 2 a shows a lamellar body in a post-synaptic ending of a Purkinje nerve cell (arrows). Note the numerous filaments (F) in the process in the center. Figs. 2b & c show fuzzy material and several lamellar bodies in neuronal cytoplasm of exposed animals.

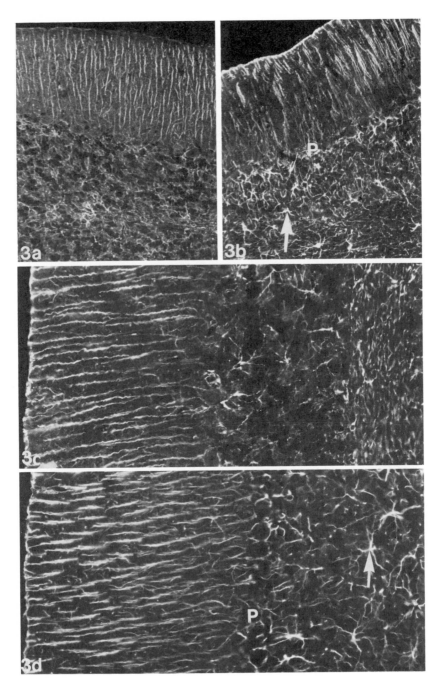

methods (Figs 3, 4). Depending on the time of exposure to electricmagnetic fields hypertrophic glial reactions became evident. There was an increased number of hypertrophic neuroglial cells in the granular cell layer too (Figs 3, 4). In some animals, even the radial glial cells appeared increased in size. Their normally delicate, branching processes were replaced by hypertrophic ones. In our experience, a postnatal exposure period of 2-3 weeks was necessary to enable demonstration of these reactive changes. Immunochemical examination using an ELISA-method confirmed the quantitative increase of the glial marker protein S-100 in the cerebellum (Table 1), while in other areas, such as frontal cortex, somatomotor cortex and hippocampus there were no net changes in the concentration of S-100 protein as calculated per wet weight. The combined use of immunohistochemical and imunochemical methods enabled us to demonstrate not only quantitative changes but also altered distribution of the glial cells within various regions. It may be concluded that the presence of glial reactive changes support our conclusion that exposure for long time periods of growing animals to electric fields of high intensity affect both neuronal and neuroglial cells in the brain. Whether this also means significant affection of brain function needs further studies.

Sciatic nerves isolated from adult frogs were in an in vitro system exposed to low current through agar bridges. The nerve extended through a three-chamber box and was immersed in a temperature-controlled, buffered and oxygenated balanced salt solution. Low current, 50 - 1000 nA, at 16 Hz for 17 h resulted in reduced number of microtubules while the filaments in the axons increased. Similar but less extensive changes could be demonstrated at 50/60 Hz. These studies are to includ different pretreatments and currents to elucidate mechanisms causing the noticed changes in the axonal cytoskeletons.

Fig. 3 Fluorescence micrographs of cerebellar vermis of rats exposed (Fig. 3 b & d) to 14 kV/m (60 Hz) for 4 weeks after birth and sham-exposed controls (Figs. 3 a & c),treated for demonstration of gliofibrillary acidic protein (GFA) in neuroglial cells. Note the increased staining in Figs. 3b & d. Purkinje cells marked P and neuroglial cells by arrows.

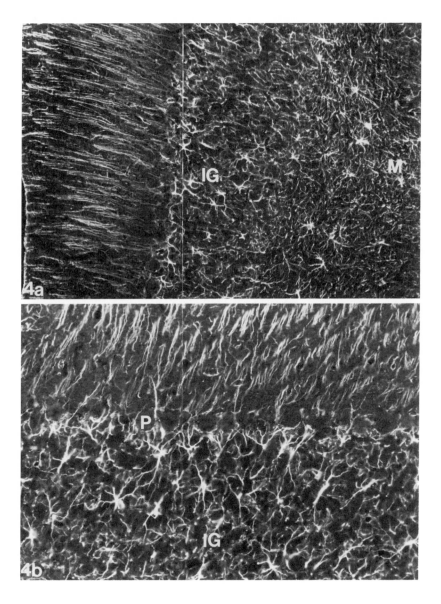

Effects of Microwave Exposure on Nervous Tissue

Microwaves may induce affection and damage on nervous tissue, either by thermal or non-thermal mechanisms (Baranski and Czerski 1976, Lerner 1980, Adey 1981). There are several reports indicating acute damage to the nervous system after microwave exposure (Albert and DeSantis 1975, Switcher and Mitchell 1977, Albert and Kerns 1981). Developmental abnormalities have also been reported and species differences demonstrated (Albert et al 1981 a, b).

Our interest in microwaves arised from these reports, as well as from the one of Aurell and Tengroth (1973) about lenticular and retinal changes secondary to microwave exposure in subjects , accidently and/or occupationally exposed. The retinal damage could experimentally be induced by microwave radiation at 55 mW/cm2 at 3.1 GHz (1.4 usec pulses, 300 Hz repetition frequency with peak intensity about 1000 times the average) (Paulsson et al 1979). Even a single exposure for one hour could induce ultrastructural changes in the retina, still demonstrable after 3.5 months . Our first studies have been extended and do presently also include analysis of brain tissue. All rabbits were exposed under far field conditions on the right side of their head, with the center of the horn directed against the right eye. The animals were not given any anaesthesia or other types of treatment during the exposure period , which lasted for one hour per day, usually repeated during three days. The core body temperature rised about 2 C. The SAR in the right temporal lobe of the brain was about 20 W/kg as calculated from measurements using a fibre optic system. The SAR of the retina in the right eye was calculated to be about 20 W/kg, based on temperature determinations useing several different measuremet systems. The animals were at variable times after the exposure processed as described above for light and electron microscopic analysis, immunohistochemical and biochemical studies.

Figs. 4a & b. Specimens treated as in Fig. 3b. Some of the E-field-exposed rats got strongly increased staining of their hypertrophic neuroglial cells. Medulla marked M and inner granular layer IG.

Minimal acute changes could be demonstrated in the retina. The retinal epitelial cells showed swelling and oedema initially. There was as well degeneration of small number of photoreceptor cells and nerve cells. These acute inflammatory reactions and the minimal cell loss was evident only the first two weeks. In the cerebral cortex on the right side scattered cells containing myelin bodies could be demonstrated. Special attention was paid to the hypothalamus, previously reported to be sensitive to microwave exposure. However, after 2-4 months and later on an increasing frequency of nerve cells were observed to contain myelin bodies and related structures, indicating nerve cell damage. Glial reactions could concomitantly be demonstrated using immunohistochemical and electronmicroscopic methods. These changes were noticed both in the right retina, the right optic nerve and in superficial parts of the right hemisphere of the brain, including the lateral hemisphere of the cerebellum. Analysis of the brain and retina from the contralateral, left side revealed no significant increase, as compared to sham exposed controls, of myelin bodies and related structures. Immunohistochemical analysis of sections from the right and left optic nerve enabled demonstration of hypertrophic neuroglial cell changes, as well as to some extent, increased number of glial cells. These changes were evident even 1.5 years after the initial exposure for one hour during three consecutive days to microwaves. Biochemical analysis of soluble proteins in the brain tissue from exposed rabbits revealed the appearance of an acidic protein (pI 4), not observed in the sham exposed. Furthermore, the relative intensity of some other acidic protein bands becamed altered. These changes were only possible to observe after 2 - 4 months.
However, all rabbits examined 9 - 18 months after the microwave exposure showed the presence of the acidic abnormal protein band as well as relative changes in concentration of several other protein bands as examined by isoelectric focusing. We interpret these changes as a result of a chronic damage, which became evident after a " silent " period of several months after the exposure. The biochemical as well as the structural data indicate increase in extent and severity with time of the changes induced. Studies are in progress using various exposure schedules and supplementary analysing methods aiming to further elucidate the extent of delayed damage to the

Table 1. Concentrations of S-100 per wet weight in various brain regions of exposed and control rabbits, determined by an ELISA method.

Area		S-100 (ug/g wet weight)
Frontal cortex	Exposed	417+13.1
	Control	417+11.8
Hippocampus	Exposed	280+21
	Control	278+7
Cerebellum anterior hemisph.	Exposed	1174+12**
	Control	1063+23

((Unpubl. data; H-A Hansson, L Rosengren & KG Haglid))

nervous system as well as to elucidate its mechanisms.

The results of these studies on experimentally microwave exposed rabbits suggested that even humans occupationally exposed to microwaves of moderate to high intensity could be at risk of brain damage. We therefore initiated a study on radar technicians working at a military base. So far, 17 male radar technicians all having several years of electromechanical work with microwave equipment, were examined clinically, as were corresponding matched controls with no history of microwave exposure. Accidental and/or occupational exposure to high levels of microwaves in the range of 1-10 GHz were reported. Clinical examination revealed an increased frequency of frontal lobe neuropsychiatric symptoms as compared to the controls. Retinal changes of the type described by Aurell and Tengroth 1973 could further be demonstrated. Analysis of the protein pattern in cerebrospinal fluid taps revealed the presence of an abnormal protein band with an isoelectric pI of 4.05. Furthermore, several other protein fractions could be measured quantitatively to be altered. The acidic protein with pI 4.05 have not been demonstrated in patients with various neurological symptoms due to tumours, injury, demyelinating or degenerative diseases or neurotoxic agents. Our preliminary data is suggestive of that the neuropsychiatric symptoms as well as the pathological protein pattern in the cerebrospinal fluid indicate that microwave exposure may induce chronic affections of nervous tissue which may become evident after a " silent period " . Preliminary studies performed on monkeys exposed to microwaves are suggestive of that such a working hypothesis is reasonable.

FUTURE RESEARCH PLANS

Our main research interest has so far been power frequency electromagnetic field effects on nervous tissue as well as effects of microwave exposure. These studies will be extended. The 50/60 Hz studies will to a larger extent than before consider the magnetic fields in addition to the electric ones. Different combinations of exposure schedules and intensities will be examined. Furthermore, more quantitative methods will be used in order to make it possible to correlate morphometric data with biochemical ones. In the microwave research field an extensive study is in progress aimed to correlate the time, intensity of exposure, and biochemical and morphological changes, in order to try to establish possible correlation between "dose" and response. Our intention is furthermore to extend the range of frequencies from the microwave field into that of radiofrequency. There is a need for more accurate data in order to evaluate the possible hazards by exposure to electromagnetic fields to the human population. Our present data are not sufficient to enable us to indicate possible mechanisms for affection of the nervous system and risks for health. A main conclusion is that long term effects after exposure to electromagnetic fields are possible to demonstrate even in cases where no or minimal acute changes were obvious. Thus, absence of acute effects does not exclude the possibility that chronic changes may be evident later, i.e. at a time when there may be no obvious relation between exposure and later evident clinical symptoms.

Acknowledgements. The presented results are based on studies done in collaboration with RW Adey, S Dyberg, E Edvardsson, KG Haglid, Y Hamnerius, AA Marino, B Nordström, E Norström, LE Paulsson, L Persson, RD Phillips, L Rosengren, B Rozell, S Stemme and U Svedin.

REFERENCES

Adey WR (1981). Tissue interactions with nonionizing electromagnetid fields. Physiol Rev 61: 435.

Adey WR (1984). Nonlinear, nonequilibrium aspects of electromagnetic field interactions at cell membranes. In Adey WR, Laurence AF (eds): "Nonlinear Electrodynamics in Biological Systems", New York: Plenum Press, p. 3.

Albert EN, De Santis M (1975). Do microwaves alter nervous system structure? Ann NY Acad Sci 247:87.

Albert EN, Kerns JM (1981). Reversible microwave effects on the blood brain barrier. Brain Research 230: 153.

Albert EN, Sherif MF, Papadopoulos NJ (1981a). Effects of nonionizing radiation on the Purkinje cells of the uvula in squirred monkey cerebellum. Bioelectromagnetics 2: 241.

Albert EN, Sherif MF, Papadopoulos NJ, Slaby FJ, Monahan J (1981b). Effect of nonionizing radiation on the Purkinje cells of the rat cerebellum. Bioelectromagnetics 2: 241.

Albert E, Cohen G, Avellino L, Kornhauser G, Yoshioka A (1984). Electron microscopic observations on rat cerebellum and hippocampus after exposure to 60 Hz electric fields. Presented at the 6th Ann Meet BEMS, Atlanta, GA, July 15-19.

Aurell E, Tengroth B (1973). Lenticular and retinal changes secondary to microwave exposure. Acta Ophthal (Kbh) 51:764.

Barándi S, Czerski P (1976). Biological effects of microwaves. Stroudsburg Pa: Dowden, Hutchinson and Ross Inc.

Becker RO, Marino AA (1982). "Electromagnetism and Life". Albany NY: State University of New York Press.

Blackman CF, Benane SG, House DE, Rabinowitz JR, Joines WT (1984). A role for the magnetic component in the field-induced efflux of calcium ions from brain tissue. Presented at the 6th Ann Meet BEMS. Atlanta Ga, July, 15-19.

Hansson HA (1981a). Lamellar bodies of Purkinje nerve cells experimentally induced by electric field. Brain Research 216: 187.

Hansson HA (1981b). Purkinje nerve cell changes caused by electric fields - ultrastructural studies on long-term effects on rabbits. Med Biol 59: 103.

Hansson HA (1984). Effects on nervous tissue of exposure
    to electromagnetic fields. In Adey WR, Leurence AF
    (eds): "Nonlinear Electrodynamics in Biological
    Systems". New York: Plenum Press, p. 65.
Lerner EJ (1980). Electromagnetic hazards. RF radiation:
    biological effects. IEEE Spectrum 18: 51.
Palay SL, Chan-Palay V (1974). Cerebellar Cortex; Cyto-
    logy and Organization. Berlin: Springer Verlag.
Paulsson LE, Hamnerius Y, Hansson HA, Sjöstrand J (1979).
    Retinal damage experimentally induced by microwave
    radiation at 55 mW/cm^2. Acta Ophthalmol 57: 183.
Portet R, Cabanes J, Pierre J, Delost H (1984). Déveloupe-
    ment du jeune lapin soumis à un champ électrique in-
    tense. C R Soc Biol 178:142.
Shepherd GM (1979). "The Synaptic Organization of the
    Brain". New York: Oxford University Press.
Sheppard AR, Eisenbud M (1977). "Biological Effects of
    Electric and Magnetic Fields of Extremely Low
    Frequency". New York : New York University Press.
Switzer WG, Mitchell D (1977). Long-term effects of 2,45
    GHz radiation on the ultrastructure of the cerebral
    cortex and on hematological profiles of rats. Radio
    Science 12: 287.

Electromagnetic Fields and Neurobehavioral Function, pages 135–151
© 1988 Alan R. Liss, Inc.

MORPHOLOGICAL CHANGES IN CEREBELLUM OF NEONATAL RATS EXPOSED TO 2.45 GHz MICROWAVES

Ernest N. Albert, Ph.D.
And
Mahmoud Sherif, M.D., Ph.D.
Department of Anatomy
The George Washington University Medical Center
Washington, D.C.

Abstract

One-day and six-day old Sprague-Dawley rats were exposed in the far field to 2.45 GHz (cw) microwaves at 10 mW/cm^2 for five consecutive days, 7 hours per day (SAR 2W/kg). Pups were euthenized one day after exposure and the cerebella processed for light and electron microscopy. Matching cerebellar sections and folia from irradiated and sham irradiated animals were examined. Light microscopic examination revealed the presence of small deeply-stained cells with hyperchromatic pyknotic nuclei within the external granular layer (EGL). The number of these pyknotic cells in the experimental animals was nearly twice that in the controls. The Nissl bodies in Purkinje cells were finely dispersed. In some experimental animals mononuclear cellular infiltration was demonstrated. Under the electron microscope the deeply-stained pyknotic small cells presented electron dense nuclei with clumped chromatin, extrusion or disintegration of the nucleus, ruptured nuclear membrane, and the vacuolization of the cytoplasm. Eventually these cells became phagocytosed by surrounding EGL cells. Most of the Purkinje cells of experimental animals showed small, disorderly arrays of rough endoplasmic reticulum (RER) instead of the typical orderly stacks of parallel arrays. These observations suggest that microwave radiation may interfere with early genesis of cerebellar microneurons and alter the metabolic status of Purkinje cells. However, this effect might be reversible.

Introduction

     The effects of high power density non-ionizing
radiation on adult mammalian brain have been reported by
many authors (Oldendorf, 1949; Minecki and Bilski, 1961;
Cholodov, 1966; Tolgskaja and Gordon, 1971). These effects
consisted of degenerative lesions in nerve cells and white
matter, hyperemia, inflammatory and glial reactions in the
brains of rabbits, rats and mice exposed to high power
density microwave irradiation and high intensity
magnetostatic fields. Exposure of Chinese hamsters to 2.45
and 1.7 GHz microwaves at low and intermediate power
densities (10, 25, and 50 mW/cm^2) resulted in
vacuolization, chromatolysis, scarcity of rough endoplasmic
reticulum (RER) and polyribosomes in neuronal somas in
hypothalamic and subthalamic nuclei (Albert and Desantis,
1975).

     Gross effects of non-ionizing radiofrequency
electromagnetic (RFEM) radiation on fetal development have
also been reported. These include occurrence of
hemorrhage, resorption, exencephaly and fetal death in
conceptuses of CF-1 mice exposed, during gestation, to 2.45
GHz microwaves at 123 mW/cm^2 (Rugh et al., 1974; Rugh et
al., 1975; Rugh and McManaway, 1976). Shore et al., (1977)
reported no effect on the litter size, but did note a
decrease in body and brain mass in rats exposed to 2.45 GHz
microwaves at 10 mW/cm^2 for five days during gestation.
Berman et al. (1978) exposed CD-1 mice to 2.45 GHz
radiation for 100 minutes daily at power densities that
ranged from 3.4 to 28 mW/cm^2. They observed a decrease in
mean body mass and an increased incidence of exencephaly
among fetuses exposed at the highest (28 mW/cm^2) power
density. Thus, the existing studies on the effects of
non-ionizing radiation on developing fetus have examined
gross teratology, body mass, litter size and uterine
resorptions, but none have addressed the question of
cellular and subcellular changes.

     Recently, this laboratory explored the effects of 2.45
GHz (10mW/cm^2) and 100 GHz (46 mW/cm^2) non-ionizing
radiation on the developing rat cerebellum. There was no
effect on the size of the cerebellum. The proportion
between the cerebellar cortical layers and the white core
was the same in both experimental and control animals but
there was a statistically significant decrease in the
relative number of Purkinje cells of rats irradiated in
utero, or during early postnatal life (Albert et al.,

1981a). However, the decrease in Purkinje cell population was insignificant when the animals were irradiated during early postnatal life and left for 40 days to recover. These findings raised questions about the mechanisms of radiation effect in rats resulting in numerical reduction of Purkinje cells. A similar study on Monkey cerebellum showed absence of any effects on Purkinje cells (Albert et al., 1981b).

It has been reported that agents interfering with normal development of cerebellar granule cells from EGL will subsequently affect the cerebellar neurones such as Purkinje cells as a result of loss of granule cells (Altman, 1972; Altman and Anderson, 1972; Jacobson, 1978). Therefore, the present study was designed to investigate the possible effects of low level non-ionizing RFEM radiation on the EGL of the neonatal rat cerebellum with special emphasis on Purkinje cells.

Materials and Methods:

Twenty-four newly born Sprague-Dawley rats were used in this study; eight pups were one-day old, sixteen were six-days old. Two separate anechoic chambers were utilized to provide exposure to RFEM radiation or sham (control) exposure. During exposure, animals were housed in plexiglass containers with internal dimensions of 19 x 11.4 x 7.6 cm. The tops and bottoms of these containers consisted of removable polystyrene grids to permit proper ventilation. Each container was positioned reproducibly on a plexiglass rack 208 cm. below a trunkated horn antenna. Sham-exposed animals were similarly housed in a separate anechoic chamber.

In an effort to define the exposure of individual subjects, a series of three field intensity measurements were made within each of the plexiglass containers. The measurements were made with and without nonexperimental subjects in the remaining containers. All measurements were made with nonperturbing, three dimensional probe (Collins S/N 57) and EIT digital receiver (S/N 1004).

It was determined that exposures varied as function of position within the container and also with time due to field perturbations produced by the movements of other animals. Consequently, although the average field intensity was 10 mW/cm^2, an animal might have received as little as 4 mW/cm^2 or as high as 30 mW/cm^2 at any instant. Utilizing the Radio-Frequency Radiation Dosimetry Handbook (Durney et al., 1977), specific absorption rate (SAR) for these rats was computed to be 2 mW/g.

Matching sets of litter mates from both groups of animals, the one-day and six day old pups, were placed in well ventilated plexiglass cages in anechoic chambers (as described above) for 3.5 hours (9:00 a.m. -12:30 p.m.). One chamber was energized so that the pups were irradiated with 2.45 GHz (cw) microwaves at 10 mW/cm^2, while the other chamber was used for sham irradiation. After 3.5 hours of irradiation, the pups were reunited with their mothers outside the anechoic chambers for 1.5 hours for feeding. At 2:00 p.m., control and experimental pups were again placed in their respective chambers and irradiated for an additional 3.5 hours (2:00 p.m. - 5:30 p.m.). The pups were then returned to the cages with their mothers until the next morning. This procedure was repeated daily for five days. Thus the young rats were irradiated for 7 hours/day for five consecutive days. On the sixth day all animals were anesthetized by pentobarbital sodium (50 mg/kg) and fixed by intracardiac perfusion. Animals used for light microscopy were perfused with 10% buffered formalin. Those for electron microscopy were perfused with weak Karnovsky's fixative containing 1% paraformaldehyde, 1.25% glutaraldehyde, 0.12% CaCl$_2$ in Cacodylate buffer. After perfusion, the brains were dissected out, the cerebella were separated and left in the fixatives for 12 hours.

For light microscopy, the cerebella were bisected in the median plane, dehydrated, double imbedded in paraffin-celloidin and serially sectioned at 10 un in the sagittal plane. Sections were stained alternatively with hematoxylin and easin and 1% thionin in Wolpole acette buffer at pH 4.8 for Nissl substance. The entire series of sections from experimental and conrol animals were matched and examined according to predetermined 5 parasagittal planes (Albert et al., 1981). This step was necessary to insure that identical areas of the cerebellar folia and EGL were examined in both experimental and control animals.

For electron microscopy, thin sagittal slices (1-2 un thick) were cut from the cerebella at the vermal and paravermal regions. Small wedges from the cortical area of matching folia were cleanly dissected and processed for electron microscopic examination.

Observations and Results:

I. Light microscopic examination of cerebella of irradiated (experimental) and sham irradiated (control) animals revealed the following:
a) Along with mitotic cells, there were many small deeply stained cells scattered among the developing normal microneuron in the EGL of both experimental and control animals. However, there was a consistently greater preponderance of these cells in the experimental animals than in controls. The deeply stained cells possessed hyperchromatic pyknotic nuclei, usually rounded and centrally placed. In some cells the nuclei were eccentric, indented or fragmented (Fig. 1). These observations are indicative of various stages of degeneration. The degenerating cells were scattered throughout the EGL. These cells were counted in 3 serial parasagittal sections at 5 different matching planes of the cerebella of both experimental and control animals. The results indicated a statistically significant increase in the relative number of pyknotic cells per folium in the irradiated animals. Their number in the experimental animals was approximately twice as much as their number in the control animals (Table).

b) In addition to the changes in the EGL cells, there was a change in the pattern of Nissl bodies of many Purkinje cells in experimental animals in comparison to controls. The Nissl bodies were in the form of finely dispersed granules instead of the compact rod shaped appearance generally seen under the light microscope in normal Purkinje cells (Fig. 2). However, tyical chromatolytic patterns were not observed.

c) Some folia of the irradiated animals were studded with mononucleated blood cells, usuallly near a capillary blood vessel in the white core. The mononucleated cells were dispersed over the internal granular layer as well. Neither extravasation of red blood cells, nor any pathological changes of the blood vessels were observed. It is noteworthy to mention that the vascular cellular infiltration was not unique to that of any specific or non-specific inflamatory conditions.

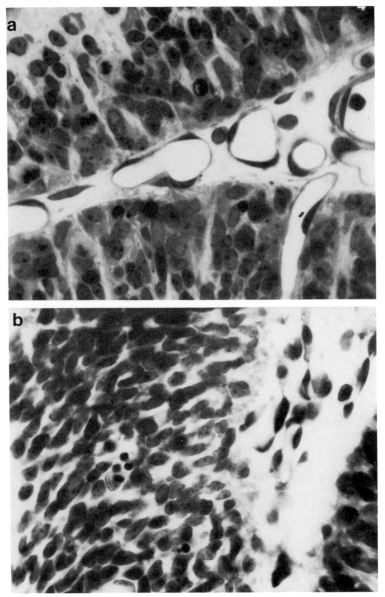

Fig. 1   Photomicrographs a & b of parasagittal sections in
         rat cerebellar cortex showing deeply stained
         degenerated cells with hyperchromatic, pyknotic
         nuclei within the external granular layer.

Effect of 2450 MHz (CW) microwaves at 10 mW/cm^2 on the external granular layer (EGL) of rat cerebella irradiated during day 1 – 5 and 6 – 10 postnatally*.

	Total No. of degenerated cells/parasagittal section.	Relative No. of degenerated cells/folia in parasagittal section.	Difference between relative No. of degenerated cells in experimental and control cerebella.	Proportion of increase of relative No. of degenerated cells in experimental animals.
Animals irradiated day 1-5. Experimental	52.1 SD+24.78	5.17 SD+1.89	2.22 SED+1.62	1:1.75
Control	27.78 SD+10.5	2.95 SD+0.81	0.001<P<0.01	
Animals irradiated day 6-10. Experimental	128.30 SD+35.01	11.76 SD+3.83	5.23 SED+3.11	1:1.80
Control	76.16 SD+19.7	6.53 SD+1.71	0.02<p<0.05	

* All values are the mean number of degenerated cells counted in parasagittal sections at different planes studied in each group.

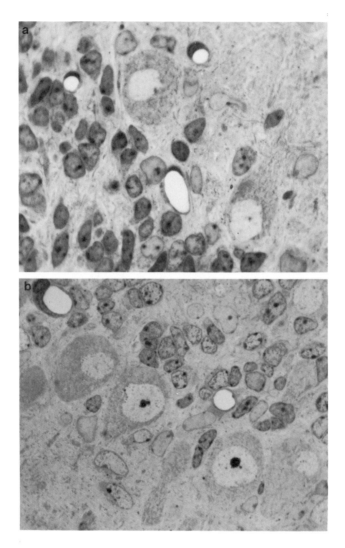

Fig. 2   Photomicrograph of cerebellar Purkinje cells
          stained with thionin. a) Purkinje cells from
          control animal showing the compact packing of rod
          shaped Nissl substance.   b)   In constrast
          Purkinje cells from irradiated animal show finely
          dispersed Nissl bodies.

II. Electron microscopic observations:

a)   The pyknotic cells observed under light microscopy presented large rounded nuclei compactly packed with homogenous electron dense material (heterochromatin), concealing any nuclear details. Some of these cells presented ruptured nuclear membrane with leakage of the nuclear contents in a dense cytoplasm. Some cells showed extrusion of the nucleus with polarized compact heterochromatin and normal appearance of euchromatin. Others presented disintegrated nucleus with vacuolated cytoplasm (Fig. 3). This is interpreted as various stages of degeneration among the neuroblasts in EGL of irradiated animals. It was not uncommon to find the degenerated cells engulfed by other surrounding EGL cells, probably glioblasts.

b)   On the other hand, most of the Purkinje cells of exposed animals mainly showed small, disorderly arrays of rough endoplasmic reticulum (RER) instead of the typical orderly stacks of parallel arrays (Fig. 4a,b). Nevertheless, such observation among Purkinje cells of irradiated animals is not suggestive of definite chromatolysis.

Discussion:

In this study, exposure of neonatal rats to 2.45 GHz (cw), 10 mW/cm^2 microwave irradiation resulted in some degenerative changes among EGL cells. The appearance of these degenerating cells is somewhat similar to those reported in rat EGL after postnatal exposure to x-ray irradiation (Altman et al., 1969; Altman and Anderson, 1972; Das, 1977). However, the incidence of such degenerating cells after exposure to non-ionizing microwave radiation is far less than that obtained by x-irradiation. On the other hand, degenerating cells were reported in EGL of the control animals as well. However, their number in the experimental animals was nearly double that in the controls. It is now generally accepted that histogenic cell death normally occurs during development of the nervous system (Jacobson, 1970; and Cowan, 1973). It is strongly contingent on conditions outside the cells that die; e.g., interaction with other cells, nutritional, hormonal and trophic influences. It seems therefore that microwave irradiation might have induced a destructive effect on the developing EGL cells which resultd in

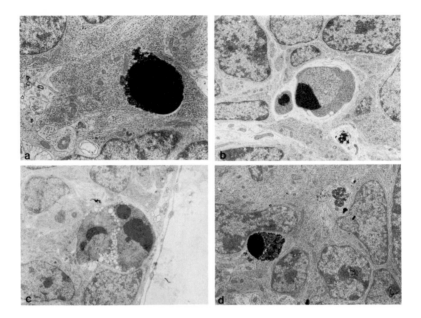

Fig. 3   Electron micrographs of the deeply stained cells
          within EGL of experimental animals.   a) Nuclei
          showing clumped chromatin.   b) Extruding nucleus.
          c) A cell with disintegrated nucleus and vaculated
          cytoplasm (arrow).   d) Phagocytosed degenerated
          cell.   (Note the ruptured nuclear membrane).

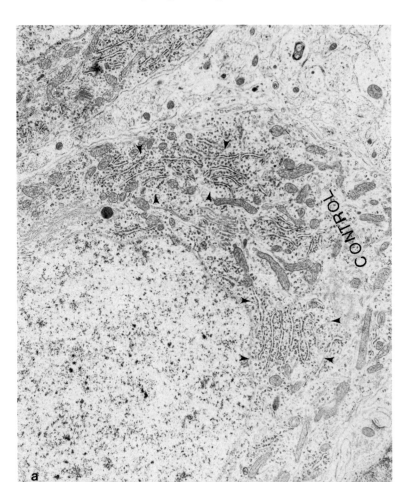

Fig. 4a   Electronmicrograph of a Purkinje cell from a
control animal. Arrows outline orderly stacks of
RER.

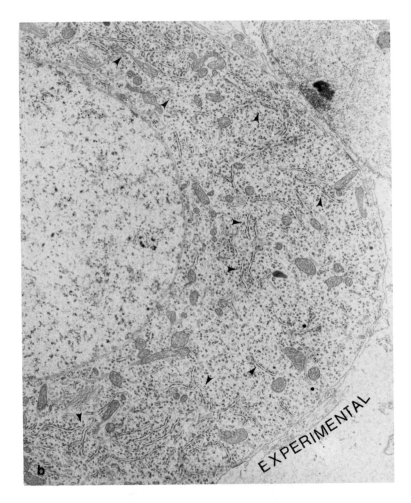

Fig. 4b Electronmicrograph of a Purkinje cell from an
          irradiated animal. Arrows point to the disorderly
          arrays of RER of the experimental animal. (Note
          the lack of the typical stacks of RER).

increased histogenic cell death in irradiated animals. However, the relative number of degenerated cells per cerebellar folium of the experimental animals is not sufficient to produce teratogenic manifestations. This view may provide a substratum to explain a variety of results ranging from decrease in body and brain mass, without any anomalies, at low power densities up to exencephaly, resorption and fetal death at higher power densities (Rugh et al., 1975; Rugh and McManaway, 1976; Berman et al., 1978). The different irradiation parameters could be the cause of these variations but the nature of the degenerative effect of radiation is still present in all the experiments conducted. Albert et al. (1981) reported a decrease in Purkinje cell population when the animals were exposed to 2.45 GHz (cw) at 46 mW/cm^2 microwave radiation in utero and during early postnatal period. The possibility that microwave radiation might have interfered with the early genesis of developing neurons may be the underlying cause behind this finding.

Examination of the cytology of Purkinje cells in the exposed cerebella revealed a change in the pattern of their Nissl substance. At the light microscopy level the tigroid substance appeared finely dispersed in the cytoplasm as if it had been disintegrated. This was confirmed at the electron microscopy level; the RER appeared in the form of a few small disordered arrays. On the contrary, the RER of Purkinje cells of control animals was in the form of orderly stacks of parallel arrays characteristic of normal Purkinje cells (Palay and Chan-Palay, 1974). This finding is in accord with Hansson (1981) who reported alteration of RER and disintegration of Nissl bodies of Purkinje cells in rabbits exposed to E field of 14 kV/m (undisturbed field, 50 Hz AC). The change in the pattern of Nissl substance and RER is indicative of alteration in the metabolic status of the cell, especially the common protein metabolic pool. Although this could be an early sign of degeneration, there was no evidence of definite chromatolytic changes. This is in favor of a reversible effect of non ionizing (microwave) radiation at low power density. This finding may provide an explanation for the results previously obtained in our laboratory (Albert et al., 1981). There was a statistically significant decrease in Purkinje cell population when the animals were sacrificed immediately after exposure to microwave radiation with specifications similar to the experiment conducted in this study.

However, the decrease in Purkinje cell number was insignificant when the animals were allowed to recover for 40 days after cessation of irradiation.

In other experiments, adult chinese hamsters exposed to 2.45 GHz electromagnetic radiation at power densities of 10, 25 and 50 mW/cm^2 displayed morphological alterations (Albert and de Santis, 1975; and Mckee et al., 1980). These changes consisted of pykosis, chromatolysis, vacuolation of cytoplasm, paucity of free ribosomes and RER in hippocampal, thalamic and hypothalamic neurons. However, these authors did to mention any change in cerebellar Purkinje cells. The morphological change reported in these studies and the findings of the present study are more or lessunique in spite of the variation of the site of change itself. This variation could be attributed to the difference in vulnerability of the various euronal systems of different species during different ages to EM radiation.

During examination of the material in this study some folia of the irradiated animals showed extravasation of some mononucleated blood cells in the vicinity of a capillary vessel in the white core. No change in the vascular walls was observed. This finding argues with the observations reported from the studies on the effect of electro-magnetic radiation on the blood-brain barrier (BBB) (Oldendorf, 1970; Frey et al., 1975; Oscar and Hawkins, 1977; Albert, 1977 and 1978). These authors suggested an increase in the permeability of blood brain barrier BBB due to irradiation. However, no opening in the tight junction between the endothelial cells of the brain vasculature was reported in spite of the increased passage of injected horse-radish peroxidase tracer through BBB of irradiated animals (Albert and Kerns, 1981).

It is evident that there is an obvious need for additional research on the mechanisms of interaction of electromagnetic radiation with the nervous system although the effect of exposure to low intensity radiation seems to be reversible.

1. Albert, E.N. and DeSantis, M., Do microwaves alter nervous system structure? A light and electron microscopic study. Annal N.Y. Acad. Sci. 247 (1975) pp. 87-108.

2. Albert, E.N., Light and electron microscopic observations on the blood-brain barrier after microwave irradiation. In: Symposium on Biological Effects and Measurements of RF/Microwaves, Ed. Hazzard D., HEW Publications (EPA) 77-8026 (1977) pp. 294-304.

3. Albert, E.N., Ultrastructure Pathology Associated with Microwave Induced Alterations in Blood-Brain Barrier Permeability. In: Open Symposium on the Biological Effects of Electromagnetic Waves, URSI, Helsinki (1978) p. 58.

4. Albert, E.N., Sherif, M.F., Papadopoulos, N.J., Slaby, F.J. and Monahan, J., Effect of nonionizing radiation on Purkinje cells of the rat cerebellum. Bioelectromagnetics 2 (1981a) pp. 247-257.

5. Albert, E.N., Sherif, M.F. and Papadopoulos, N.J. Effects of non-ionizing radiation on the Purkinje cells of the uvula in squirrel monkey cerebellum. Bioelectromagnetics (1981b) 2:258-264.

6. Albert, E.N. and Kerns, J.M., Reversible microwave effects on the blood-brain barrier. Brain Res., 230 (1981) pp. 153-164.

7. Altman, J., Anderson, W.J. and Wright, K.A., Early effects of X-irradiation of the cerebellum in infant rats: Decimation and reconstitution of the external granular layer. Exp. Neurol., 24 (1969) pp.196-216.

8. Altman, J., Postnatal development of the cerebellar cortex in the rat. II. Phases in the maturation of Purkinje cells and of the molecular layer. J. Comp. Neurol. 145 (1972) pp. 399-464.

9. Altman, J. and Anderson, W.J., Experimental reorganization of the cerebellar cortex. I. Morphological effects of elimination of all microneurons with prolonged X-irradiation started at birth. J. Comp. Neurol. 146 (1972) pp. 355-406.

10. Berman, E., Kinn, J.B. and Carter, H.B., Observations of mouse fetuses after irradiation with 2.45 GHz microwave. Health Phys. 35 (1878) pp. 791-801.

11. Cholodov, J.A. Vliganii electromagnitnych i magnitnych polgeg na centralnuju sistemu. Medgiz. Moskva, 1966 (The influence of electromagnetic and magnetic fields on the central nervous system). Cited by Baranski, S. and Czerki, P. "Biological Effects of Microwaves". Dowden, Hutchinson and Ross, Inc. Stroudsburg, Penn. Sylvania (1976) p. 98.

12. Cowan, W.M., Neuronal death as a regulative mechanism in the control of cell number in the nervous system. Development and Aging in the Nervous System (M. Rockstein, ed.), Academic Press, New York (1973) pp. 19-41.

13. Das, G.D. Experimental analysis of embryogenisis of cerebellum in rat. I. Subnormal growth following X ray irradiation on day 15 of gestation. J. Comp. Neurol. 176 (1977) pp. 419-434.

14. Frey, A., Feld, S.R., and Frey, B. Neural function and behavior: Defining the ralationship. Biological effect of non-ionizing radiation, Ed. Tyler, P., Ann. New York Acad. Sci. 247 (1975) 433-439.

15. Hansson, H.A. Lamellar bodies in Purkinje nerve cells experimentally induced by electric field. Brain Res. 216 (1981) pp. 291-282.

16. Jacobson, M. Developmental Neurobiology. Plenum Press, New York and London, 2nd ed. (1978) pp. 281-282.

17. Mineki, L. and Bilski, R. Zmiany histopathologiczne w narzadach wewnetrznych myszy possawanych dzialaniu mikrofal (pasmo S). Histopathologic lesions in the internal organs of mice exposed to microwave (S band). Med. Pracy 12 (1961) p.337.

18. McKee, A.E., Dorsey, C.H., Eisenbrandt, D.L. and Woollen, N.E. Ultrastructural observations of microwave-induced morphological changes in the central nervous system of hamsters. Bioelectromagnetics 1 (1980) p. 206.

19.   Oldendorf, W.H. Focal neurological lesions produced by microwaves irradiation, Proc. soc. Exp. Biol. Med., 72 (1949) p. 432.

20.   Oldendorf, W.H. Measurement of brain uptake of radiolabeled substances using a tritiated water internal strand. Brain Res. 24 (1970) pp. 372-276.

21.   Oscar, K.J. and Hawkins, T.D. Microwave alterations of the blood brain barrier system of rats. Brain Res. 126 (1977) pp. 281-293.

22.   Palay S.L., Chan-Palay V., "Cerebellar Cortex, Cytology, and Organisation". New York, Heidelberg, Berlin: Springer-Vergas, 1974, pp. 25-8.

23.   Rugh, R., Ginns E.I., Ho H.S., Leach W.M., Are microwaves teratogenic? In "Biological Effects and Health Hazzards of Microwave Radiation". Proc. Int. Symp., Poland, Polish Medical Press, 1974.

24.   Rugh, R., Ginns, E.I., Ho H.S., Leach M.W., Response of the mouse to microwave radiation during oestrous cycle and pregnancy, Rad. Res., 62 (1975) pp. 225-236.

25.   Rugh, R., McManaway M., Anesthesia as an effective agent against the production of congenital anomalies in mouse fetuses exposed to electromagnetic radiation, J. Exp. Zool., 197 (1977) pp. 363-372.

26.   Shore M.L., Felten R.P., Lamanna A., The effect of repetitive prenatal low-level microwave exposure on development in the rat. In Hazzard D. (ed.): Proc. Symp. Biol. effects of Measurement Radio frequency/Microwaves, U.S. Dept. of H.E.W., Rockville, Md., 1977.

27.   Tolgskaya, M.C. and Gordon, Z.W. Morfologitcheskoje izmenenija pri deistvii elektromagnitnych voln radiochastat (eksperimentalnye issledovania). "Morphologic changes induced by electromagnetic radiofrequency waves. Experimental investigations". Izd. Medicina. Moscow. 1971. Cited by Baranski, S. and Czerki, P. "Biological Effects of Microwaves". Dowden, Hutchinson & Ross, Inc. Stroudsburg, Pennsylvania (1976) p. 97.

Electromagnetic Fields and Neurobehavioral Function, pages 153–177
© 1988 Alan R. Liss, Inc.

MICROWAVE EFFECTS ON THE CARDIOVASCULAR SYSTEM: A MODEL FOR
STUDYING THE RESPONSIVITY OF THE AUTONOMIC NERVOUS SYSTEM TO
MICROWAVES

D. I. McRee, Ph.D., M. J. Galvin, Ph.D.,
C. L. Mitchell, Ph.D.
Laboratory of Behavioral and Neurological
 Toxicology, NIEHS
P.O. Box 12233
Research Triangle Park, NC 27709

This chapter presents an overview of research to evaluate the effects of microwave radiation on the cardiovascular system. Results will be presented which indicate that
the reported effects are not due to direct influence on the
myocardium or its neural components but one triggered by
the autonomic nervous system to maintain homeostasis. Therefore, the cardiovascular system may represent a very useful
model for investigating changes in responsivity of the autonomic nervous system to electromagnetic fields.

INTRODUCTION

Soviet and Eastern European literature is replete with
references to microwave effects on the autonomic (vegetative) nervous system (Petrov 1970; Presman and Levitina
1962; Presman and Levitina 1963; Presman 1970, Drogichina et
al., 1966). Indeed, alterations in the autonomic regulation
of the cardiovascular system following exposure to microwaves has according to Presman (1970) been "most convincing-
ly demonstrated" even in cases where the intensity is presumably non-thermal. In contrast the United States' literature is quite controversial on this subject. Most studies
have used power densities which produce thermal effects for
short exposure duration, and apparently, no studies on the
effect of long-term, low-level, microwave exposures on the
automonic nervous system has been done by U.S. investigators.

A large number of investigators have studied the effects
of microwave radiation on the cardiovascular system. Some
researchers have reported changes in the cardiovascular

system in studies using in vitro or in vivo preparations while other investigators have reported no alterations using basically the same biological preparations.

Isolated heart preparations from several different species have been used to study direct effects of microwaves on the heart. In those studies which reported changes, the most prominent effect was a chronotropic one. Tinney et al. (1976) and Reed et al. (1977) observed bradycardia when either isolated rat or turtle hearts were exposed to 960 MHz CW microwaves at specific absorption rates (SARs) between 1 and 10 W/kg. At higher SARs tachycardia was observed which the authors attributed to tissue heating. Reed et al. (1977) reported that when both parasympathetic and sympathetic blocking agents were added to the perfusate, microwave radiation (SAR=1.5-2.5 W/kg) had no significant effect on heart rate. When atropine alone (a parasympathetic blocking agent) was applied in combination with microwaves, the heart rate increased. When propranolol hydrochloride (a sympathetic beta-site blocking agent) was applied in combination with microwaves, the heart rate decreased more than when the blocking agent was absent. Frey and Seifert (1968) reported effects of pulsed 1.425 GHz microwaves on isolated frog hearts. The peak power density used was 60 mW/cm^2. Since the pulse rate was one per second and the pulse width was 10 msec, the average power density was approximately 0.6 μW/cm^2. When the pulse was synchronized at 200 msec after the P wave, about the time the QRS complex occurred, tachycardia was observed. However, in a similar but not identical study, Liu et al. (1976) found no significant changes in the rates of frog hearts irradiated in situ with pulsed 10.0- or 1.42-GHz microwaves. Clapman and Cain (1975) observed no effects of microwave radiation on the isolated frog heart exposed to 3.0- or 1.5-GHz pulsed radiation.

More recently Yee et al. (1984) studied the effects of 2.45 GHz CW microwave radiation on the beating rate of isolated frog hearts. The purpose of their study was to measure the effects of microwaves on isolated frog hearts using a variety of recording techniques. The techniques used were 3-M KCl glass filled electrodes, ultrasound, tension transducer, metal wire plus glass electrodes filled with Ringer's solution, and glass electrodes filled with Ringer's solution only. They found no effects of microwave on the beating rate of frog hearts using ultrasound, tension-transducer, or Ringer's solution. Bradycardia was measured using 3-M KCl

electrodes and metal wire plus glass electrodes filled with
Ringer's solution. All the exposures were performed using a
temperature controlled waveguide exposure chamber at an SAR
of 8.55 W/kg. Yee et al. (1984) concluded that the bradycardia may have been due to an induced-current artifact of
the high concentration of KCl and the metal wire electrode.

Investigations to study the effects of partial or whole-
body exposure of live animals have produced varying results.
Presman and Levitina (1962; 1963) exposed various regions of
rabbits to 2.45 GHz and 3.0 GHz continuous wave (CW) and
pulsed wave (PW) microwave radiation. The exposures were
carried out both dorsally and ventrally for 20 minutes at
power densities of 7-12 mW/cm^2 CW and 3-5 mW/cm^2 PW. Dorsal
exposure resulted in tachycardia, and ventral exposure produced bradycardia. They also reported that the chronotropic
effect of PW radiation was more pronounced than for CW radiation. Kaplan et al. (1971) in an attempt to replicate
these results reported an absence of effects when the heads
of rabbits were dorsally exposed to 2.4 GHz microwave radiation at a power density of 10 mW/cm^2 for 20 minutes. They
also irradiated the head to a power density of 80 mW/cm^2
which resulted in increased body temperature and ultimately
an increase in heart rate. Chou et al. (1980) exposed rabbits dorsally and ventrally to 2.45 GHz for 20 minutes to
continuous wave (CW) at 5 mW/cm^2, to pulse waves (PW) of 1-
micro-second width at a repetition rate of 700 pps at an
average power density of 5 mW/cm^2 and at a peak power density of 7.1 W/cm^2 and to CW microwaves at a power density
of 80 mW/cm^2. The only effect observed was an increase in
heart beat rate at 80 mW/cm^2.

Dorsal exposures of anesthetized rats to 2.45 GHz
microwave radiation were conducted at a power density of 80
mW/cm^2 (Cooper et al., 1962). The exposure continued until
the rectal temperature reached 40.5°C. The average duration
of exposure was 12 minutes. The cardiac output, heart rate
and arterial blood pressure increased at the hyperthermic
level of 40.5°C.

Phillips et al. (1975) exposed rats one at a time in a
multimodal resonating cavity (microwave oven) having a frequency of 2.45 GHz. The animals were exposed for 30 minutes
at SARs of 0, 4.5, 6.5, or 11.1 W/kg. Rats exposed to 4.5
W/kg exhibited an initial transient increase in colonic and
skin temperatures but no alterations in other function. The

group irradiated at 6.5 W/kg had greater elevations in colonic and skin temperatures immediately after exposure followed by overcompensation and lower than normal colonic temperatures for approximately 3 hours. Metabolic rate was depressed in these animals for 3 hours. Bradycardic developed within 20 minutes after exposure and continued for approximately 3 hours. The animals exposed to 11.1 W/kg responded similarly to those exposed to 6.5 W/kg, but the changes were more severe and lasted longer. In addition the ECG tracings of these rats showed transient abnormalities including irregular rhythms and incomplete heart block.

A number of Eastern European studies on industrial exposure of workers to microwave radiation have reported cardiovascular effects (Drogichina et al. 1966; Medvedev 1980; Sadchikova and Nikonova 1971; Yakovleva 1968). Bradycardia, in addition to other cardiovascular changes, were described. For example, Drogichina et al. (1966) have described autonomic and cardiovascular disorders during chronic exposure to microwaves (2 mW/cm^2, frequency not specified). The populations were a group of 100 persons who worked in a microwave field and were observed for 10 years. In the early exposure period, there were mild asthenic manifestations. After a prolonged exposure, the workers exhibited a number of cardiovascular abnormalities. The data from this study provides support for the concept that microwave radiation can alter the cardiovascular system. However, it is not reasonable to speculate that this microwave-induced bradycardia represents a risk factor to the healthy cardiovascular system since the magnitude of the decrease was very small. However, in a diseased state, microwave radiation may have a more pronounced effect on the cardiovascular system.

The purpose of this chapter is to report results of studies in our laboratories on the effects of microwave radiation on the cardiovascular system. These studies include results from exposures of spontaneously beating rat atria, cat hearts in situ, and whole animals (rats). The results will be discussed in terms of the possibility of using the cardiovascular system as a model for investigating the effects of microwaves on the autonomic nervous system.

EXPERIMENTS

Atria Experiments

The details of this research have been reported previously (Galvin, et al., 1982). The objective of the experiment was to determine the effects of microwaves on the chronotropic and inotropic function of the heart. Chronotropic changes are those effects that influence the heart rate. Inotropic changes are those effects that modify contractility (force of contraction). Male sprague Dawley rats weighing between 250 and 300 g were used. The rats were euthanized by decapitation, the heart immediately removed, and the atria isolated and suspended in a glass tube. Force and rate were continuously recorded from the time the glass tubes were placed into the temperature controlled waveguide exposure chamber (Fig. 1) to the end of the experiment. Experiments were conducted at two different temperatures, 22 and 37°C, and at two different dose rates, 2 and 10 W/kg. The frequency of the microwaves was 2.45 GHz, and the delivery mode was continuous wave radiation. For each experiment atria from two rats were used. The atria from one rat was placed in the exposed tube, and the atria from another rat was placed in the control tube (see Fig. 1).

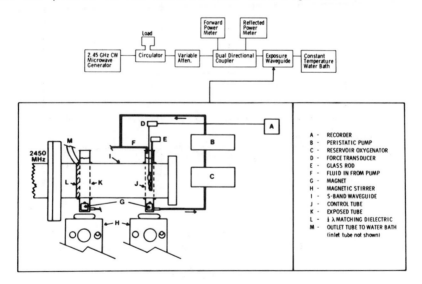

Fig. 1. Schematic of microwave exposure system for exposing isolated spontaneously beating rat atria.

Following a 20- to 30-minute equilibration, the initial rate and force of contraction were determined for each atrial preparation. The atria located in the exposure waveguide tube were then irradiated for a 30-min period. During this time, developed contractile force (mg) and rate (beats-per-min) were recorded for both the exposed and control (non-exposed) atria at the moment radiation began, and 1, 2, 5, 10, 15, 20, 25 and 30 min after the onset of exposure. At the completion of the exposure period, a 30-min recovery period was allowed during which measurements were recorded

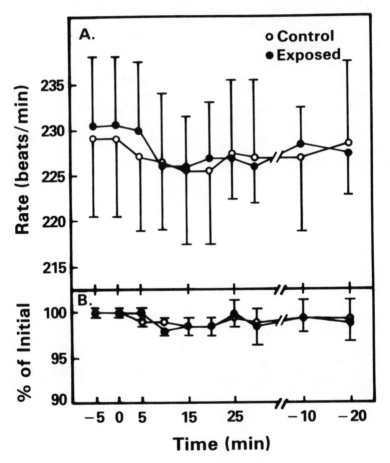

Fig. 2. The effect of microwave radiation on the contraction rate of isolated rat atria exposed at 2 W/kg at 37 $\pm$ 0.1°C. Each data point is the mean $\pm$ SE for six to eight animals. A, contraction rate; B, percent of initial contraction rate.

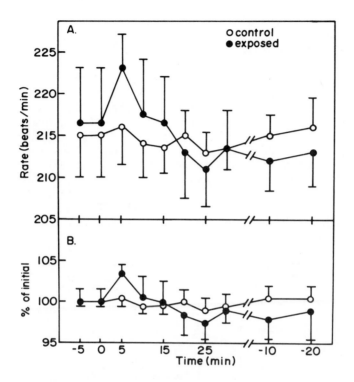

Fig. 3. The effect of microwave radiation on the contraction rate of isolated rat atria exposed at 10 W/kg
at $37 \pm 0.1^{\circ}C$. Each data point is the mean $\pm$ SE
for six to eight animals. A, contraction rate; B,
percent of initial contraction rate.

immediately after termination of exposure and at 10-min intervals. The control atria were treated in an identical
manner except they received negligible microwave irradiation.

The effect of microwave radiation on the rate of contraction of isolated rat atria maintained at $37^{\circ}C$ is depicted in Figure 2A and 3A at 2 W/kg and 10 W/kg, respectively.
At 2 W/kg, the rate for both exposed and control atria averaged 230 beats per min (Fig. 2), while at 10 W/kg the rate
was 215 beats per min (Fig. 3). The percent of initial rate
is presented in Figure 2B and 3B. Neither group showed significant variation from 100 percent. The average developed
tension was 640 mg for all three groups and was not influenced by either microwave dose. Furthermore, no data point

for the exposed atria was significantly different from the corresponding control value for any of the actual (force and rate) or calculated (percent of initial rate) values.

The effect of microwave radiation on atrial rate at 22 + 0.1°C is presented in Figure 4A and 5A, for 2 W/kg and 10 W̄/kg, respectively. As expected, the atrial rate was much lower due to the lower temperature. The average rate at 2 W/kg was 102 (see Fig. 4) beats per minute, while at 10 W/kg, it was 106 (Fig. 5) beats per min. Again there was no significant difference in rate between the exposed and the control atria at either SAR. The percent of the initial rate is shown in Figure 4B and 5B. Neither group showed significant variation from 100 over the 90-min period. The average developed tension was 1,200 mg for all three groups over the 90-min experimental period.

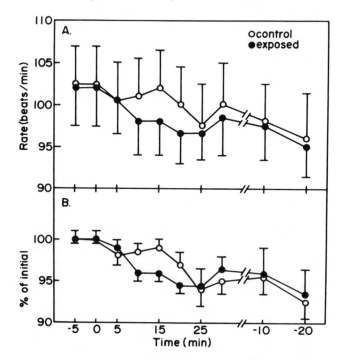

Fig. 4. The effects of microwave radiation on the contraction rate of isolated rat atria exposed at 2 W/kg at 22 + 0.1°C. Each data point is the mean + SE for six to eight animals. A, contraction rate; B, percent of initial contraction rate.

The results of these experiments show that there were no effects of 2.45-GHz CW microwave radiation on the rate of contraction (beat-rate) nor on the contractile force if the temperature is maintained at a constant level. These findings demonstrate that the microwaves used in this study have no direct influence on the myocardium or its neural components.

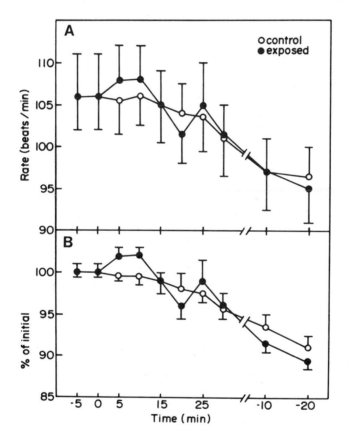

Fig. 5. The effects of microwave radiation on the contraction rate of isolated rat atria exposed at 10 W/kg at $22 \pm 0.1^{\circ}$C. Each data point is the mean $\pm$ SE for six to eight animals. A, contraction rate; B, percent of initial contraction rate.

Cat Heart Experiment

The results of this experiment has been reported previously by Galvin and McRee (1981). This study examined the
effects on cardiac function of direct microwave irradiation
of the exposed intact heart. Mean arterial blood pressure
(MABP), heart rate (HR), cardiac output (CO), and the release of creatine phosphokinase (CPK) were evaluated in
cats whose hearts were exposed for 5 hours to 2.45-GHz radiation with and without myocardial ischemia. Myocardial
ischemic hearts were used in order to determine if damaged
hearts were more sensitive to microwave radiation than a
normal healthy heart. Plasma CPK activity was measured
because studies have shown that agents which influence the
degree of myocardial damage generally affect the level of
CPK activity in the plasma (Maroko et al., 1971).

Cats of either sex weighing 2.7 - 3.4 kg were anesthetized with pentobarbitol sodium (30 mg/kg). A mid-sternal
thoracotomy was then performed, and the exposed pericardial
sac was retracted, allowing for exposure of the anterior
surface of the heart. Myocardial ischemia was induced in
some of the cats by occlusion of the coronary artery. A
schematic of the apparatus used for exposing the cat myocardium is shown in Figure 6. A dielectrically loaded waveguide (RG-49/U) was positioned 2 cm from the cardiac surface.
The SAR of the heart was computed from the slopes of the

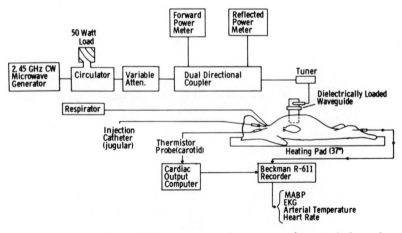

Fig. 6. Schematic of the system for exposing cat hearts
to microwaves.

time-temperature profiles of irradiated myocardium. These profiles were obtained by using a Vitek thermistor probe implanted 2-3 mm into the heart tissue of cats which had been killed and cooled to room temperature (McRee 1974). The SAR for all exposures was 30 W/kg for 5 hours. In the nonexposed cats the waveguide was positioned above the heart but the microwaves were not turned on. The cats were placed on a 37°C water-type heating pad throughout the experimental period.

A relatively stable hemodynamic pattern was exhibited by all four groups of animals over the 5-hour observation period. Table 1 summarized the MABP, HR, and CO data. Cats not subjected to coronary artery ligation and not exposed to microwaves (sham) exhibited no significant changes in MABP, HR, or CO over the 5-h experimental period. These parameters were not altered in the exposed group. The nonexposed myocardial ischemic (MI+ sham) cats had hemodynamic values comparable to the sham group and were not significantly different from the initial values at any sampling period. There was no significant interaction between microwave radiation and ischemia on the measured cardiovascular indices. The values for MABP, HR, and CO, approximately

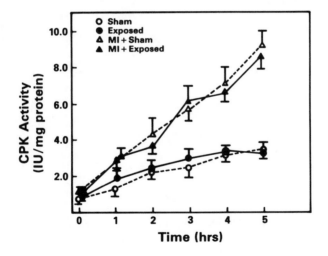

Fig. 7. Plasma creating phosphokinase (CPK) activities expressed as means + SE for 7-11 animals in each group. Initial activities were similar for all 4 groups of cats.

Table 1. Hemodynamic consequences of microwave radiation during myocardial ischemia

Group	n	Time, hours					
		0	1	2	3	4	5
		Mean arterial blood pressure, mmHg					
Sham	7	125	125	128	132	133	130
		+6	+3	+5	+6	+6	+8
Exposed	7	132	132	135	139	139	137
		+3	+5	+5	+8	+8	+6
Myocardial ischemia + sham	8	126	118	119	124	124	118
		+5	+5	+5	+6	+6	+7
Myocardial ischemia + exposed	11	135	118	120	129	129	124
		+6	+5	+5	+5	+5	+5
		Cardiac output, ml·min^{-1},kg^{-1}					
Sham	7	130	138	148	136	134	140
		+08	+10	+16	+18	+10	+14
Exposed	7	150	148	136	132	130	132
		+10	+14	+18	+16	+14	+18
Myocardial ischemia + sham	.8	145	142	150	132	130	130
		+12	+10	+10	+16	+8	+16
Myocardial ischemia + exposed	8	140	136	124	128	132	128
		+12	+12	+10	+10	+10	+10
		Heart rate, beats/min					
Sham	7	126	115	117	124	125	125
		+6	+6	+4	+7	+7	+4
Exposed	7	122	117	120	123	122	123
		+4	+5	+5	+4	+4	+5
Myocardial ischemia + sham	8	123	111	121	123	122	124
		+5	+6	+6	+6	+5	+7
Myocardial ischemia + exposed	11	126	113	120	125	122	119
		+6	+7	+4	+4	+6	+4

Values shown are means ± SE for each group of cats. n, no. of cats in each group.

120 mmHg, 124 beats/min, and 130 ml·min^{-1}, kg^{-1}, respectively, for both exposed and MI + exposed groups at 5 h, were not significantly different from their respective pre-exposure values.

The plasma CPK activities are depicted for the four experimental groups in Figure 7. The initial values for the groups were similar, having a value of approximately 1.0 IU/mg protein. In the sham group this value increased to approximately 3.0 IU/mg protein over the 5-h experimental period. The exposed group exhibited a similar increase, which was not significantly different from the sham value at any sampling time. In contrast, both the MI + sham and MI + exposed groups exhibited significant increases in plasma CPK activity at 3, 4, and 5 h compared with the appropriate sham group. The final values were three times those of the sham-operated groups. The similar increase in CPK activity for both microwave-exposed groups in comparison to the appropriate sham further indicates that microwave radiation at this SAR has no measurable effect on normal or ischemic myocardium.

In summary, this study provides data on the effect of microwave radiation on the myocardium in situ. In contrast to some previous studies, these data were obtained under

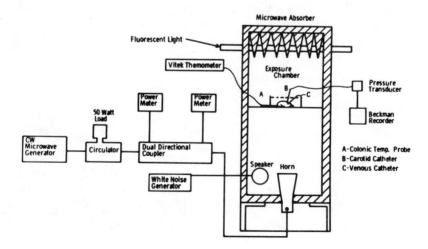

Fig. 8.   Schematic of monitoring and exposure systems for measuring microwave effects on cardiac function.

conditions of a known specific absorption rate and with the
site or irradiation limited to cardiac tissue. No effects
of microwaves on cardiac function were observed in normal
cats, nor was the course of acute myocardial ischemia affected by microwave radiation at the dose rate and frequency
used in these experiments. These findings demonstrate that
direct exposure of the intact heart to microwave radiation
has no effect on the myocardium or its neural components.

Ventral Exposure of Rats

In this study the influence of acute (6 hr) exposure to
2.45-GHz (CW) microwave radiation of incident power density
of 10 mW/cm^2 on certain cardiovascular indices was examined

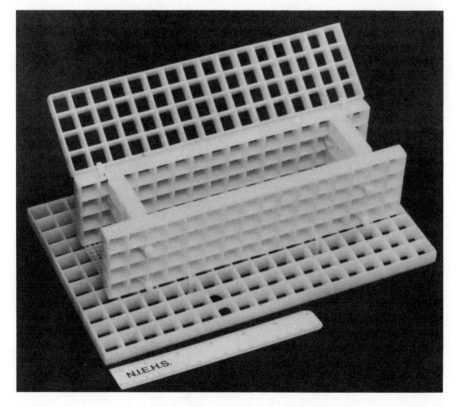

Fig. 9.   Exposure cage used for exposure of rats in unanesthetized state while monitoring cardiac function.

in unanesthetized male Sprague-Dawley rats weighing 250 +
25 g. Under methoxy-flurane anesthesia, a catheter was inserted into the right femoral artery which was used for monitoring blood pressure and heart rate. Colonic temperature
was monitored via a Vitek thermistor probe, inserted rec-
tally to a depth of 5 cm. The rat was subsequently placed
into a ventilated restraining cage which was located inside
an anechoic box (Fig. 8 and 9). The temperature and humidity in the box were maintained at 22.5°C and 60% respectively during the experimental period by placing the entire
exposure apparatus in a large environmental chamber.

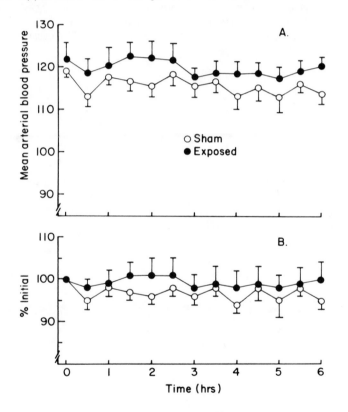

Fig. 10. The effects of microwave radiation on the mean
arterial blood pressure of rats exposed to 10
mW/cm² at ambient temperature of 22.5°C. A,
mean arterial blood pressure; B, percent of initial blood pressure.

The incident power density was measured using an NBS Model B electromagnetic field probe. The power density measured in the restraining cage varied less than ± 10 percent. The average, whole-body, specific absorption rate (SAR) was measured using a calorimetric technique (McRee and Davis, 1984). The SAR was determined to be 2.3 W/kg for an incident power density of 10 mW/cm^2.

The experiment included 10 replications (each replication included one exposed and one sham rat) which resulted in 10 animals per group. The mean arterial blood pressure for the sham and microwave exposed rats is depicted in Figures 10A (absolute value) and 10B (percent of initial). Both groups of rats exhibited a similar MABP at time 0, and

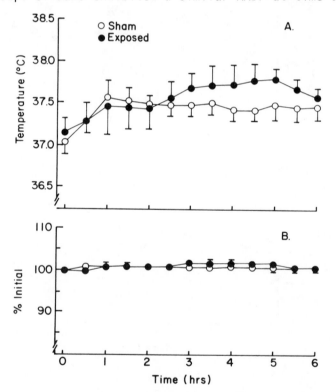

Fig. 11. The effects of microwave radiation on the colonic temperature of rats exposed to 10 mW/cm^2 at ambient temperature of 22.5°C. A, colonic temperature; B, percent of initial colonic temperature.

it remained stable throughout the 6 hour exposure period. Ventral microwave exposure had no influence on this parameter.

In Figure 11, the colonic temperature is shown as absolute (11A) and percent of initial (11B) values. As with the blood pressure data, no differences were noted between the sham and microwave exposed rats. Both groups had initial colonic temperatures of approximately 37°C and were unchanged throughout the 6 hour experimental period.

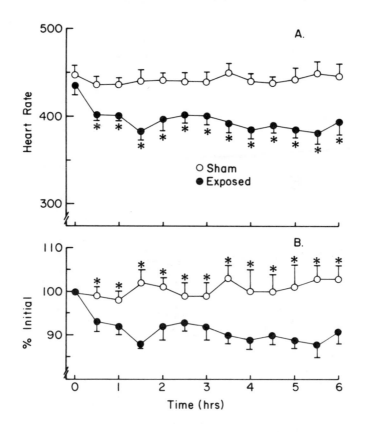

Fig. 12.   The effects of microwave radiation on the heart rate of rats exposed to 10 mW/cm^2 at an ambient temperature of 22.5°C. A, heart rate; B, percent of initial heart rate. *p<0.01 compared to the appropriate sham value.

The heart rate data for the 2 groups of rats are shown in Figure 12. Both groups exhibited comparable heart rates at time 0, (i.e., 450 vs. 440 beats/min for the sham and exposed rats respectively). However, by 60 min after the onset of exposure, the exposed rats exhibited a significantly lower heart rate than the sham exposed rats ($p \leq 0.01$). This reduction in heart rate, although small, persisted

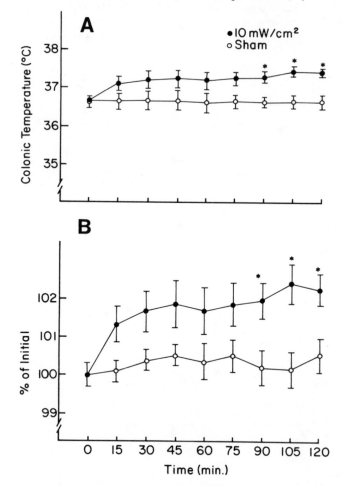

Fig. 13. The effect of microwave radiation on colonic temperature of the rats exposed to 10 mW/cm^2 at an ambient temperature of 27°C. A, colonic temperature; B, percent of initial colonic temperature. *$p<0.01$ compared to the appropriate sham values.

throughout the remainder of the 6 hour exposure period. When calculated as a percent of initial heart rate (Fig. 12B), the sham-exposed rats had heart rates between 98 and 100 percent of initial, while the exposed rats exhibited heart rates between 90 and 95 percent of initial during the 6 hour exposure periods. An additional group of rats was

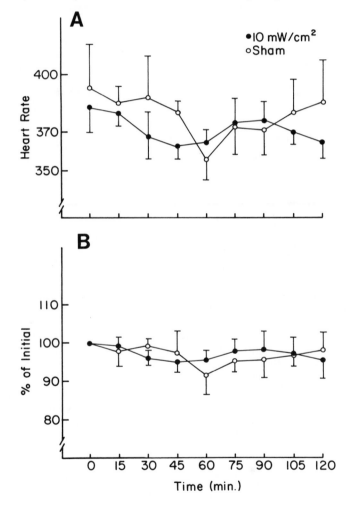

Fig. 14. The effects of microwave radiation on the heart rate of rats exposed to 10 mW/cm^2 at an ambient temperature of 27°C. A, heart rate; B, percent of initial heart rate.

exposed to determine if the rats would recover from the microwave-induced bradycardia. In this group, the microwaves were turned off after a 2 hour exposure and monitored for an additional 2 hours. The rats exhibited bradycardia 1 hour after the start of exposure; however, heart rate returned to initial pre-exposure levels within 2 hours after termination of microwave irradiation (data not shown).

Experiments have just been completed in our laboratory in which rats were exposed ventrally to the same conditions described above (2.45 GHz and 10 mW/cm^2) but at an ambient temperature of 27°C. No significant change in heart rate was observed although a slight increase (less than 1°C) in colonic temperature was measured (Figs. 13 and 14). This would indicate that the metabolic rate was not changed enough to result in a change in heart rate. Also, it should be noted that the resting heart rate at an ambient temperature of 22°C (Fig. 12) is higher than at an ambient temperature of 27°C (thermal neutral value for rats) (Fig. 14).

DISCUSSION

Although some earlier studies reported that direct exposure of isolated hearts to microwave radiation produced changes in beating rate, more recent studies using 2.45-GHz CW microwaves have shown no change in beating rate if temperature is carefully controlled, and the technique for measuring the beating rate does not produce alterations. Yee et al. (1984) used a waveguide exposure system which allowed accurate control of temperature to show that no change in beating rate was found if an ultrasound probe, tension transducer, or Ringer's solution glass electrode were used, whereas bradycardia was measured using 3-M KCl glass electrodes or a metal wire inserted in the Ringer's solution electrode. They state that their results indicate that the bradycardia could be due to electrode artifacts resulting from intensification of the electromagnetic fields at the electrode tip.

In our study using the spontaneously beating rat atria, a waveguide system similiar to that used by Yee et al. (1984) was used for accurate temperature control. A tension transducer located outside the waveguide which could not interfere with the electromagnetic field or beating rate was used to measure the beating rate. No change in beating rate was observed for SAR's of 2 and 10 W/kg as long as

temperature was controlled. In our investigation directly
exposing the intact heart of cats, the results demonstrated
that direct irradiation of the innervated heart at a specific absorption rate of 30 W/kg at 2.45-GHz had no effect
on the ionotropic or chronotropic actions of the heart. No
change in the temperature of the beating heart was measured
at this high absorption rate. This result was probably due
to the large volume of blood circulating through the heart
which carried the heat away very rapidly. From the information presented in our experiments and those of Yee et al.
(1984), it is our opinion that CW microwave radiation does
not have a direct effect on the myocardium or its neural
components. We believe, therefore, that the cardiovascular
effects observed by others in vivo may be due to microwave
effects on the autonomic nervous system.

The maintenance of constancy, or homeostasis, is primarily the function of the endocrine system and the autonomic nervous system. If microwave exposure does not have
a direct effect on the cardiovascular system, then the response of the cardiovascular system could be due to the
adjustment of metabolism to compensate for the energy being
absorbed. In the description of our work on the ventral
exposure of unanesthetized rats, a bradycardia was reported.
This reduction in heart rate may represent a compensatory
response to the energy being absorbed by the rat.   For the
10 mW/cm^2 exposure intensity the specific absorption rate
was approximately 2.0 W/kg. Though not sufficient to induce a measurable change in colonic temperature, it represents a thermal input of approximately 30 percent of the
resting metabolic rate (Durney et al. 1978). These studies
were conducted at an ambient temperature of 22°C which is
approximately 5° lower than the thermal neutral temperature
of the rat (i.e. the temperature where the resting metabolic
rate is lowest). Thus, during these experiments the rat is
doing additional metabolic work in order to generate heat
to maintain thermal homeostasis. The input of approximately
2.0 W/kg of heat via microwaves thus reduces the metabolic
heat requirement. This could result in a reduction in the
resting metabolic rate at 22°C. It has been shown that as
the metabolic rate decreases, there can be a concomitant
decrease in heart rate (Elizondo 1977; Wang and Hudson
1971). Although this explanation ignores all the other
homeostatic adjustment processes which were invoked to maintain thermal balance, the animal in compensating for the
microwave thermal load, may reduce metabolic rate, which in

turn is accompanied by a reduction in heart rate.

Several investigators have exposed animals to 2.45-GHz radiation at a power density of 80 mW/cm^2 (Kaplan et al. 1971; Chou et al. 1980; Cooper et al. 1962). The first two studies used rabbits and the third study used rats. In all three cases an increased heart rate was observed. This increased heart rate would be expected at this power density due to the high thermal stressing of the animal and an increase in metabolic rates to dissipate this stress.

In summary, the results indicate that the response of the cardiovascular system is not a direct response on the heart itself but one triggered by the autonomic nervous system to maintain homeostasis. Depending on the ambient temperature, specific absorption rate, and duration of exposure, it is possible that a bradycardia, no change, or tachycardia could be observed when exposure to microwave occurs.

These studies leave unanswered, however, the question concerning changes in the responsivity of the autonomic nervous system following long-term exposure to microwaves. We suggest the cardiovascular system represents an especially useful model for investigating changes in responsivity of the autonomic nervous system for several reasons:

1. There is a highly integrated pattern of antagonistic effects of sympathetic and parasympathetic actions on the heart, whereas control of blood pressure is due almost entirely to sympathetic control of vascular resistance. Thus, by examining both cardiac and vascular changes, one can obtain insight into whether an effect is predominantly sympathetic, parasympathetic, or non-specific.

2. The organization of central control of the cardiovascular system is reasonably well understood, and therefore, provides approaches toward separating central affects from those acting directly on the peripheral systems.

3. Cardiac muscle represents one of the few effector cells in which junctional autonomic transmission can be studied.

4. One can study the cardiovascular system both in vivo and in vitro with relative ease. Thus, one can deter-

mine whether or not the effects, if any, are mediated directly on the effector tissue, through changes at the post-synaptic neuroeffector junction, or require central mechanisms.

It would seem, therefore, that a careful and systematic analysis of changes in cardiovascular function induced by microwaves utilizing techniques useful in examining autonomic responsivity such as pre and post ganglionic stimulation, denervation, and/or pharmacological agonists and antagonists would add valuable insight to the effects of microwave exposure on the autonomic nervous system.

REFERENCES

Adair ER, Adams BW (1982): Adjustment's in metabolic heat production by squirrel monkeys exposed to microwaves. J. Appl. Physiol: Respirat. Environ. Physiol. 52: 1049-1058.

Chou CK, Han LF, Guy AW (1980): Microwave radiation and heart-beat rate of rabbits. J. Microwave Power. 15(2): 87-93.

Clapman RM, Cain CA (1975): Absence of heart rate effect on isolated frog heart with pulse modulated microwave energy. J. Microwave Power. 10: 411-419.

Cooper T, Pinakatt T, Jellinek M, Richardson A (1962): Effect of reserpine on circulation of the rat after microwave irradiation. Am. J. Physiol. 202: 1171-1174.

Drogichina EA, Konchalovskaya NM, Glotova KV, Sadchikova MN, Snegova GV (1966): Autonomic and cardiovascular disorders during chronic exposure to super-high frequency electromagnetic field. Gigiegena truda i professional'nyye Zabolevnija. 7: 13-17 (Russian).

Durney CH, Johnson CC, Barber PW, Massoudi H, Iskander MF, Lords JL, Ryser DK, Allen SJ, Mitchell JC (1978): Radiofrequency radiation dosimetry handbook. 2nd ed. Report SAM-TR-78-22. Brooks Air Force Base, San Antonio: USAF School of Aerospace Medicine.

Elizondo R (1977): Temperature regulation in primates. International Review of Physiol. 15: 71-107.

Frey, AH, Seifert E (1968): Pulse modulated UHF energy illumination of the heart associated with change in heart rate. Life Sciences 7: 505-512.

Galvin MJ, Dutton MS, McRee DI (1982): Influence of 2.45-GHz CW microwave radiation on spontaneously beating rat atria. Bioelectromagnetics 3: 219-226.

Galvin MJ, McRee DI (1981): Influence of acute microwave radiation on cardiac function in normal and myocardial ischemic cats. J. Appl. Physiol: Respirat. Environ. Exercise Physiol. 50(5): 931-935.

Ho HS, Edwards WP (1977): Oxygen-consumption rate of mice under differing dose rates of microwave radiation. In: Biological Effects of Electromagnetic Waves. Edited by D. R. Justesen and A. W. Guy. Radio Science 12(65): 131-138.

Kaplan IT, Metlay W, Zaret MM, Birenbaum L, Rosenthal SW (1971): Absence of heart-rate effects in rabbits during low-level microwave radiation. IEEE Trans. Microwave Theory and Tech. 19: 168-173.

Liu LM, Rosenbaum FJ, Pickard W F (1976): Insensitivity of frog heart rate to pulse modulated microwave energy. J. Microwave Power. 11: 255-232.

Maroko PR, Kjekshus BE, Sobel BE, Watanabe T, Corel JW, Ross J, Braunwald E (1971): Factors influencing infarct size following experimental coronary artery occlusions. Circulation 43: 67-78.

Medvedev VP (1980): Cardiovascular diseases in persons with a history of exposure to the effect of an electromagnetic field of extra-high frequency. Gigi. truda i profesional'nyye Zabolevaniia 17: 6-9 (Russian).

McRee DI (1974): Determination of the absorption of microwave radiation by a biological specimen in a 2450 MHz microwave field. Health Phys. 26: 385-390.

McRee DI, Davis HG (1984): Whole-body and local dosimetry in rats exposed to 2.45-GHz microwave radiation. Health Phys. 46: 315-320.

Petrov IR (1970): "Influence of Microwave Radiation in the organism of man and animals." NASA TT-F-708, Feb. 1972. National Technical Information Service, Springfield, VA.

Phillips DR, Hunt EL, Castro RD, King NW (1975): Thermoregulatory, metabolic, and cardiovascular response of rats to microwaves. J. Appl. Physiol. 38: 630-635.

Presman AS (1970): "Electromagnetic Fields and Life." New York-London: Plenum Press, p. 116-119.

Presman AS, Levitina NA (1962): Non-thermal action of microwaves on cardiac rhythm. Communication I. A study of the action of continuous microwaves. Bull. Exp. Biol. Med. (USSR) 53: 36-39.

Presman AS, Levitina NA (1963): Non-thermal action of microwaves on the rhythm of cardiac contractions in animals. Communications II. Investigation of the action of impulse microwaves. Bull. Exp. Med. (USSR) 53: 154-157.

Reed JR, Lords JL, Durney CH (1977): Microwave irradiation of the isolated rat heart after treatment with ANS blocking agents. Radio Science 12(65): 161-165.

Sadchikova MN, Nikonova KV (1971): Comparative evaluation of health of persons working in an environment influenced by microwaves of various intensities. Gigi. truda i professional'nyye Zabolevanii 9: 10-15 (Russian).

Tinney CK, Lords JL, Durney CH(1976): Rate effects in isolated turtle hearts induced by microwave irradiation. IEEE Trans. Microwave Theory Tech. 24: 18-24.

Wang LC, Hudson JW (1971): Temperature regulation in normothermic and hibernating eastern chipmunk Tamias striatus. Comp. Biochem. Physiol. 38: 59-90.

Yakovleva MI (1968): Effect of superhigh-frequency electromagnetic fields on conditioned reflex regulation of cardiac and respiratory activity. J. Higher Nervous Activity 18: 418-423 (Russian).

Yee KC, Chou CK, Guy AW (1984): Effect of microwave radiation on the beating rate of isolated frog hearts. Bioelectromagnetics 5: 263-270.

Electromagnetic Fields and Neurobehavioral Function, pages 179–201
© 1988 Alan R. Liss, Inc.

MICROWAVE CHALLENGES TO THE THERMOREGULATORY SYSTEM

Eleanor R. Adair

John B. Pierce Foundation and Yale University

New Haven, Connecticut

INTRODUCTION

The organs and systems of the body that accomplish
thermoregulation in endothermic species are normally
dedicated to other functions, with the probable exception
of the eccrine sweat glands. Thus, while the skeletal
musculature normally moves the body about in the world,
makes postural adjustments, etc., high-frequency contractions of the same muscle fibers (shivering) generate extra
heat to combat hypothermia. Also, the circulatory system,
which normally functions to supply nutrients to the cells
and carry off the waste products of metabolism, will
distribute heat by differential changes in blood flow.
Under certain circumstances, these changes in blood flow
will selectively bring heat from deep in the body to the
skin surface (vasodilation) for dissipation to the environment. Whether or not these organ systems are mobilized
for thermoregulation depends on whether the local temperature of certain critical regions of the central nervous
system (CNS) deviates significantly from a set or neutral
level. This becomes a critical issue when an endotherm is
exposed to microwaves because the thermal gradients in body
tissues during irradiation may differ from those that
result from exercise or in the presence of conventional
sources of heat.

Many discrete CNS sites have been identified as having
thermoregulatory function; these sites harbor neurological
elements that are sensitive to changes in their own temperature, either warming or cooling. The most important site

appears to be the medial preoptic/anterior hypothalamic area of the brainstem (PO/AH). This region has been dubbed the "central thermostat" of endothermic species because it not only exhibits great thermosensitivity but also is involved with the integration of input signals from many other thermosensitive sites and the generation of an output signal for the mobilization of thermoregulatory effector responses. Included among the extra-hypothalamic thermosensitive sites are the posterior hypothalamus, midbrain, medulla, spinal cord, deep abdominal structures and, most importantly, the skin. All of these regions may be involved in the mobilization of thermoregulatory responses when an endotherm is exposed to a microwave field. Whether a particular site will be stimulated directly (i.e., by electromagnetic energy deposited therein) or indirectly (i.e., by convective or conductive heating) will depend on many parameters of the radiation, notably the frequency, polarization, and intensity.

Some researchers currently hold the belief that the deposition of energy in body tissues during exposure to microwaves is unique and that the physiological mechanisms that distribute and eliminate the heat generated may be different from those mobilized during exposure to conventional heat sources or during exercise (Elder and Cahill, 1984; Lerner, 1984). The thesis to be defended in this paper is that the thermoregulatory system functions in the presence of electromagnetic fields in exactly the same manner as it does in the presence of environmental sources of radiant or convective heat; further, the response hierarchy (order in which responses are mobilized) is normal and the magnitude of the effector response is a function of the total incident energy integrated over the exposed surface of the body, even during partial-body exposure. A corollary to this thesis, also to be demonstrated, is that the PO/AH plays a minimal role in the generation of appropriate thermoregulatory responses during heating of the whole body by microwaves.

In defense of this thesis, several different experiments from our laboratory will be described. All experiments involved the use of adult male squirrel monkeys (Saimiri sciureus) as subjects and acute exposures to 2450-MHz continuous wave (CW) microwaves (unilateral planewave) in an anechoic chamber. This frequency is well above whole-body resonance for these experimental animals;

indeed, because the radiation may penetrate 1.5 to 2.0 cm below the skin surface, it has the potential to produce a high rate of energy deposition (i.e., an electrical hotspot) in the center of the head, close to the PO/AH thermoregulatory center. Hotspots have been predicted under such conditions by theoretical models (Burr, et al., 1980; Kritikos and Schwan, 1979) and localized regions of above-normal temperature have been demonstrated in tissue-equivalent spheres exposed to microwave fields (Burr and Krupp, 1980). If a "thermal hotspot" existed in the PO/AH region, it would be expected to stimulate vigorous changes in thermoregulatory effector responses.

For purposes of this discussion, a "thermal hotspot" may be defined as a localized rise in tissue temperature that exceeds the general rise in temperature of the body core (e.g., as measured in the colon). Some evidence against the formation of thermal hotspots in the brain, even under conditions most favorable for their occurrence, has recently been presented (Adair, et al., 1984). Monkeys were chronically implanted with teflon re-entrant tubes in the PO/AH so that the probe of a Vitek Electrothermia Monitor (Bowman, 1976) could be inserted to measure PO/AH temperature while the conscious animal was exposed to microwaves. At a thermoneutral ambient temperature (T_a) of 34 °C, during 10-min microwave exposures at power densities from 4 to 20 mW/cm², the temperature of the PO/AH did not rise significantly higher than that of the body core (measured in the colon). Further, the increment in PO/AH temperature seldom exceeded 0.3 °C in the presence of the microwave field whenever the monkeys were actively controlling T_a themselves.

The Thermoregulatory Profile

Basic knowledge of the normal thermoregulatory responses of the species in question is essential to the analysis of changes in thermoregulation that may occur during microwave irradiation. Endotherms are capable of generating heat in their bodies, of conserving heat, and of dissipating heat to the environment by radiation, convection, and evaporation. The particular thermoregulatory mechanism that may be operative at any given time will depend in large measure on the prevailing T_a. The graphical illustration of response mobilization as a function of

T$_a$ is known as the thermoregulatory profile, an example of which appears in Figure 1.

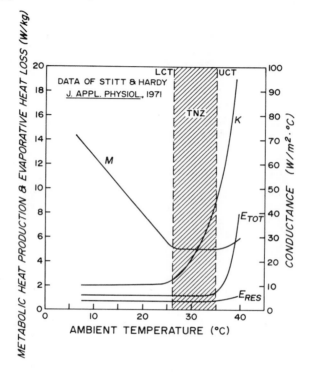

Figure 1. Thermoregulatory profile of restrained squirrel monkey (<u>Saimiri sciureus</u>) across a range of environmental temperatures from 10 to 39 °C. M = metabolic heat production (W/kg); K = conductance (W/m²·°C); E$_{tot}$ = total evaporative heat loss (W/kg); E$_{res}$ = respiratory evaporative heat loss (W/kg); LCT = lower critical temperature; UCT = upper critical temperature. The region between LCT and UCT is called the thermoneutral zone (TNZ). Data adapted from Stitt and Hardy, J Appl Physiol, 31:48-54 (1971).

The figure summarizes steady-state data for squirrel monkeys equilibrated to a wide range of T$_a$ under still air conditions (Stitt and Hardy, 1971). At T$_a$ below the lower critical temperature (LCT), metabolic heat production (M) is elevated to maintain a normal body temperature in the face of environmental cold stress. The lower the T$_a$, the higher is M, while the mechanisms of heat loss remain at low levels. Within the thermoneutral zone (TNZ), which encompasses T_a between the LCT and the upper critical temperature (UCT), M is at the resting level and thermoregulation is accomplished by changes in vasomotor state or thermal conductance (K). For the squirrel monkey, changes in K represent the major mechanism of heat loss from T_a = 26 to 35 °C; the peripheral vessels of the tail vasodilate at about T_a = 26 °C (Lynch, et al., 1980) and those of the hands and feet at about T_a = 33 °C (Lynch and Adair, 1978). Above the UCT, thermoregulation in endotherms is accomplished by the evaporation of water during sweating or panting. Certain endotherms (e.g., the rodents) have very limited evaporative capability and must rely on behavioral maneuvers (e.g., seeking shade, spreading saliva or other fluids over the body surface) to thermoregulate in warm environments. The squirrel monkey exhibits limited evaporative heat loss (E) in the form of eccrine sweating from the palms and soles (Machida, et al., 1967; Stitt and Hardy, 1971) but not elsewhere on the body surface. If T_a exceeds the UCT by more than a few °C or if a substantial amount of radiofrequency energy is deposited in their bodies, squirrel monkeys will rapidly become hyperthermic unless they are able to escape from these hostile conditions (Adair, 1985). Indeed, the upturn in the M function at T_a above the UCT is attributed, in part, to struggling in the chair in an attempt to escape (Stitt and Hardy, 1971). It is also attributable to the speeding up of response processes as tissue temperature rises, the so-called Q_{10} effect (Bligh and Johnson, 1973). It is important to recognize that although these animals are inferior to man in their ability to lose heat from the body through sweating, they show a significant evaporative heat loss response with a reliable threshold that provides a useful model for the examination of the thermoregulatory consequences of microwave exposure in thermoneutral and warm environments.

Inspection of Figure 1 reveals that the particular thermoregulatory response that may be altered when a squirrel monkey is exposed to a microwave field will depend on the T_a to which the animal is equilibrated prior to and during the exposure. Thus, at T_a = 15 °C, only M will be altered when microwave energy is absorbed because the other available responses (vasomotor and evaporative) are at low ebb. The thesis of this paper states in effect that there is an equivalence between T_a and microwave intensity; i.e., exposure at higher and higher power densities will be akin to exposure to warmer and warmer environments. Thus, for an animal equilibrated to T_a = 15 °C, if the microwave intensity is sufficiently high to reduce M to the resting level of 5 W/kg, further increases of intensity should initiate an increase in K, i.e., initiate vasodilation of the tail vessels. This is the next response in the hierarchy that is triggered when T_a increases.

Thermoregulatory Adjustments to High Intensity Microwaves

Experimental verification of the above prediction has been provided by recent experiments conducted by Candas (Candas, et al., in press). Squirrel monkeys were equilibrated for 90 min to a cool environment (T_a = 20 °C) to elevate M. They were then exposed to microwaves for two 30-min periods that were separated by a 70-min period for re-equilibration. In any given experiment, the power densities of the two exposures were different, either 30 and 35 mW/cm² or 40 and 45 mW/cm². At a whole-body rate of energy absorption (SAR) of 0.15 (W/kg per mW/cm²), these power densities were the equivalent of roughly 90 to 135 percent of the resting M of the monkeys.

Candas' results showed that each microwave exposure induced a rapid decrease in M, a finding that confirmed earlier reports not only for monkeys but for other mammals (Phillips, et al., 1975; Ho and Edwards, 1977; Adair and Adams, 1982). All power densities reduced M to the resting level (i.e., that normally observed in the TNZ), but at least 15 to 20 min of exposure was necessary to complete this reduction. Further, when the microwave field was extinguished, M did not begin to increase immediately, but, instead, gradually returned to the pre-exposure level over a period that depended on the power density of the preceding microwave exposure. Sometimes, when power density equalled or exceeded 40 mW/cm², more than 20 min was required to restore a stabilized level of M.

And what of the other thermoregulatory responses during these periods of microwave irradiation? Figure 2 shows the mean colonic (T_{co}) and tail skin (T_{tl}) temperatures of two monkeys, before, during, and after the 30-min microwave exposures at each of the four power densities. Each curve represents the mean of 3 experiments. The T_{co}

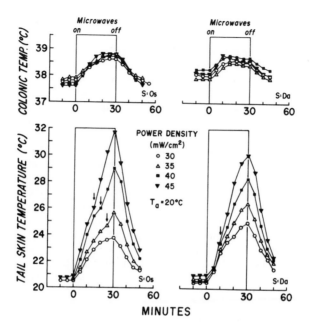

Figure 2. Colonic and tail skin temperatures of two monkeys (Os and Da) before, during, and after 30-min exposures to 2450-MHz CW microwaves at four different power densities. All tests were conducted at an ambient temperature (T_a) of 20 °C. Arrows indicate onset of vasodilation in the peripheral vessels of the tail. Data adapted from Candas, et al., Bioelectromagnetics, in press.

responses, while different for the two monkeys, reflected the activity of the peripheral vasomotor system, particularly of the tail. Monkey Os showed elevations in T_{co} that were proportional to the power density and that stabilized during the last 10 min of the microwave exposure. The T_{co} of monkey Da rose during the first 10-15 min of the exposure and then either remained constant or fell slightly. The lower part of Figure 2 shows that T_{tl} underwent large increases during all microwave exposures and exhibited a discontinuity of slope partway through the exposure. Early on, the increase of T_{tl} was of an exponential nature, but then, instead of tending toward a stable level, T_{tl} increased its rate of rise dramatically (as indicated by the arrows) even though the power density was constant. This increase of slope represents the initiation of active vasodilation of the tail vessels, as warm blood from the body core was brought close to the skin surface. The initiation of this response served to arrest, and even reduce, the rise in T_{co} of monkey Da that was well under way during the microwave exposure. When the irradiation was terminated, the tail vessels rapidly vasoconstricted again.

On the basis of these results, we may conclude that if the intensity of an imposed microwave field is sufficiently high to saturate (or reduce to resting level) an ongoing autonomic thermoregulatory response, the next response in the normal hierarchy may be mobilized to continue the thermoregulatory defense. Exactly the same result is obtained when the ambient temperature rises (Fig. 1). Thus, these results provide strong evidence for the equivalence between absorbed radiofrequency energy and dry heat loads imposed by radiant or convective sources in the environment.

Restricted Exposure of the Body

We have conducted two series of experiments to explore the thermoregulatory consequences of exposing only a limited part of the body to the microwave field. During the experiments, the monkey was restrained inside a ventilated Styrofoam box at a T_a of 20 °C. Rectal (colonic) and four representative skin temperatures were measured continuously as was oxygen consumption from which M was calculated. A three-panel screen covered with 20-cm pyramidal microwave absorber was interposed between the horn antenna and the animal's box inside the anechoic chamber. During the first series of experiments, a 30 x 30 cm aperture was cut in the center panel of the screen so that only the monkey's head received substantial irradiation, the remainder of the body being screened fairly effectively, given the limits imposed by diffraction. During the second series, the original aperture was closed and a new aperture, 30 cm wide and 45 cm high, was cut just below the location of the original in the center panel of the screen. Under these conditions, the body from the neck down received substantial irradiation while the head was screened.

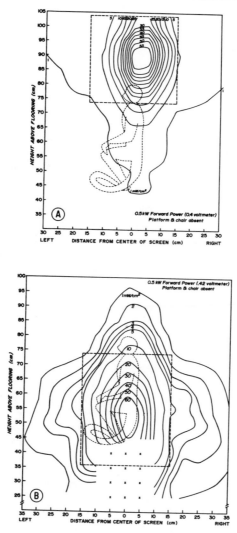

Figure 3. Contour maps of field intensity across a 61 x 86 cm plane orthogonal to the K vector and centered on the antenna boresight 1.42 m from the front edge of the transmitting antenna within the anechoic chamber. A three-panel screen interposed between antenna and monkey had a 30 x 30 cm aperture to expose monkey's head (Panel A) or a 30 x 45 cm aperture to expose monkey's body (Panel B). Dashed figure in each panel shows location of animal in the plane of measurement. Forward power = 0.5 kW.

Extensive field measurements across a plane that passed through the center of the monkey's location, orthogonal to the direction of propagation of the microwave field, indicated steep gradients of power density near the center of each aperture, but fair uniformity over the remainder (screened portion) of the body. The contour plot in Figure 3A shows that the power density measured at the location of the head, when the body was screened, was about 10 dB greater than the whole-body average; the corresponding contour plot in Figure 3B shows that the power density measured at the head, when the head was screened, was about 10 dB less than the whole-body average.

The experiments were designed to determine the threshold power density, during 10-min microwave exposures, that would reliably reduce M from the equilibrated level that is characteristic of T_a = 20 °C. In each series, three experimental tests were conducted on each of three monkeys; the results were compared with published data (Adair and Adams, 1982) for unilateral planewave (i.e., whole-body) exposure of the same animals at the same T_a and exposure duration.

Representative experiments from each series are presented in Figure 4. Exposure of the head alone (Fig. 4A) initiated reliable reductions in the M of an animal at T_a = 20 °C but the power densities, measured at the location of the head, had to be very high. In general, for a comparable reduction of M, the field strength had to be about 10 times that required when the whole body was exposed. On the other hand, when the trunk and extremities were exposed and the head screened (Fig. 4B), the threshold power density for a reduction of M (mean value = 6-8 mW/cm²) was only slightly higher than that determined during whole-body exposure (mean value = 4-6 mW/cm²). It should be emphasized that in all cases the specified power densities were measured at the location of the monkey's head.

The mean reduction in M (W/kg) during the second 5 min of each 10-min microwave exposure, relative to the last 5 min of stabilization immediately preceding that exposure, was calculated for all the experiments of both series. These delta M values are plotted in Figure 5 against power density. However, the power density in this case is not that measured at the location of the head, as was the case

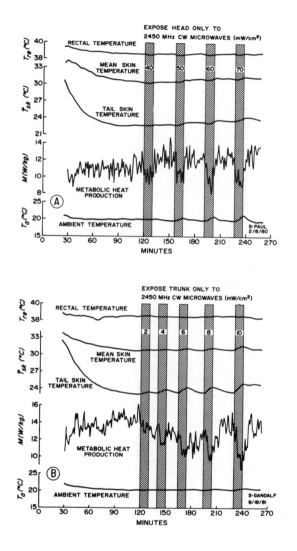

Figure 4. Representative experiments on individual monkeys equilibrated to an ambient temperature (T_a) of 20 °C to determine effects on metabolic heat production (M) of 10-min exposures of the head alone (Panel A) or trunk alone (Panel B) to 2450-MHz CW microwaves. Also shown are rectal (T_{re}), weighted mean skin ($\bar{T}_{sk}$), and tail skin (T_{tl}) temperatures.

in Figure 4, but, instead, that averaged over the total cross-sectional area of the body as determined from the contour plots (Figure 3). Also shown in the figure are comparable data of Adair and Adams (1982) for unrestricted exposure of the whole body. It is clear that the three sets of data are adequately described by the same function. This finding indicates that during partial-body exposure, any changes that may occur in autonomic thermoregulatory responses will depend upon the integral of energy absorption by the whole body, not upon energy deposited in some restricted locus of the body. A similar finding has been reported for behavioral thermoregulatory responses (Adair, in press); the aggregate emphasizes the importance of conductive and convective thermal transfer within the body and the major role played by the circulatory system during thermoregulation in the presence of electromagnetic fields. A logical extension of these findings is that the potential for the formation of "thermal hotspots" in CNS regions of importance to thermoregulation may be less than has been anticipated on theoretical grounds (Kritikos and Schwan, 1979).

Role of the Hypothalamic Thermoregulatory Center

The PO/AH is the CNS region of greatest importance to the control of thermoregulatory processes in endotherms. We have demonstrated that an increase of 0.2-0.3 °C in the temperature of this region may be associated with the threshold for a change in thermoregulatory behavior when a 2450-MHz microwave field is present (Adair, et al., 1983). Maximal penetration of the squirrel monkey head by radiation of this frequency, together with possible focussing of the radiation, has the potential for an enhanced rate of local energy deposition, and therefore selective local heating, perhaps in the region of the PO/AH. We have developed a technique for a chronic brain implant that allows for both measurement and control of PO/AH temperature so that we may determine the role played by this thermosensitive region in the mobilization and control of the thermoregulatory responses of animals exposed to microwaves.

Each of several squirrel monkeys has been stereotactically implanted with a pair of sealed teflon tubes in the medial preoptic nucleus of the hypothalamus (PO/AH). Each tube, one of which is illustrated in Figure 6, was 1.1 mm

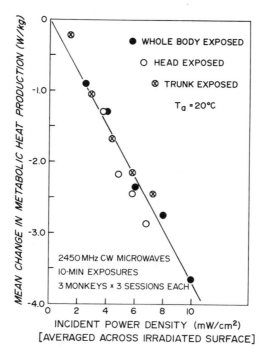

Figure 5. Mean change in metabolic heat production (W/kg) from stabilized level during 10-min exposures to 2450-MHz CW microwaves as a function of the incident power density averaged across the irradiated surface when the whole body or selected parts of the body were irradiated. Each point is the mean of 3 sessions on 3 monkeys. Ambient temperature (T_a) was 20 °C in all experiments.

I.D. and had a wall thickness of 0.12 mm. The tubes were centered 2.5 mm apart and were anchored to the skull with nylon screws and dental acrylic. During experiments that were conducted post-surgically, one tube (called a thermode) was connected, as shown in the figure, to a perfusion system so that temperature-controlled, light silicone oil could be pulled through the tube whenever a vacuum was applied to the system outlet. This procedure produced a rapid step change in the temperature of local PO/AH tissue that was related directly to the temperature of the circulating oil. Gradual changes in PO/AH temperature were produced by slow manipulations of the temperature of the

oil. The PO/AH temperature was measured by the probe of a
Vitek Electrothermia Monitor (Bowman, 1976) inserted into
the second tube.

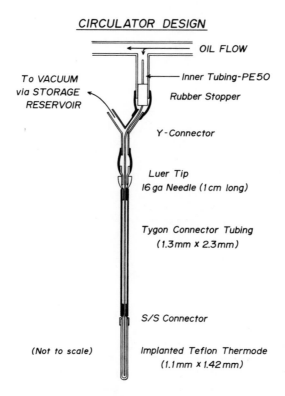

CIRCULATOR DESIGN

Figure 6. Schematic diagram (not drawn to scale) of the
circulation of temperature-controlled silicone oil through
an implanted teflon thermode tube to produce localized
heating or cooling of brain tissue (PO/AH) during exposure
to microwave fields.

During the experiments, a monkey was restrained inside
a climate-conditioned Styrofoam box that was located in the
far field of a horn antenna. The T_a inside the box was
34.5 - 35.5 °C, very close to the temperature (LCT) at
which heat loss through sweating may be mobilized (cf.
Figure 1). In addition to the PO/AH temperature, we also
measured rectal temperature and four skin temperatures
(abdomen, tail, leg, foot) from which a weighted mean skin

temperature was calculated (Stitt, et al., 1971). A Plexiglas hood over the animal's head collected the expired air which was drawn outside the chamber at 7 L/min for analysis of oxygen content. M was calculated from oxygen consumption assuming a RQ of 0.83. Thermoregulatory sweating from the foot was assessed from changes in dew-point temperature of air drawn at 1.9 L/min through a Lucite boot that enclosed the right foot. Since sweating in the squirrel monkey can be emotional as well as thermo-regulatory, it is essential to measure M as well as sweat-ing rate. The animal was always equilibrated to the prevailing ambient temperature (90-min minimum) before initiation of any microwave exposure or other experimental maneuver.

A representative experiment on one monkey, illustra-tive of both the experimental protocol and typical results, appears in Figure 7. A total of 20 such experiments was conducted. All experiments involved four 10-min treatments or episodes that were separated by sufficient time for re-stabilization of all measured variables. The first episode was an unrestricted exposure of the whole body to microwaves at one of three power densities (10, 15, or 20 mW/cm²). The second episode involved ramp heating of the PO/AH, at a rate similar to that recorded during the preceding microwave exposure. The third episode repeated the microwave exposure of episode one with the addition of simultaneous ramp cooling of the oil that perfused the thermode. This maneuver prevented the passive rise in PO/AH temperature that would normally have accompanied microwave exposure. The fourth episode, a control for the rate of rise of PO/AH temperature, involved a step increase in PO/AH temperature via thermode in the absence of micro-wave exposure. The step increase in this case was of identical magnitude to the ramp increase in the second episode.

Figure 7 shows that a 10-min unrestricted exposure of one monkey to microwave irradiation at a power density of 15 mW/cm² raised the PO/AH temperature by about 0.7 °C. Increments of approximately the same magnitude occurred in rectal temperature, while a sharp rise in the temperature of foot skin indicated an augmentation of vasodilation in this locus. No change occurred in M, already at the resting level (cf. Figure 1), but a small amount of sweat-ing was initiated, as indicated by the increase in dewpoint

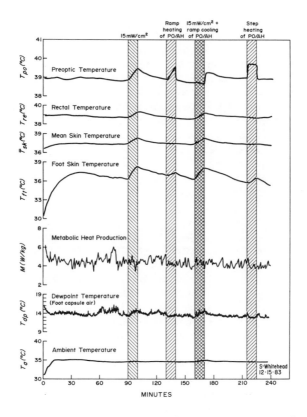

Figure 7. Representative experiment on one monkey equilibrated to an ambient temperature (T$_a$) of 35 °C to demonstrate the different thermoregulatory responses that result
from preoptic heating via thermode vs preoptic heating (or
supressed heating) that occurs passively during 10-min
exposures to 2450-MHz CW microwaves. See text for details.

temperature of the air passing through the foot capsule.
Ramp heating of the PO/AH during episode two produced very
different responses: a slight fall in rectal temperature,
no remarkable change in skin temperature, and no sweating.
On the other hand, while ramp cooling of the PO/AH during
microwave exposure (episode three) prevented the rise of
PO/AH temperature, all other responses to microwave irradiation were the same as in episode one. That some heating
of extra-PO/AH brain tissue occurred during episode three
is evident from the sharp increase in PO/AH temperature

that was recorded when thermode cooling ceased. Episode four demonstrated that the rate at which PO/AH temperature rises is probably not a significant factor. The results of this experiment imply that heating of the hypothalamic thermoregulatory center is not essential to the mobilization of appropriate autonomic thermoregulatory responses during microwave exposure; indeed, the responses observed during microwave exposure are very different from those observed when the PO/AH alone is heated. The same conclusions are warranted by the results of the partial-body experiments (head screened) described earlier in this paper.

A summary of the results of eight such experiments on the same monkey appears in Figures 8 and 9. The range of T_a was 34.5 to 35.5 °C and that of power density was 10 to 20 mW/cm². In each figure, the change in relevant thermoregulatory responses is plotted against the change in preoptic (PO/AH) temperature, which was a direct function of either power density or thermode temperature. Figure 8 contrasts the responses to microwaves with the responses to ramp or step heating of the PO/AH produced by the thermode. At this T_a, microwave irradiation heats the skin, raises the rectal temperature, and initiates sweating from the foot. Comparable increments of preoptic temperature, in the absence of microwave irradiation, produce no change in skin temperature, a slight fall in rectal temperature, and modest or no sweating. Thus, the thermoregulatory response to an elevation of preoptic temperature is very different in the two cases.

That the PO/AH plays a minimal role in thermoregulation during microwave irradiation is exemplified by the data summarized in Figure 9. It is clear that the rectal temperature rises, M changes minimally, and some sweating is initiated, whether or not the PO/AH temperature is allowed to rise during microwave exposure. But, one may ask, can a single thermode exert adequate bilateral control over the temperature of the PO/AH? In the squirrel monkey, the medial preoptic nuclei are centered 1 mm lateral to the midline and line the walls of the IIIrd ventricle, just above the optic chiasm. A teflon thermode of 1.34 mm O.D., centered in one preoptic nucleus, must encroach upon the contralateral preoptic nucleus, both physically and thermally.

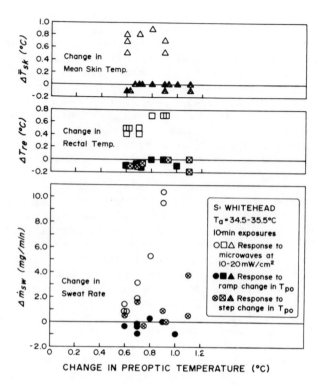

Figure 8. Summary of thermoregulatory response changes of one monkey from equilibrated levels as a function of the change in preoptic (PO/AH) temperature that occurred during 10-min exposures to 2450-MHz microwaves or to thermode heating. The responses to microwaves are contrasted with those to localized thermode heating of the brain. The ambient temperature (T_a) was 34.5 - 35.5 °C in all experiments.

It is of interest to note in Figure 9 that the highest sweat rates were associated with an elevated M, a condition that occurred in two experiments when PO/AH temperature rose by 0.9 °C. Most probably, the excess rise in PO/AH temperature was itself due to the elevated M, as the animal moved in the chair in an attempt to escape the imposed thermal stress. Figure 1 indicates that M should be at the resting level at T_a = 35 °C and that M should begin to rise only at higher T_a. This datum, in itself, supports the thesis of this paper that the thermoregulatory system functions in the presence of electromagnetic fields in exactly the same manner as it does in the presence of environmental sources of radiant or convective heat and that an equivalence can be drawn between T_a and microwave intensity.

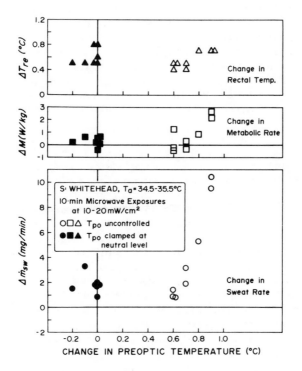

Figure 9. Summary of thermoregulatory response changes of one monkey from equilibrated levels as a function of the change in preoptic (PO/AH) temperature that occurred during 10-min exposures to 2450-MHz microwaves. Responses when the PO/AH temperature (T_{po}) was prevented from rising, by cooling an implanted thermode, are contrasted with those when the PO/AH temperature rose passively. The ambient temperature (T_a) was 34.5-35.5 °C in all experiments.

Summary and Conclusions

The results of several kinds of experiments have been introduced as evidence in support of the thesis that the thermoregulatory system of endotherms functions no differently in the presence of microwaves than it does in the presence of conventional sources of thermal energy. The thermoregulatory profile, unique for each species, provides the framework for the argument. The results of our experiments have demonstrated the equivalence between T_a and microwave intensity as they influence individual responses of heat production and heat loss. This equivalence, in turn, allows the prediction of specific alterations in thermoregulatory responses when microwaves are present. Predictions of this kind are possible because the hierarchy of autonomic responses available to any given species is always the same. This fact should provide some comfort to those who profess concern about the uniqueness of absorbed radiofrequency energy and its fate within the body.

Additional comfort can be derived from the demonstration that changes in thermoregulatory responses in the presence of microwaves depend upon the integral of energy absorption by the whole body, not upon energy deposited in some restricted locus such as the PO/AH. It is clear that the circulatory system plays a major role in the distribution of energy deposited during such exposures, a fact already emphasized by others (Burr and Krupp, 1980; Way, et al., 1981; Stolwijk, 1983; Krupp, 1983). This fact does not negate the presence of electrical hotspots as predicted on theoretical grounds (e.g, Kritikos and Schwan, 1979) or as demonstrated dosimetrically (e.g., Guy, 1971), but it does deemphasize their importance as potential deterrents to the efficient mobilization of thermoregulatory responses.

The utility of the thermoregulatory profile in research of the kind described here cannot be overemphasized. Accurate profiles have been determined for most of the commonly-used laboratory animals as well as for human beings. In the broader sense, such profiles should serve as fundamental data to the design of any experiment in which microwaves may be present. For example, the normal "room temperature" for clothed human beings lies well below the LCT of most laboratory species and such a T_a may exert a substantial influence over diverse behavioral responses, drug effects, etc. as well as basic thermoregulatory responses (Adair, et al., 1983). This paper has demonstrated that by considering the thermoregulatory profile, microwave challenges to the thermoregulatory system assume their proper position within the fundamental science of thermal physiology.

ACKNOWLEDGMENTS

Data from my laboratory that are reported in this paper were collected with support from AFOSR Grant 77-3420 and Air Force Contract No. F-33615-82-K-06700. During his tenure in my laboratory, V. Candas was supported in part by grants from NATO and the Philippe Foundation. The conduct of all experiments has been greatly aided by the expert technical assistance of B.W. Adams and G.M. Akel. R.O. Rawson designed and constructed the thermode perfusion system. The consultation and encouragement of J.D. Hardy is gratefully acknowledged.

REFERENCES

Adair ER (1985). Thermoregulation in the squirrel monkey. In Coe, C, Rosenblum, L (eds): "Handbook of Squirrel Monkey Research," New York, Plenum Press, pp 219-252.

Adair ER (In press). Microwave irradiation and thermoregulatory behavior. In D'Andrea, J, Monahan, J (eds): "Proceedings of a Workshop on the Behavioral Effects of Microwave Radiation Absorption."

Adair ER, Adams BW (1982). Adjustments in metabolic heat production by squirrel monkeys exposed to microwaves. J Appl Physiol: Respirat Environ Exercise Physiol 52:1049-1058.

Adair ER, Adams BW, Akel GM (1984). Minimal changes in hypothalamic temperature accompany microwave-induced alteration of thermoregulatory behavior. Bioelectromagnetics 5:13-30.

Adair ER, Casby JU, Stolwijk JAJ (1970). Behavioral temperature regulation in the squirrel monkey: changes induced by shifts in hypothalamic temperature. J comp physiol Psychol 72:17-27.

Adair ER, Spiers DE, Stolwijk JAJ, Wenger CB (1983). Technical note: On changes in evaporative heat loss that result from exposure to nonionizing electromagnetic radiation. J Microwave Power 18:209-211.

Bligh J and Johnson KG (1973). Glossary of terms for thermal physiology. J. Appl Physiol 35:941-961.

Bowman RR (1976). A probe for measuring temperature in radio-frequency-heated material. IEEE Trans Microwave Theory Tech 24:43-45.

Burr JG, Cohoon DK, Bell EL, Penn JW (1980). Thermal response model of a simulated cranial structure exposed to radiofrequency radiation. IEEE Trans Biomed Engr 27:452-460.

Burr JG, Krupp JH (1980). Real-time measurement of RFR energy distribution in the Macaca mulatta head. Bioelectromagnetics 1:21-34.

Candas V, Adair ER, Adams BW (In press). Thermoregulatory adjustments in squirrel monkeys exposed to microwaves at high power densities. Bioelectromagnetics.

Elder JA, Cahill DF, eds. (1984). "Biological Effects of Radiofrequency Radiation," Research Triangle Park, US Environmental Protection Agency.

Guy AW (1971). Analysis of electromagnetic fields induced in biological tissues by thermographic studies on equivalent phantom models. IEEE Trans Microwave Theory Tech MTT-19:205-214.

Ho HS, Edwards WP (1977). Oxygen-consumption rate of mice under different dose rates of microwave radiation. In Justesen DR, Guy, AW (eds): "Biological Effects of Electromagnetic Waves," Champaign, IL Am Geophys Union (Maxiprint) pp 131-138.

Kritikos HN, Schwan LP (1979). Potential temperature rise induced by electromagnetic field in brain tissues. IEEE Trans Biomed Engr 26:29-34.

Krupp JH (1983). In vivo temperature measurements during whole-body exposure of Macaca mulatta to resonant and non-resonant frequencies. In Adair ER (ed): "Microwaves and Thermoregulation," New York, Academic Press, pp 95-107.

Lerner EJ (1984). The drive to regulate electromagnetic fields. IEEE Spectrum March:63-70.

Lynch WC, Adair ER (1978). Ambient and hypothalamic temperatures alter vasomotor thresholds in squirrel monkey. In Houdas Y, Guieu JD (eds): "New Trends in Thermal Physiology," Paris, Masson pp 130-132.

Lynch WC, Adair, ER, Adams BW (1980). Vasomotor thresholds in the squirrel monkey: effects of central and peripheral temperature. J Appl Physiol: Respirat Environ Exercise Physiol 48:89-96.

Machida H, Perkins E, Hu F (1967). The skin of primates XXXV. The skin of the squirrel monkey (Saimiri sciurea). Am J Phys Anthropol 26:45-54.

Phillips RD, Hunt EL, Castro RD, King NW (1975). Thermoregulatory, metabolic, and cardiovascular responses of rats to microwaves. J Appl Physiol 38:630-635.

Stitt JT, Hardy JD (1971). Thermoregulation in the squirrel monkey (Saimiri sciureus). J Appl Physiol 31:48-54.

Stitt JT, Hardy JD, Nadel ER (1971). The surface area of the squirrel monkey in relation to body weight. J Appl Physiol 31:140-141.

Stolwijk JAJ (1983). Evaluation of thermoregulatory response to microwave power deposition. In Adair ER (ed) "Microwaves and Thermoregulation," New York, Academic Press pp 297-305.

Way WI, Kritikos H, Schwan H (1981). Thermoregulatory physiologic responses in the human body exposed to microwave radiation. Bioelectromagnetics 2:341-356.

Electromagnetic Fields and Neurobehavioral Function, pages 203–218
© 1988 Alan R. Liss, Inc.

THERMOREGULATORY RESPONSES IN THE RHESUS MONKEY DURING
EXPOSURE AT A FREQUENCY (225 MHz) NEAR WHOLE-BODY RESONANCE

W. Gregory Lotz and Jack L. Saxton

Naval Aerospace Medical Research Laboratory
Pensacola, Florida 32508

A major thrust of our research on the biological effects of nonionizing electromagnetic fields has, until recently, been directed toward characterizing endocrine function in mammals exposed to microwave radiation. Alterations in circulating levels of corticosterone, growth hormone, and thyrotropin were observed in rats exposed for up to 2 hr to 2450 MHz fields of moderate intensity (Lotz and Michaelson, 1978; Michaelson et al., 1977). Similar findings have also been reported and reviewed by other investigators (Lu et al., 1980). Glucocorticoid stimulation by microwaves was also observed in rhesus monkeys exposed to 1290 MHz pulsed fields of 38 mW/cm^2 (4.1 W/kg) for 8 hr (Lotz and Podgorski, 1982). In both rats and monkeys, the endocrine changes were concomitant with increases in deep body temperature. The data from these various experiments were consistent with the hypothesis that the cortisteroid response was controlled by the central nervous system (CNS) in an integrative manner in responding to the imposed heat load.

In a subsequent set of experiments with rhesus monkeys exposed to 225 MHz, a frequency near whole-body resonance for the monkey, the rise in rectal temperature (T_{re}) was much faster and larger than at 1290 MHz. In an effort to understand this pronounced body heating at the resonant frequency, we shifted our emphasis from endocrine physiology to thermoregulatory physiology. The studies to be reported in detail here deal with the body temperature, vasomotor, and metabolic responses to 225 MHz radiofrequency (RF) exposure of the rhesus monkey.

MATERIALS AND METHODS

Five male rhesus monkeys, Macaca mulatta, 6.5 to 8.5 kg, were used in these experiments. The animals were housed in standard metal primate cages in a room adjacent to the exposure room. They were fed a standard laboratory diet (Wayne Monkey Chow, Allied Mills, Chicago, IL) and provided water ad libitum. The light cycle in the cage rooms was 16:8 hr light:dark with the lights on from 0600 to 2200. Ambient temperature (T_a) in these rooms was between 21 and 25 °C. The monkeys were born and raised in the Naval Aerospace Medical Research Laboratory monkey colony, and had been used previously in other microwave/RF radiation studies of a similar nature. The subjects were accustomed to restraint and to the experimental apparatus used.

The animals were restrained during each experiment in a chair built of rigid and foamed (Styrofoam) polystyrene. The anechoic chamber (3.3 x 3.3 x 6.7 m) used for the experiments has been described in detail previously (Lotz, 1985). The irradiation setup was also as previously described, with 225 MHz continuous wave RF exposure provided by a military radio set and cavity-type amplifier. The subject was facing the horn antenna at a distance of 240 cm from the mouth of the antenna, with the electric field oriented parallel to the long axis of the body. Power densities were measured in the absence of the animal and restraint chair with a Narda Model 8608 system, and the values reported represent the mean over the region occupied by the animal. Average specific absorption rates were 0.285 $(W/kg)/(mW/cm^2)$ as determined by Olsen and Griner (1982) in a tissue equivalent rhesus monkey model exposed in the same facility.

The restraint chair was enclosed in a secondary Styrofoam box, a microchamber, to allow for better control of ambient conditions. Conditioned air was pumped through this microchamber by a Vista temperature/humidity controller at a rate of 300 CFM. Air flow across the monkey (from front to back) ranged between 0.2 to 0.5 m/sec, with the highest velocity in the region of the tail. The relative humidity (RH) was monitored in the input air duct, and the temperature was continuously monitored in the mixed air of the return duct between the microchamber and the temperature/humidity controller. Ambient temperature was controlled within $\pm$ 0.5 °C, and RH was controlled within $\pm$ 5%.

Body temperatures [rectal, tail skin (T_t), and inner thigh skin (T_{le})] were continuously monitored using Vitek Model 101 Electrothermia Monitors. The rectal probe was covered with a polyethylene sheath and inserted 10 cm past the anus. The skin temperature probes were attached by inserting the Vitek probe tip through the side of a 1-cm diameter doughnut-shaped piece of Plexiglas and taping the doughnut in place so that the probe tip itself was not covered by tape. Inner thigh skin temperature was selected because of its reported strong correlation to mean skin temperature ($\overline{T}_{sk}$) in the rhesus monkey (Johnson and Elizondo, 1974). The correlation between $\overline{T}_{sk}$ and T_{le} in the work of Johnson and Elizondo was for a broad range of T_a. This correlation has not been shown to hold during microwave heating, and T_{le} was therefore considered only to be a preferred second location (besides tail) for monitoring skin temperature.

Exhaled air was captured with a Plexiglas hood (20 cm in diameter) that was placed over the monkey's head. This air was exhausted from the chamber and analyzed for oxygen (O_2) and carbon dioxide (CO_2) concentrations with Beckman Model 755 (paramagnetic) and 864 (infrared) analyzers, respectively. The intake for this "open" system came from around the monkey's neck. The system was tested in the absence of an animal with smoke and calibration gases to see that no exhaled air was lost when flow rates were between 6 and 10 L/min. Data from the temperature probes, the respiratory gas analyzers, and the ambient temperature probe were sampled four times per minute by a Hewlett Packard Model 9835 computer. These four subsamples were averaged, and the minute-by-minute record was numerically and graphically recorded. Metabolic rate (M) was also calculated from the O_2 data after corrections for flow rate and standard temperature and pressure were made. In previous work on this project, we did not have the capability to measure CO_2, and M was calculated assuming RQ = 0.83. For the experiments reported here, RQ was determined each minute, and averaged 0.82. However, the calculations for M were made with RQ = 0.83, since the software was not changed to correct for this slight difference.

Two experimental protocols were used in this study. Both protocols began with a 120-min preexposure equilibration period after the monkey was placed in the chair and the instrumentation was attached. Both protocols were also conducted at two ambient temperatures, 20 and 26 $^{\circ}$C. These temperatures were selected from the data of Johnson and Elizondo (1979) to provide one T_a (26 $^{\circ}$C) in the thermoneutral zone of the rhesus monkey, and one (20 $^{\circ}$C) that would be a cold stimulus. The reported thermoneutral zone for the rhesus is about 25 $^{\circ}$ to 30 $^{\circ}$C. We found that in our system it was difficult to maintain stable (i.e., equilibrated without vasodilation) T_t when T_a = 28 $^{\circ}$C, so we selected 26 $^{\circ}$C as a suitable alternative T_a within the thermoneutral zone. Relative humidity was 50% at 26 $^{\circ}$C and 65% at 20 $^{\circ}$C.

The two protocols differed in the presentation of the RF exposure. One was designed to determine the lowest power density in brief exposures at which the measured responses changed from preexposure levels, and was called the step-acute exposure. In the step-acute experiment, repetitive 10-min RF exposures at successively higher power densities were separated by recovery periods. The recovery period was variable in length between 10 and 60 min because it was extended until T_t returned to within 0.3 $^{\circ}$C of the preexposure value. Tail temperature was used for the determinations of the length of the recovery period because it showed the largest increases during RF exposure. Rectal temperature was always within 0.1 $^{\circ}$C of the preexposure value by the end of the recovery period. Power densities of 1.2, 2.5, 5.0, 7.5, and 10.0 mW/cm^2 were used. A vasodilation response was considered to have occurred when T_t showed marked increases in the rate of rise, or when T_t continued to rise after the irradiation stopped. An increase in the rate of rise of T_t was considered to meet this criterion when the rate more than doubled abruptly during exposure, e.g., from 0.1 to 0.2 $^{\circ}$C/min (passive) to more than 0.5 $^{\circ}$C/min (vasodilation). Step-acute exposures were conducted twice for each monkey at each ambient temperature. The results of these two replicate experiments were averaged for later analysis.

The second protocol was designed to evaluate steady-state thermoregulatory adjustments during RF exposure. Following the 120-min preexposure period, the monkey was exposed for 120 min to a single power density, and data were collected for an additional 10 to 60 min after exposure. The five monkeys were each exposed once in this protocol to 0 (sham), 2.5, 5.0, 7.5, and 10.0 mW/cm^2 at 20 $^\circ$C, and to 0(sham), 1.2, 2.5, 5.0, and 7.5 mW/cm^2 at 26 $^\circ$C. The monkeys were generally retested once per week. The replication of the step-acute experiments with each subject had indicated that the responses for each individual monkey were reproducible. The data from successive preexposure periods with a particular animal were also consistent. Thus, even though the limitations of a single replication of a given set of conditions were recognized, we decided to limit steady-state experiments to only one exposure for each animal at each power density and temperature. The sequence of the presentation of power densities for each animal was determined by a Latin-square design.

Metabolic rate data were analyzed statistically using one-way analysis of variance (ANOVA) for repeated measures, followed by Tukey's Highly Significant Difference (HSD) test for multiple comparisons (Kirk, 1968). The 0.05 level of significance was the criterion for a difference to be considered significant. For step-acute experiments, the mean M for the 10-min exposure at a given power density for each animal (2 sessions) was used as the test value. For baseline comparison to an unexposed period, the mean M for the 10-min period immediately preceding the associated exposure step was used. The data were converted to percent of preexposure [100 x (exposure M/preexposure M)] for each exposure level, and the ANOVA and Tukey's tests were then applied to these ratio data. For the steady-state exposures, the same tests were applied to the data of all exposure levels, including sham exposure, to test for differences between the values recorded during the last 30 min of the exposure period.

RESULTS

The results of a representative step-acute experiment at 20 $^\circ$C with monkey 62 are shown in Fig. 1. The experiment proceeded until vasodilation of the tail skin occurred during exposure to 7.5 mW/cm^2. The increases in T_t at lower power densities did not meet the criteria established as indicating vasodilation. The power density at which tail vasodilation occurred was reproducible for each monkey in the duplicate experiments, and depended on T_a, as expected.

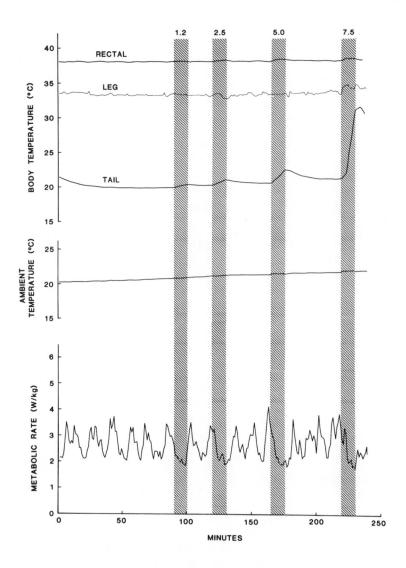

Fig. 1. Results of representative step-acute experiment at 20 °C with monkey 62, showing rectal, inner thigh (leg) skin, tail skin, and ambient temperatures, and metabolic rate. The hatched regions indicate the 10-min exposures at the power density shown at the top.

Table 1. No. of monkeys showing vasomotor response[a] in 10 min

Ambient Temperature ($^{\circ}$C)	Power Density (mW/cm^2)			
	2.5	5.0	7.5	10.0
26	0	4	5	b
20	0	0	2	5

[a]Response indicated by tail vasodilation as defined in text.

[b]Not determined.

A summary of the vasomotor response data for step-acute experiments is shown in Table 1. These data suggest that the lowest power density that stimulated a vasomotor response was about 5 mW/cm^2 at a T_a of 26 $^{\circ}$C. Although T_{le} was somewhat erratic, it was also elevated during the 7.5 mW/cm^2, suggesting that the vasomotor response observed in Fig. 1 was generalized to other body surface areas as well as the tail.

The metabolic response during step-acute experiments was partially masked by the large, pulsatile variation in M in the absence of RF exposure. These pulses in M were seen for each monkey, and were reproducible. In the experiment shown in Fig. 1, it is clear that no M spike began during RF exposures of 2.5 mW/cm^2 or higher. In other experiments, as well as this one, RF exposure reliably suppressed these pulses, leading to a lower mean value of M during the 10-min exposure periods at a T_a of 20 $^{\circ}$C for 5.0 mW/cm^2 or greater power densities. The ANOVA indicated that the effect of exposure was significant (F = 6.44, df = 4,16; p = 0.003). Tukey's HSD test revealed that the differences among means were significant for 7.5 and 10.0 mW/cm^2 exposures. For a T_a of 26 $^{\circ}$C, the M ratio (percent of preexposure) was also significantly altered by exposure (F = 9.71, df = 2,8;

p = 0.007). The effect at a T_a of $26^{\circ}C$ was for 5.0 mW/cm^2. Based on these data, a power density in the range of 5 to 7.5 mW/cm^2 was required to cause a significant decrease in M during 10-min RF exposures.

Fig. 2 shows the results of a representative steady-state experiment at 20 $^{\circ}C$ and 7.5 mW/cm^2. A successive initiation of metabolic adjustments and vasomotor shifts was observed. Both responses, once initiated, were sustained throughout the exposure. As expected, the recruitment of the vasomotor response occurred earlier in the exposure for higher power densities. The prompt rise in T_{re}, as well as in skin temperatures, that can be seen after the onset of exposure in both Fig. 1 and 2 was also characteristic of all the animals. Mean values of T_{re}, T_t, and T_{le} during the last 30 min of the steady-state exposures are shown in Table 2. The mean T_t was lower than T_a at a T_a of 20 $^{\circ}C$ because of the distribution of temperatures within the microchamber, with the area around the tail being colder than the mean T_a. Mean M values for these same periods are shown in Fig. 3. The mean M during RF exposure at T_a = 20 $^{\circ}C$ was reduced from the sham level toward the level of M (preexposure or sham) at T_a = 26 $^{\circ}C$. Although the variability due to the pulsatile nature of M in these animals again limits the interpretation of the data, the effect of RF exposure in suppressing M pulses is apparent in Fig. 2. The reductions in mean M between sham and exposure conditions of steady-state experiments at a T_a of 20 $^{\circ}C$ were found by ANOVA to be significant (F = 4.45, df = 20, p = 0.013). Tukey's HSD indicated that these significant differences were at 7.5 and 10.0 mW/cm^2. There were no significant differences in M among any exposure conditions at a T_a of 26 $^{\circ}C$.

A comparison of T_{re} and T_{le} changes at the two ambient temperatures is shown in Fig. 4. The mean increase in these temperatures was much larger at 20 $^{\circ}C$ than at 26 $^{\circ}C$ primarily because the baseline or preexposure temperature was lower at 20 $^{\circ}C$. Final steady-state temperatures during RF exposure were comparable in most cases, as seen in Table 2. It is interesting that the relative relationship of changes in T_{re} and T_{le} is inverted when comparing the two ambient temperatures, i.e., the increase in leg skin temperature (ΔT_{leg}) was greater than the increase in rectal (ΔT_{re}) when T_a = 26 $^{\circ}C$, but at a T_a of 20 $^{\circ}C$, ΔT_{re} was greater than ΔT_{leg}.

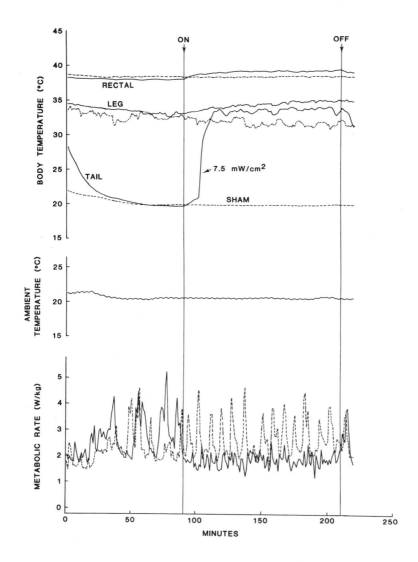

Fig. 2. Results of a representative steady-state experiment at 20 °C with monkey 62, showing the same parameters as for Fig. 1. The data for the sham exposure are shown with a dashed line, and the data for the 7.5 mW/cm² exposure are shown with a solid line. The vertical lines mark the beginning and end of the 120-min exposure.

Table 2. [a]Steady-state body temperatures during RF exposure

Power Density (mW/cm²)	Ambient Temperature (°C)	Rectal Temperature (°C)	Thigh Skin Temperature (°C)	Tail Skin Temperature (°C)
0(sham)	26	38.3 ± 0.1[b]	34.8 ± 0.3	26.2 ± 0.2
1.2	26	38.4 ± 0.2	34.9 ± 0.7	31.1 ± 1.5
2.5	26	38.7 ± 0.1	35.0 ± 0.6	34.4 ± 0.6
5.0	26	39.0 ± 0.1	35.3 ± 0.4	35.6 ± 0.7
7.5	26	39.5 ± 0.2	35.4 ± 0.7	35.7 ± 0.5
0(sham)	20	37.7 ± 0.1	32.8 ± 0.8	19.6 ± 0.1
2.5	20	38.7 ± 0.2	33.8 ± 0.9	22.5 ± 2.7
5.0	20	38.9 ± 0.1	34.6 ± 0.4	31.7 ± 2.1
7.5	20	39.0 ± 0.2	34.8 ± 0.5	30.7 ± 1.9
10.0	20	39.5 ± 0.2	34.8 ± 0.5	31.8 ± 2.1

[a]Last 30 min of 120-min exposure.

[b]Mean ± SE, n = 5.

DISCUSSION

When we first observed increases that were larger than expected in the rectal temperature of rhesus monkeys exposed to 225 MHz, the cause of such increases was unclear (Lotz, 1985). Limited control of the ambient environment was suggested as a possible contributing or confounding factor in such increases, and definitive data on the thermoregulatory responses were clearly needed. The data from the present experiments demonstrate the initiation of metabolic and vasomotor adjustments in rhesus monkeys exposed to 225 MHz. These responses are appropriate to

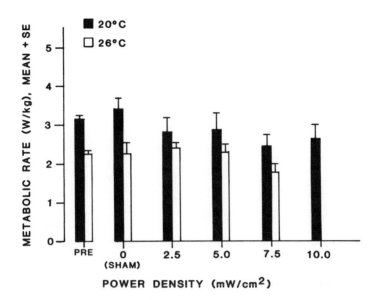

Fig. 3. Means and SE for metabolic rates of five rhesus
monkeys during the last 30 min of the 120 min steady-state
exposures at either 20 or 26 °C. The values for the last 30
min of the preexposure periods are indicated above PRE on
the abscissa.

reduce the stored heat in the animal and show relationships
in progressive recruitment, dependence upon T_a, and
dependence upon the magnitude of the imposed RF heating
that are all similar to the relationships known to exist for
other thermal stimuli, e.g., a warm environment (Johnson and
Elizondo, 1979). Nevertheless, the observed increases in
T_{re} during exposure were still larger and more prompt than
those observed at a higher RF frequency, 1290 MHz (Lotz,
1985; Lotz and Podgorski, 1982). Further comparisons of
thermoregulatory responses during exposure to other
frequencies, particularly 1290 MHz where the T_{re} comparisons
were made, are needed to confirm this finding.

The most extensive investigations of thermoregulatory
responses in microwave exposed animals have been done by
Adair and her colleagues. The results of the present study

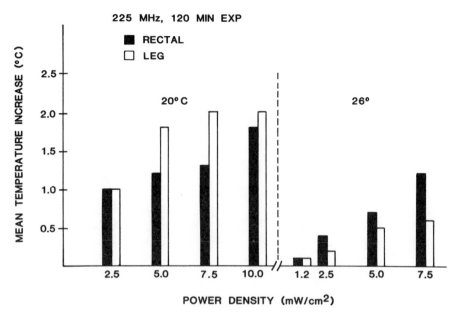

Fig. 4. Mean increase in rectal and inner thigh (leg) skin temperatures of five rhesus monkeys during exposure to 225 MHz radiation at either 20 or 26 °C. The values shown are the differences between the means of the last 30 min of the preexposure and exposure periods.

agree in general with the findings of Adair and Adams (1980, 1982), but show differences that are probably species and frequency related. The vasomotor and metabolic responses observed in the rhesus monkey exposed to 225 MHz were quite similar to the same responses reported by Adair and Adams in the squirrel monkey exposed to 2450 MHz. In both species, the thermoregulatory responses to microwave/RF exposure were similar to the responses to other thermal stimuli. In both species, RF exposure in a cold T_a caused recruitment of adjustments in metabolism first, followed by a vasomotor response. At a thermoneutral T_a, metabolic adjustments were absent, or very small. The power density required to elicit a particular response was dependent on T_a for both species. However, Adair and Adams (1982) reported that the decrease in the metabolic rate of the squirrel monkey during prolonged exposure to microwaves in the cold was approximately equal to the whole-body SAR. In our experiments, the metabolic rate change in the rhesus monkey was, except at the lowest intensities, always less than the average SAR. This difference is probably due to the lower M of the rhesus monkey in both thermoneutral and cold conditions. In the rhesus monkey, we found M during the preexposure period at a T_a of 20 ^oC to be about 38%, or 0.87 W/kg, higher than the corresponding M at a T_a of 26 ^oC. In the squirrel monkey, M was 3-4 W/kg higher at a T_a of 20 ^oC than at a T_a of 26^oC (Adair and Adams, 1982). Thus, the rhesus has less capacity to reduce M to offset the radiant energy absorbed.

Another difference between the results of our study and the results of the work by Adair and Adams is the magnitude of the rectal temperature increases seen during exposures that stimulated similar thermoregulatory adjustments. One straightforward explanation for the relatively large increases in T_{re} of rhesus monkeys exposed to 225 MHz is the internal distribution of absorbed energy. At 225 MHz, the RF energy penetrates more than at higher frequencies, resulting in substantially greater direct heating of the body core than occurs at shorter wavelengths (Olsen et al., 1980; Olsen and Griner, 1982). Perhaps this primary heating of the core is not adequately redistributed to keep the T_{re} lower during exposure, even though the autonomic recruitment of thermoregulatory responses appears to be prompt and appropriate to reduce stored heat in the body.

The results of our T_{le} measurements were not as helpful in addressing the question of thermal distribution within the body as we expected. Leg skin temperature was somewhat erratic, apparently due to technical problems associated with using a Vitek probe for skin temperature when the monkey's leg moved around. Nevertheless, it was surprising to see that ΔT_{le} was less than ΔT_{re} at any T_a, as it was at a T_a of 26 ^oC, and that this relationship shifted with T_a. At frequencies well above whole-body resonance, the increases in surface temperature in both rhesus and squirrel monkeys substantially exceed the increases in core temperature during RF exposure (Lotz, unpublished observations; Adair and Adams, 1980). At the higher frequencies, deep body temperature is not raised as effectively as at resonant frequencies. One experimental approach to test the concept of primary internal heating would be to expose the monkeys at a frequency substantially below whole-body resonance. Since lower frequencies would also provide deep heating of internal tissues, similar thermoregulatory relationships to those observed at 225 MHz might be expected. However, if the responses are uniquely related to the resonance condition, then they would not be reproducible with other penetrating frequencies below resonance.

The RF-induced shift in metabolic rate observed in these experiments has a character that suggests prompt and sustained sympathetic nervous system (SNS) action as a part of the response. While no direct evidence exists of such SNS involvement, two features of the metabolic response are consistent with this hypothesis. One such feature is the rapid nature of the response. Metabolism is under the partial control of the endocrine system, but certain components of this endocrine control, e.g., thyroid hormones, do not change in the short time in which pronounced changes in M occur during RF exposure. To achieve such rapid changes in M as we observed, the SNS may have a distinct involvement in the response, since it is important in the control of chemical thermogenesis (Landsberg, et al., 1984). The second feature of the M adjustments that suggests SNS involvement is the RF-damping of apparent pulses in M that were normally seen during preexposure and sham exposure periods. These pulses may be related to emotional activity of the animal, but the data indicate a degree of regularity to the pulses in M, particularly at a T_a of 20 $^{\circ}$C, that is greater than what seems to be associated with psychological factors. Subjective observation of the monkeys on the TV monitor during the experiments did not reveal any apparent emotional disturbance or restlessness that would explain these pulses in M. No evidence of shivering was noted, either. The magnitude of the spikes in M appears to be correlated with T_a, being greater in the cold, and the reduction in M during RF exposure at 20 $^{\circ}$C is primarily due to a suppression of the spikes, with little reduction in the baseline (trough) level of M. Hansen et al. (1982) observed rapid fluctuations in the circulating catecholamine levels of chair-restrained rhesus monkeys. The most common periodicity in these catecholamine fluctuations was 6 to 13 min/cycle as determined by spectral analysis. This periodicity is similar to the apparent periodicity of the variations in M noted in our monkeys. Experiments in which circulating catecholamine levels and metabolic rate are both measured in monkeys exposed to RF energy might provide a better evaluation of this hypothesis.

In summary, these experiments have demonstrated vasomotor and metabolic responses in rhesus monkeys exposed to 225 MHz. The thermoregulatory adjustments have thresholds of exposure intensity that are dependent on ambient temperature. Recruitment of the two responses was progressive in a manner similar to that known to exist for exposure to warm ambient temperatures. However, increases in rectal temperature were larger than those observed for similar heat loads imposed by higher frequency microwave exposure, suggesting that the heat produced directly in internal tissues by such long wavelength radiation is not fully redistributed by the circulation during exposure, even in a cool environment.

ACKNOWLEDGMENTS

The technical assistance of ENS Michael Golightly, Mr. Steve Woodson, and Mr. Robert Upchurch is gratefully acknowledged. We also thank Mr. Chuck Mogensen and Mr. Robert Barrett for assistance in manuscript preparation.

Opinions or conclusions contained in this report are those of the authors and do not necessarily reflect the views or the endorsement of the Navy Department. This research was supported by the Naval Medical Research and Development Command under Project No. MF58.524.02C-0009, Accession No. DN277076. The animals used in this study were handled in accordance with the principles stated in the "Guide for the Care and Use of Laboratory Animals," Institute of Laboratory Animal Resources, National Research Council, DHEW, NIH Publication No. 85-23, 1985, and The Animal Welfare Act of 1966, as amended.

REFERENCES

Adair ER, Adams BW (1980). Microwaves induce peripheral vasodilation in squirrel monkey. Science 207: 1381.
Adair ER, Adams BW (1982). Adjustments in metabolic heat production by squirrel monkeys exposed to microwaves. J Appl Physiol 52: 1049.

Hansen BC, Schielke GP, Jen K-LC, Wolfe RA, Movahed H, and Pek SB (1982). Rapid fluctuations in plasma catecholamines in monkeys under undisturbed conditions. Am J Physiol 242: E40.

Johnson GS, Elizondo RS (1974). Eccrine sweat gland in Macaca mulatta: Physiology, histochemistry, and distribution. J Appl Physiol 37: 814.

Johnson GS, Elizondo RS (1979). Thermoregulation in Macaca mulatta: a thermal balance study. J Appl Physiol 46:268.

Landsberg L, Saville ME, and Young JB (1984). Sympathoadrenal system and regulation of thermogenesis. Am J Physiol 247:E181.

Kirk RE (1968). Experimental Design: Procedures for the Behavioral Sciences. Belmont: Wadsworth.

Lotz WG (1985). Hyperthermia in radiofrequency exposed rhesus monkeys: A comparison of frequency and orientation effects. Radiat Res 102: 59.

Lotz WG, Michaelson SM (1978). Temperature and corticosterone relationships in microwave-exposed rats. J Appl Physiol 44: 438.

Lotz WG, Podgorski RP (1982). Temperature and adrenocortical responses in rhesus monkeys exposed to microwaves. J Appl Physiol 53: 1565.

Lu S-T, Lotz WG, and Michaelson SM (1980). Advances in microwave-induced neuroendocrine effects: the concept of stress. Proc IEEE 68: 73.

Michaelson SM, Guillet R, Lotz WG, Lu S-T, and Magin RL (1977). Neuroendocrine responses in the rat and dog exposed to 2450 MHz (CW) microwaves. In Hazzard DG (ed): "Symposium on Biological Effects and Measurement of Radiofrequency/Microwaves," HEW Publication (FDA) 77-8026, Washington: USDHEW, p 263.

Olsen RG, Griner TA (1982). Electromagnetic dosimetry in a sitting rhesus model at 225 MHz. Bioelectromagnetics 3: 385.

Olsen RG, Griner TA, and Prettyman GD (1980). Far-field microwave dosimetry in a rhesus monkey model. Bioelectromagnetics 1: 149.

Electromagnetic Fields and Neurobehavioral Function, pages 219–234
© 1988 Alan R. Liss, Inc.

MICROWAVES AS REINFORCING EVENTS IN A COLD ENVIRONMENT

M. J. Marr, J. O. de Lorge, R. G. Olsen, and M. Stanford

Naval Aerospace Medical Research Laboratory
Pensacola, Florida 32508

The experimental analysis of operant behavior maintained by thermal reinforcement began with the work of Carlton and Marx (1957) and Weiss (1957) in which heat generated by infrared radiation served as a maintaining event in a cold environment for a selected operant. Since that time numerous studies have demonstrated such effects with a variety of species. (See, e.g., the review by Satinoff and Henderson, 1977.)

The present study represents an initial effort to explore the properties of microwave radiation as a thermal reinforcer with the rhesus monkey. As a program of research, the experimental analysis of microwave-maintained responding has several goals. Our immediate goal was to develop procedures that would support responding with microwave irradiation. Most studies of operant behavior in the context of microwave radiation have established contingencies wherein the radiation could serve as a negative reinforcer. That is, organisms were trained under conditions where avoidance or escape of irradiation was the reinforced behavior (Levinson et al, 1982). Such procedures emphasize the possible noxious, if not dangerous properties of microwave exposure. The present study examined contingencies wherein the presentation of a microwave signal served to maintain a behavior; the irradiation thus functioned as a positive reinforcer.

If operant behavior can be maintained by the presentation of microwave radiation, comparisons between that consequence and properties of more conventional reinforcing events represent an extensive area for experimental analysis. The present paper focused on the shaping, acquisition, and maintenance of schedule control under conditions of intermittent reinforcement.

METHOD

Subjects

Four male rhesus monkeys, Macaca mulatta, who were individually caged were maintained on free-feeding of Wayne Monkey chow supplemented with fruit. Water was continuously available in the home cages. The animals were approximately 4 years old and weighed an average of 4.5 kg at the beginning of training. The animals were obtained from the breeding colony at the Naval Aerospace Medical Research Laboratory. They were all experimentally naive, and had been maintained on a 12:12 lighting cycle.

Apparatus

The experimental chamber was an aluminum-lined room, cavity, instrumented with an environmental control unit that produced and maintained temperatures as low as -10 $^{\circ}$C. Relative humidity was not measured but estimated relative humidity was maintained between 80 and 95% dependent on the laboratory relative humidity. The room was 2.43 m high by 2.54 m wide by 2.25 m long and had a glass window in one wall. The window was covered with a standard copper insect screen to reduce microwave transmission. A black curtain was placed on the outside of the window to prevent the animal seeing the experimenter. A 150 watt ceiling light provided chamber illumination and a 15 watt lamp placed on a wooden panel to the left of the animal was used as a signal of the presence of microwave radiation. A relay was also affixed to the wooden panel and provided audible feedback during responses that displaced the response lever 80 mm with a force of 0.147 N.

Through one wall of the cavity protruded the waveguide and a low-gain transmission horn (10-12 db). A Styrofoam chair (illustrated in Figure 1) with a teflon response lever attached was placed in the center of the chamber directly in front of the horn. The chair was situated so that the restrained monkey would face the observation window and be frontally irradiated primarily at chest height, although the low gain horn distributed a broad pattern and the metal walls insured that at least some irradiation came from virtually all angles of the room.

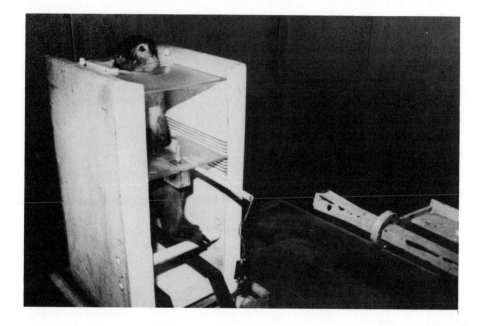

Fig. 1. A rhesus monkey in the Styrofoam chair located in the exposure chamber. The transmission horn is seen on the right of the figure.

The microwave source, an oscillator (HP-8350A) and kW amplifier (MCL Inc), was connected by a waveguide (WR-112) to the chamber and provided continuous wave (CW) energy at a frequency of 6.4 GHz at an intensity, as measured mid-torso of a seated monkey, of 50 mW/cm^2 with a Narda probe, Model 8633. This irradiation power produced a specific absorption rate (SAR) of 12 W/kg in a saline monkey model whose surface was 69.5 cm from the horn (the distance all subjects were positioned from the horn).

Control and recording equipment were located in the room adjoining the chamber.

Procedure

Sixty-minute sessions were conducted daily with each animal. A typical session began with a 15 min pre-session, "cool-down," period when the animal was placed in the chamber and the response lever was non-functional. The house light was off and the room temperature set at $0 \pm 0.5^{\circ}C$. The house light was turned on as the session started. During training a successive approximation technique was used to shape the lever response. Each reinforcement event was the presentation of a 2 sec burst of microwaves accompanied by the signal light. A lever response would produce the reinforcer and audible click. Responses during reinforcer presentations had no consequences. During the course of training the response lever was covered with surgical tape to enhance its discriminability. After each animal learned to respond on the lever the schedule of reinforcement was gradually changed from a fixed ratio of one reinforcer per response (FR 1) to FR 20. Schedule manipulations differed for each of the animals.

After it was shown that all animals had learned to respond on schedules greater than FR 1 several manipulations in the experimental conditions were instituted. These changes included eliminating the microwaves, eliminating the visual signal, and eliminating both the microwaves and the visual signal during portions of the session.

RESULTS AND DISCUSSION

Shaping

The shaping of lever pressing with microwave presentations required no special techniques beyond those ordinarily used, as for example, with food. It is essential for shaping that a subject exhibit sufficient activity from which target behaviors can be selectively reinforced. This may be a problem with organisms that tend to become inactive in a cold environment. The restraining chair was a significant aid in the shaping of the target behavior. The subject was unable to move about in the chamber thereby preventing it from moving to a location distant from the source of the microwave signals, the light stimulus, and the lever. In addition, behaviors, e.g., attempts to escape, which would be incompatible with the selected operant were rapidly extinguished. Inactivity in the chair was occasionally a problem with some animals, but, just as in the case of food deliveries, frequent presentations of microwave signals at the beginning of a shaping session generally enhanced activity to a level where the method of successive approximations was successful within one or two sessions.

Acquisition and Control of Ratio Responding

One animal, AOO, was trained to respond on an FR 3 schedule of microwave reinforcement but ceased to respond thereafter. Attempts to retrain with different session lengths, reinforcer duration and rearrangements of various other contingencies failed. This animal exemplified one end of the spectrum of success in this experiment.

Figure 2 illustrates the development of schedule control in animal 136 beginning with the second session and continuing through session 15. Sessions are indicated on the upper left of each cumulative record along with the schedule value (e.g. FR 5). During session 5 after the ninth reinforcement a counter malfunction occurred preventing reinforcement. Approximately 100 extinction responses were emitted before the counter was repaired and the animal's behavior was recovered by gradually increasing the ratio size back to FR 5.

The development of behavior in an animal responding at higher rates is seen in Figure 3. Monkey 132 responded sporadically in the initial session but by the end of the second session responses were very frequent and by the fifth session this animal was responding well on an FR 20 schedule.

The development of responding in the highest rate animal is illustrated in Figure 4. Monkey 142 was responding on an FR 10 schedule by the end of the second session and by the end of the tenth session this animal

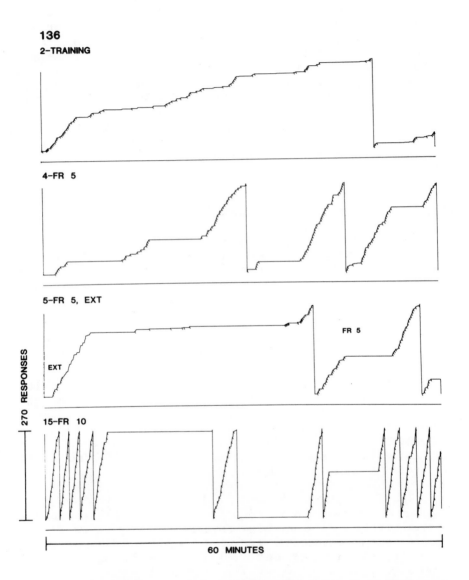

Fig. 2. Cumulative records of monkey 136 from four different one-hour sessions. Lever responses are indicated on the ordinate and time is indicated on the abscissa. Hash marks denote microwave presentations. The session number is shown in the upper left of each record.

continued responding throughout the entire session on an FR 20 schedule. Schedule control improved throughout additional sessions as seen in the third record of Figure 4.

The highly consistent performance of Monkey 142 provided a stable baseline to investigate the controlling properties of the microwave signal and the light stimulus. To evaluate these, sessions were split into three 20-min phases. During the first and third phases both the

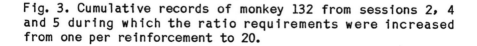

Fig. 3. Cumulative records of monkey 132 from sessions 2, 4 and 5 during which the ratio requirements were increased from one per reinforcement to 20.

microwave signal and the light stimulus were presented after each FR 20 performance. In the middle 20-min phase, in different sessions, the microwave signal, or the light, or both were eliminated. All other conditions remained the same.

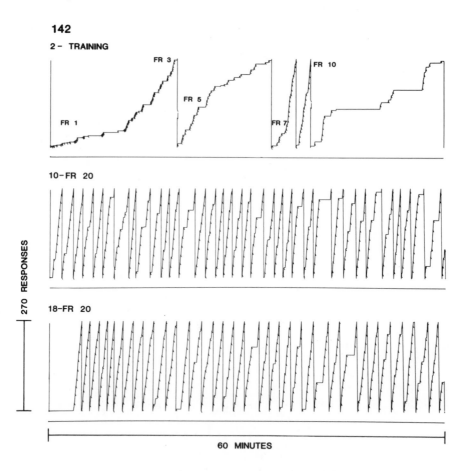

Fig. 4. Cumulative records of the highest rate animal, monkey 142. Sessions 2, 10 and 18 are shown as the ratio requirements are increased from one to 20.

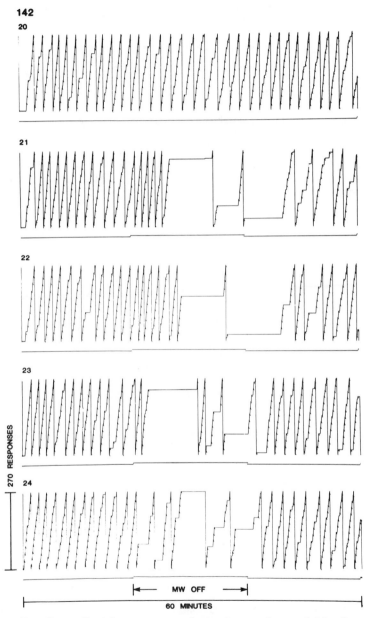

Fig. 5. Cumulative records of monkey 142 for five consecutive sessions. In sessions 21-24 the microwaves did not occur in the middle 20-min portion of the session.

Cumulative records of the performance under these conditions are shown in Figures 5 and 6. Figure 5 shows the effects of elimination of the microwave signal but retention of the light. Responding was maintained for up to 10 min during this phase, but disruption ensued. Recovery of responding occurred in the final 20 min phase with the restoration of the microwave signal.

Removal of the light stimulus while maintaining the microwave signal resulted in little change in performance as seen in Figure 6. Removal of both the microwave signal and the light stimulus during the middle 20 min of the session again resulted in disruption of responding also shown in Figure 6.

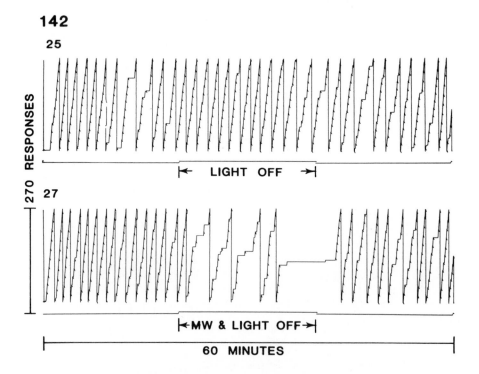

Fig. 6. Cumulative records of monkey 142 for session 25 when the light stimulus was removed and for session 27 where both the microwaves and the light stimulus were removed during the middle 20-min portion of a session.

Figures 7-10 show data characterizing the performance of Monkey 142 under the above conditions. Under conditions in which the microwave signal was not presented the number of ratios completed per min dropped to about half the control value. This reduction in the number of ratios emitted is also reflected in the overall rate as shown in Figure 8. Overall rate tells us relatively little about the pattern of responding engendered by the contingencies, however. Ratio responding is characterized by an initial

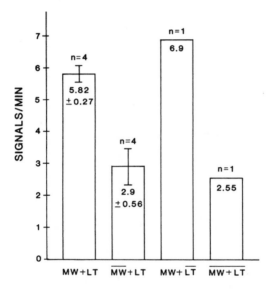

Fig. 7. Ratios or signals per min under various experimental conditions for monkey 142. MW + LT: The microwave signal (MW) and accompanying visual stimulus (LT) occurred after each fixed ratio (FR 20) performance. $\overline{\text{MW}}$ + LT: No microwaves presented, but light stimulus presented. MW + $\overline{\text{LT}}$: Microwave signal presented, but no light presented. $\overline{\text{MW}}$ + $\overline{\text{LT}}$: No microwaves or light presented. Values displayed are the arithmetic means. The bars represent ± one S.D. with the last four control sessions comprising the MW + $\underline{\text{LT}}$ condition and an additional four sessions comprising the $\overline{\text{MW}}$ + LT condition. Only one session each was conducted under the MW + $\overline{\text{LT}}$ and $\overline{\text{MW}}$ + $\overline{\text{LT}}$ conditions.

pause followed by a sustained high rate. Under small ratios (e.g., FR 20) the performance as measured in both time and response rate shows little variability from one ratio completion to another. Figures 9 and 10 show these performance features under control conditions. The running rate is here expressed as run time per completed ratio (Figure 10) to allow comparisons with pause time. When the microwave radiation was eliminated both mean values and variability in pause time and run time increased considerably. Such changes are characteristics of fixed-ratio extinction (Ferster and Skinner, 1957).

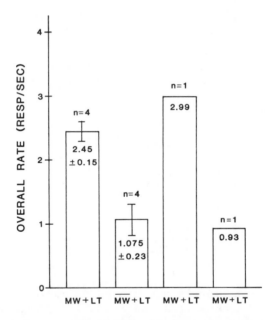

Fig. 8. The overall rate (total responses/total time) under various conditions for monkey 142. See Figure 7 for details.

Complete cessation of responding was not expected in the absence of microwave irradiation for at least two reasons. First, schedules of intermittent reinforcement establish a behavioral momentum such that changes in responding may not occur for some time after extinction conditions are imposed (see, e.g. Nevin, 1974). Second, in these procedures extinction conditions were followed by reinstatement of microwave availability. Eventually this could have lead to anticipatory responding prior to the onset of this reinstatement. Nevertheless, that microwave irradiation was essential to effect control of schedule performance in this subject seems clear.

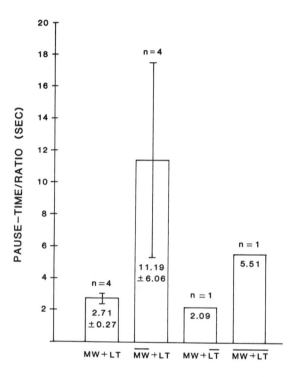

Fig. 9. The pause time per ratio under the various conditions for monkey 142. The pause time was measured from the time of availability of the schedule to the first response in the ratio. The time of availability of the ratio was measured from the beginning of a session or the offset of the last signal (or equivalent time in the case of the MW + LT condition). See Figure 7 for further details.

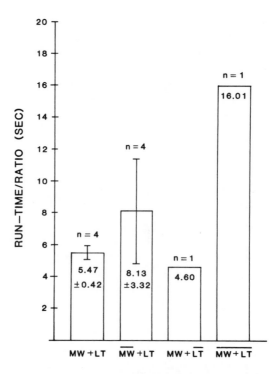

Fig. 10. The run time per ratio under the various conditions for monkey 142. The run time was measured as the time from the first response to the completion of the ratio. See Figure 7 for further details.

CONCLUSIONS

The development of performance under a schedule of intermittent reinforcement is a significant step in the assessment of the reinforcing properties of microwave radiation. Intermittent schedule performances represent perhaps the most powerful expressions of the characteristic effects of reinforcement. (see, e.g., Morse, 1966 and Zeiler, 1979). Because of their enormous cross-species and cross-reinforcer generality and the stability and diversity of rates and patterns of responding that can be engendered, schedules provide rich sources of variation to access the multi-dimensional aspects of microwave signals. Despite differences in consumatory behaviors and satiability factors, as well as uncertainties in the selection of optimal signal parameters, the results of the present study indicate that characteristic schedule performance can be developed and maintained by standard procedures derived from and utilizing more conventional reinforcers such as food.

Although it was clearly shown that microwave irradiation can serve as a positive reinforcer for rhesus monkeys in a cold environment, the demonstration was not always easily accomplished. Macaque monkeys are not very susceptible to cold environments and some, e.g., the Japanese macaque, have been shown to maintain thermal balance for one hour periods at ambient temperatures as low as 5 ^{o}C (Tokura et al, 1975). Behaviors such as shivering and huddling may compete with the lever response, thereby increasing the difficulty in training animals in this setting. There are many unanswered questions regarding the microwave parameters essential to the development and maintenance of performance at a given ambient temperature such as appropriate power density and duration of presentation. Our choice of these was empirical. That is, we initially irradiated animals with different pulse durations to insure that the duration was sufficient to be attended to but not long enough to become aversive.

This study can only be considered a starting point for more extensive investigations. Planned are parametric manipulations of intensity and duration of the microwave signal, investigation of shaping techniques and schedule contingencies, and, of particular interest, concurrent core-temperature measures for correlation with behavioral variables and reinforcement contingencies.

REFERENCES

Carlton PL, Marx RA (1957). Heat as a reinforcement for operant behavior. United States Army Medical Research Laboratory Technical Report No. 229 Fort Knox.
Ferster CB, Skinner BF (1957). "Schedules of Reinforcement." New York: Appleton-Century-Crofts.
Levinson DM, Grove AM, Clarke RL, Justesen DR (1982). Photic cueing of escape by rats from an intense microwave field. Bioelectromagnetics 3: 105.

Morse WH (1966). Intermittent reinforcement. In Honig WK (ed): "Operant Behavior: Areas of Research and Application," New York: Appleton-Century-Crofts, p. 52.

Nevin JA (1974). Response strength in multiple schedules. J Exp Anal Behav 21:389.

Satinoff E, Hendersen R (1977). Thermoregulatory behavior. In Honig WK, Staddon JER (eds): "Handbook of Operant Behavior," New Jersey: Prentice-Hall, p. 153.

Tokura H, Hara F, Okada M, Mekata F, Ohsawa W (1975). A comparison of thermoregulatory responses in the japanese macaque (Macaca fuscata) and the crab-eating macaque (Macaca irus) during cold exposure. Jap J Physiol 25: 147.

Weiss B (1957). Thermal behavior of the subnourished and pantothenic acid-deprived rat. J Comp and Physiol Psychol 50: 481.

Zeiler M (1977). Schedules of reinforcement: the controlling variables. In Honig WK, Staddon JER (eds): "Handbook of Operant Behavior," New Jersey: Prentice Hall, p. 201.

ACKNOWLEDGMENTS

Opinions or conclusions contained in this report are those of the authors and do not necessarily reflect the views of the endorsement of the Navy Department. This research was supported by Naval Medical Research and Development Command under Work Unit No. MR0000101-7035 and while the first author was participating in the U.S. Navy-ASEE Summer Faculty Research Program for 1984.

The animals used in this study were handled in accordance with the principles stated in the "Guide for the Care and Use of Laboratory Animals," Institute of Laboratory Animal Resources, National Research Council, DHEW, NIH Publication No. 80-23, 1980.

Appreciation for their respective contributions is extended to Robert C. Barrett, Brenda L. Cobb, Anna Johnson and Chuck R. Mogensen.

Electromagnetic Fields and Neurobehavioral Function, pages 235–264

MICROWAVE AND INFRARED RADIATIONS AS
SENSORY, MOTIVATIONAL, AND REINFORCING STIMULI

Don R. Justesen

Behavioral Radiology Laboratories, Veterans Administration Medical Center, Kansas City, Missouri; University of Kansas School of Medicine, Kansas City, Kansas

INTRODUCTION

In this review, I attempt to integrate data from my laboratory with findings of other investigators to the end of identifying unresolved questions with respect to sensory, motivational, and reinforcing properties of microwave radiation. Most of the pertinent findings in the literature are based on irradiation of mice, rats, and infrahuman primates but, to illuminate the critical factor of generality, I draw also on experimental observations of human beings from psychophysical studies. To lend contextual meaning to the microwave case, data based on infrared radiation of human and infrahuman subjects also are summarized.

DEFINITIONS

The diverse, multidisciplinary audience addressed by the proceedings in which this review appears begs the need for definitions of key terms, behavioral and physical. The term *aversive* is problematic because its origin is tightly linked to that of the terms *avert, aversion, avoid,* and *avoidance*, which, in the behavioral context of stimulus-and-response, are properties of the responding organism. Yet one often sees the likes of "aversive stimulus" in the behavioral literature. To evade the anthropomorphic implication that painful stimuli avoid the organism, I opt for the pristine, *Webster III* connotation: The organism has an aversion to painful stimuli, and if escape from or avoidance of a stimulus by an organism is observed, it is the organism, not the stimulus, that is averting.

Motivation is another problematic term, especially in the specification of the *motivational sign* of an affective stimulus. Again I opt for pristine, which is to say, common-language definitions. A stimulus is motivating if it arouses and impels the quiescent organism to act. The motivational sign is positive if the act is an approach to the stimulus; negative, if the act is escape from or avoidance of the stimulus.

In defining *reinforcement*, I favor the Skinnerian over the Pavlovian characterization. Both *negative* and *positive* *reinforcers* are defined empirically by Skinner (1938) as stimuli that enhance the probability of recurrence of a specified behavior—the *operant* response—they follow. Unless a stimulus increases the rate of emission of the operant it follows, it is not a reinforcer. A positive reinforcer is that which is *added* to—results from—the operant response. A negative reinforcer is an otherwise prevailing stimulus that is *subtracted* from—eliminated by—the operant response.

Unlike many contemporary experimental psychologists, I make a fine but important distinction between the construct and operational meanings of motivation and those of reinforcement. Although the stimulus that impels the organism to act has a high probability of serving as a reinforcer, I think it necessary on grounds of evidence to allow for the probability that some highly motivating stimuli under certain conditions do not have reinforcing properties in the sense of engaging an adaptive response. (Indeed, a central argument in my review is that data from behavioral studies of microwave irradiation force consideration of a contrary proposition: That highly thermalizing radiation of the mammal can motivate arousal and activity but fail to reinforce an adaptive escape response.)

My distinction of motivation and reinforcement rests on yet another distinction: that of the *experimentally naive* as opposed to the *experimentally sophisticated* animal. I concur with the mainstream assumption that almost any strongly motivating stimulus *can become* a reinforcer by fiat of special training in the stead of which the naive animal becomes experimentally sophisticated—is "shaped" or conditioned to do what the experimenter wants it to do. But I discern two plausible outcomes in the case of the naive animal that does not receive the special training: The highly motivating stimulus may or may not reinforce an adaptive response. Examples of the positive category are flight from fire and loud noise, the reflexive withdrawal of a limb from a localized (punctate, thermal, or electrical) stimulus, and the closing of the eyelids on presentation of intense light. Exemplification of the negative category is a primary objective of my review, and examples based on experimental evidence are presented in detail in later paragraphs.

One of the five anonymous reviewers of my review cautioned me to clarify what I mean by *microwaves*, to qualify depth of penetration into biological tissues as a function of frequency, and to indicate how data based on studies of microwave irradiation of small animals--mice and rats--can be generalized to the human being. Although never defined by the arbiters of the technical lexicon, the microwaves are commonly construed as electromagnetic fields that range in frequency from 300 MHz to 300 GHz. Within the microwave spectrum, penetration of mammalian tissues by an electromagnetic field is inversely related to frequency. The special case of whole-body *resonance*--maximal absorption of incident energy--is associated with maximal depth of penetration of the body, and it is frequency dependent. Resonance occurs in the mouse at frequencies near 2500 MHz; in the rat, near 700 MHz; and in adult man, near 100 MHz. (In each species, depending on its mass, its geometry, and its orientation in the field, the whole-body-resonant frequency ranges considerably. In addition, body parts, such as head, limbs, and digits exhibit resonant absorption at higher frequencies than those of the intact body (Durney, et al, 1978.)

Many experiments reported in the behavioral literature were performed at or near the resonant frequency of the species studied. Granted that resonance of the human body as a whole occurs at frequencies in the *shortwave* (30 to 300 MHz) band, not at the higher frequencies at which microwave irradiation has been used in most studies of much smaller experimental animals, the part-body human resonances definitely fall within the microwave spectrum. The overlapping resonances at microwave frequencies do not guarantee a high degree of generality to the human being of the infrahuman behavioral response to microwave irradiation, but they do argue against a presumption of the absence of generality. Moreover, the data on whole-body resonances of small animals in microwave fields do augur for caution in respect of

human, whole-body resonance in shortwave fields, which are
the dominant radio fields in the urban environment, having
their origin in thousands of commercial VHF-TV and FM transmitters. I note, too, that the relation between off-reson-
ant-to-resonant frequency and relative depth of penetration
by a shortwave or microwave field is not an invariant function across species large and small, but is best interpreted
qualitatively as a useful rule-of-thumb.

SENSORY PROPERTIES OF MICROWAVE AND INFRARED RADIATIONS

Psychophysical Data

Absolute thresholds. Although small and fragmented,
the existing base of comparative data on sensory properties
of microwave and infrared radiations as thermal stimuli
reveals several commonalities (Cook, 1952; Hendler and Hardy, 1960; Hendler et al, 1963; Justesen et al, 1982; Schwan
et al, 1966; Vendrik and Voss, 1958; Eijkman and Vendrik,
1961). For example, the findings on absolute thresholds of
cutaneous warming of human observers, which were reviewed
earlier by Michaelson (1972) and more recently by Stevens
(1982) and me (Justesen, 1983), are in agreement on the
following counts: a) The "raw feel" imparted by a supra-
threshold microwave field is a warmth indistinguishable from
that induced by infrared radiation; b) spatial summation--
reduction of threshold as area of irradiated skin in-
creases--reaches asymptote within a few tens of square cen-
timeters; c) temporal summation--reduction of threshold as
the period of irradiation increases--reaches asymptote within six to ten seconds; and d) those loci of the body that
are more sensitive to infrared--e.g., the forehead as compared with the dorsal surface of the torso--also are more
sensitive to microwave irradiation.

There are two noteworthy differences between infrared
and microwave irradiations as cutaneous thermal stimuli.
Unlike that of infrared, the absolute threshold in detection
of microwave irradiation is frequency dependent: Thresholds
decrease with increasing frequency until an asymptote is
reached near 20 Ghz. And second, the sensation of warmth
induced by microwaves at frequencies well below 20 GHz is
highly persistent, having endured after termination of irradiation for tens of seconds to minutes (cf, eg, Hendler et
al, 1963; Schwan et al, 1966, with Justesen et al, 1982).
The duration of this "afterglow" has not been studied

systematically, but it appears within limits to be a positive function of wavelength, intensity, and length of exposure to the microwave field.

Integral-dose vs irradiance thresholds. Most psychophysical studies of human and infrahuman sensitivity to microwave and infrared fields were performed before the systematic introduction of dosimetry and dose-determinate exposure systems to the radiobiological laboratory in the late 1960s and early 1970s (see, eg, Justesen and King, 1970; King et al, 1971; Justesen et al, 1971a; Justesen, 1975; Guy, 1971, 1983; Gandhi, 1974, 1975). Threshold data usually were based on and limited to irradiant measures of the incident field as specified in units of milliwatts per centimeter squared (mW/cm^2). Because irradiance is a time rate at which energy is *incident* on some target, and because the biological target in a microwave field presents complex and variable scattering properties (eg, Guy, 1971; Gandhi, 1974, 1975; Durney et al, 1978), the actual quantities of energy absorbed at thresholds of detection seldom have been measured or even estimated. To date, only one archival report (Justesen et al, 1982) has presented dosimetrically anchored comparative data on human irradiance thresholds of microwave and infrared radiations.

The ventral forearm of each of six adult observers was exposed aperiodically for 10-s periods to a continuous-wave (CW), 2450-MHz microwave field. The mean area of skin exposed to the field approximated 100 cm^2. Four of the six observers also yielded threshold data on detection of a CW infrared field during identically timed exposures of the forearm. The averaged threshold irradiance in detection of microwaves (27 mW/cm^2) was nearly 16 times higher than that of the infrared (1.7 mW/cm^2). The dosimetric measurements, on saline models of the forearm, revealed that the infrared energy was virtually perfectly absorbed; in contrast, more than half the microwave energy was scattered. Even so, sensations of warming required much more microwave than infrared energy: on average, 10 vs 1.8 joules (J). The greater depth of penetration into tissues by a microwave field at 2450 MHz [$\approx$2 cm for the e^{-1} value (Durney et al, 1978)] as compared with that of far infrared [<1 mm (Adair and Adams, 1980)], other factors being equal, implies more diffuse absorption of energy, and thus a greater quantity needed to heat the superficially situated thermal receptors to a detectable elevation of temperature (Fig. 1).

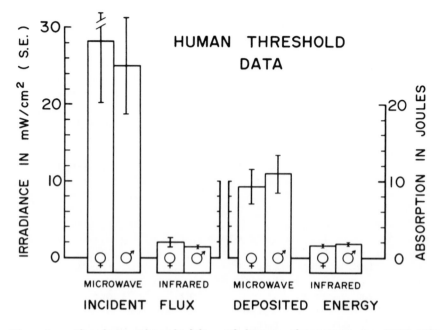

Fig. 1. Absolute thresholds of human observers to 2450-MHz microwave and far-infrared radiation of the ventral forearm are shown as means (±SE). Thresholds of incident energy are specified in mW/cm²; of absorbed energy, in joules. (Redrawn from Table I, Justesen et al, 1982.)

The data presented in Fig. 1 indicate that irradiance thresholds differed considerably among the human observers. For the four subjects that yielded data on both forms of radiant energy, the thresholds of microwave detection ranged from 15 to 44 mW/cm²; those of infrared detection, from 1.45 to 2.55 mW/cm². That the variability is primarily an expression of individual differences, not of error-of-measurement, is attested by the high intercorrelation between the respective irradiance thresholds of the four observers: r = .97 (at 2 df, P <.02, single-tail distribution). Two of the observers were women and, given the evidence of marked individual differences in thresholds, it is possible that the smaller areas of the female forearm exposed to the field were responsible (88 and 94 cm² vs 119 and 132 cm² for the men). Student's t test was performed on means of both sets of threshold data, but neither the microwave nor the infrared thresholds differed reliably as a function of sex (both *t*s <1.4 at 2 *df*, *P*s >.10). These findings are consonant with data on spatial summation reported by others (eg, Hendler et al, 1963; Schwan et al, 1966; Stevens et al 1974), ie, as the surface area of irradiated skin approaches 100 cm², spatial summation of absolute thresholds reaches asymptote.

Generality of absolute thresholds. The quantities of 2450-MHz energy absorbed at the threshold of detection ranged from 6 to 16 J among the six observers. Although based on exposure of the forearm, these integral doses compare favorably with threshold quantities associated with the rat's detection of a 2450-MHz field during whole-body exposure as determined by the technique of conditional suppression (King et al, 1971). The integral doses of three animals during discrete, 60-s periods of multipath radiation in a 2450-Mhz field averaged 31 J and ranged from 14 to 59 J; because detection of the field was evident *within* the 60-s periods, the virtual integral doses of energy at thresholds of detection were smaller, indicating well-overlapping absolute sensitivities of the sampled human beings and the rats at the indicated frequency.

Difference, pain, and terminal thresholds. There is a dearth of data on difference--incremental or decremental--thresholds of microwave irradiation. So, too, for terminal thresholds, and understandably so: Any attempt to determine the field intensity at which no further increase produced a discernible change in sensation would be an exercise in intense pain. Cook reported (1952) that the threshold of pain in human observers required a 30-s exposure of the ventral forearm to a 3-GHz field at an averaged irradiance of 2,500 mW/cm², which is nearly two orders of magnitude above the threshold of just-detectable warming at 2.45 GHz (Justesen et al, 1982).

Unrestricted exposure of a body in attempts to establish pain or terminal thresholds would pose a high probability of thermal insult. The mammalian threshold of thermal pain lies in the range of 45 to 47 °C (eg, Lowenstein and Dallenback, 1930; Hardy et al, 1952; Cook, 1952; Hellon and Mitchell (1975), which is *higher* than the temperature at which, for relatively short durations (tens of seconds), irreversible damage can occur to mammalian cells: ≈43 °C (*cf* Hardy et al, 1952; Kluger, 1979; Carroll et al, 1980; Guyton, 1981). Fortunately, and doubtless the reflection of millennia of mammalian evolution, the superficially absorbed infrared radiations admit to three adaptive properties at high intensities: One, direct injury to subdermal tissues does not occur; two, compared with microwave radiation, the higher elevations of superficial skin temperature per unit irradiance are more likely to trigger centrally mediated vasodilatation of peripheral vessels, which promotes dispersion of thermalized energy via circulatory convection; and three, if the infrared field is sufficiently intense, a rapid rise of cutaneous temperature to a painful level will occur. And localized pain, as opposed to generalized thermal discomfort, can result in rapid, reflexive retreat by the organism. In contrast, deeply penetrating microwaves have the potential to produce direct injury to subdermal tissues before the threshold of pain is reached (cf Carroll et al, 1980, with Adair, 1983a).

RADIANT ENERGIES AS MOTIVATIONAL AND REINFORCING STIMULI

Motivational Properties of Thermal Stimuli

As noted earlier, a stimulus possesses motivational properties if it impels the organism to act. A detectable radiant stimulus may not be motivating--may be neutral--or it may carry a positive or negative sign. Moreover, the motivational sign of a given radiant stimulus is not wholly an intrinsic property of the stimulus but is contextually interdependent. In a thermally "preferred" environment, by definition, motivation to change the temperature of that environment is absent. In a cold environment, the organism is motivated to approach a source of thermal stimulation. And in a hot environment, the organism is motivated to withdraw from a source of thermal stimulation (see, eg, Hardy, 1970).

It is a psychophysiological truism that an environmental temperature above or below the thermopreferendum of a species will motivate comfort-seeking behavior. Assumed also by most behavioral thermophysiologists (cf Satinoff, 1978, with Adair, 1983b) is the view that hypo- or hyperthermal stimulation not only will motivate the organism but will reinforce the response that engages the preferred temperature. However, to equate motivational potential with reinforcing efficacy is a transgression of logic and operant methodology. The logical fault is that motivation and reinforcement are not identities and therefore cannot be equated. The methodological fault is that reinforcement is an empirical construct: A thermal stimulus is validated as a reinforcer solely by demonstration under a given set of conditions that it has increased the probability of an adaptive (ie, thermopreferential) operant response.

Although the motivational potential of a stimulus does not vouchsafe its efficacy as a reinforcer, the evidence strongly supports the proposition that a stimulus must motivate an organism if it is to succeed as a operant reinforcer (Bolles, 1967). Motivation is thus a necessary but not a sufficient condition for operant reinforcement. Given the efficacy of radiant energies as motivational stimuli--the imposition of an intense infrared or microwave field on a quiescent mouse, rat, or monkey, for example, almost invariably results in increased activity and in exploratory and grooming behaviors (e.g., Murgatroyd and Hardy, 1970; Carroll et al, 1980; Levinson et al, 1982, 1985; Bruce-Wolfe and Adair, 1985)--one may turn to the literature for data that bear on the question of reinforcement.

Infrared and Microwave Radiations as Reinforcers

Infrared radiation as a positive reinforcer. The classical studies of positive reinforcement by infrared radiation were independently reported in the same year, 1957, by Weiss and by Carlton and Marks. In both studies, rats in a cold environment could activate infrared irradiation for a few seconds by depression of a lever. Stable, repetitive responding at the lever was observed, which indicates that the lamps' radiant energy--which included both luminous and non-luminous components--was positively reinforcing. Later, in confirming and extending these findings, Laties and Weiss (1960) found that experimentally naive rats in a cold environment, when given protracted (16-h) periods of access to a lever, learned to press it for brief periods of radiation by a conventional infrared lamp.

More recently, Stern et al (1979) deployed infrared radiation as a candidate positive reinforcer and 2450-MHz microwaves as a background stimulus in assessing operant behavior of the rat. The studies were performed in a cold-air environment, and the chamber in which each of several rats performed was equipped with a lever and an infrared lamp. Each depression of the lever activated the lamp for a fixed period. The lamp's radiant energy was found to reinforce the lever-pressing response, but the higher the level of the microwave background, the smaller the proportion of total time per session that individual rats activated the lamp. Although microwave radiation was not programmed as a reinforcer, Stern et al's data indicate unequivocally that non-contingent, microwave-induced heating can function as a reliable source of motivational stimulation.

The results of the studies by Weiss (1957), Carlton and Marks (1957), Laties and Weiss (1960), Stern et al (1979), and many other investigators (see the reviews by Satinoff and Hendersen, 1977; and Cabanac, 1983), have been taken as evidence that infrared radiation *per se* is a positive rein- forcer in a cold environment, an assumption questioned by Satinoff and Hendersen. These authors note in reviewing the literature on infrared-motivated, operant behavior that such behavior is based almost wholly on use of conventional infrared lamps. At question is the source of stimulus control: Does the infrared field as such suffice as a rein- forcing stimulus? or does the flux of visible photons emit- ted by a lamp function as the discriminative stimulus? Granted that an environment below an animal's preferred temperature will motivate it to seek a warmer environment, visible light will be emitted concomitantly with infrared radiation by the conventional lamp, unless the lamp is operated well below its rated wattage, and this light could be the stimulus that controls the operant response. To the attentive animal, a synchronous flux of luminous energy during periods of excitation of the infrared lamp would define the temporal boundaries of the infrared field.

Murgatroyd and Hardy (1970) also reported an attempt to reinforce the rat's lever-pressing response by infrared radiation, an archival report that is singular for this species in being based on control--elimination--of artifactual luminous stimulation. The investigators inter- posed a quartz filter between infrared lamp and rat in proximity to both. Even in a cold-air environment, and even after the rats were rendered nude by shaving of the pelt, great difficulty was encountered in training them stably to press a lever, each depression of which activated the lamp for a discrete period. Only after extensive training, did the rats display efficient thermoregulatory behavior. The absence of a luminous stimulus may have been responsible for the slow acquisition, but the response-stimulus contingency was susceptible to a source of tthermal confounding: The proximal quartz filter might have been heated sufficiently to act as a secondary radiator of infrared radiation during periods of inactivation of the infrared lamp.

Infrared radiation as a negative reinforcer. Lipton (1968, 1969), Lipton and Marotto (1969), and Lipton et al (1970) reported that rats can be trained to emit an operant response that results in a brief period of *inactivation* of an intense infrared field. The reports of Lipton and colleagues are illustrative of work by other investigators (eg, Baldwin and Ingram, 1967; Carlisle, 1970) in which infrared radiation has been programmed as a negative reinforcer of free-operant behavior. Of note is that none of the investigations in which infrared radiation was programmed as a negative reinforcer controlled for luminous flux as a potential discriminative stimulus. In a control experiment, Lipton et al (1970) did use a small, red-coated, incandescent lamp in lieu of an infrared lamp to determine whether luminous stimulation without heating would result in aversion by the rat. No evidence of aversion was observed.

I know of no archival reports of experimentation on controlled- or free-operant behavior in which the experimentally naive animal has been observed for adventitious acquisition of escape from infrared radiation in the absence of luminous cues. Vivid to my recall, however, is the frustration besetting one of my doctoral preceptors, Prof. Paul B. Porter of the University of Utah, who attempted near-daily during the summer of 1957 to reinforce negatively a series of two-choice discriminations by rats. An animal could escape from the field of an infrared lamp by choosing--pushing down and running over--one of two doors at each of several choice points in a linear maze. Prof. Porter used a Variac transformer to reduce current to the lamp, which controlled for luminous emissions, then compensated for the reduced power level by manually maneuvering the lamp in proximity to an animal as it moved through the maze, the cover of which was an open-wire mesh.

Over much time and many trials, each of a large number of rats would push against one or the other or both doors at a choice point, but acquisition of a sequential discrimination (eg, an errorless left-right-left-right sequence) never took place. During any given set of trials, a rat was as likely to err (to push first against a locked door) as it was to succeed (to push first against an unlocked door). The radiant stimulus was strongly motivating, as evidenced by the rats' rapid locomotion to each choice point when the infrared field was applied. Although the lamp was immediately withdrawn and extinguished after a correct entry to a doorway, none of the rats acquired the discrimination. Eventually, because his rats were sustaining burns, Prof. Porter abandoned the infrared lamp and motivated his rats by electric current via a metal grid that served also as a floor to the maze. Rats under motivation by the electric shock rapidly acquired the sequential discrimination.

Given a less demanding task, such as a discrete lever-pressing response, it is highly probable that, in time, a rat could be trained by successive approximations to escape from the radiations of an infrared source in the absence of a luminous cue. But the investigator would require an infrared source and an operant chamber that permitted highly selective activation and inactivation of irradiation, to avoid residual heating of animals by structures in the exposure milieu. The walls and floor of a conventional operant chamber will readily absorb, convect, and re-radiate infrared energy, which would elevate temperatures of floor and air, and which, in turn, would confound stimulus control. Unknown is whether adventitious acquisition ("autoshaping") of a lever-pressing escape response by the naive mammal will occur to infrared radiation under ideal conditions of stimulus control--no discriminative stimulation by luminous or other sensory cues--as it does to motivational footshock (eg, Weiss, 1968, 1971a, b, c; Sklar and Anisman, 1979; Carroll et al, 1980; Visintainer et al, 1982; Levinson et al, 1982; Laudenslager et al, 1983).

Microwave radiation as a negative reinforcer. In 1980, Carroll et al reported that none of 20 experimentally naive rats acquired a simple operant (locomotor-place) response (Fig. 2) that would have reduced energy dosing in a multi-path, 918-Mhz field from 60 mW/g to levels as low as 2 mW/g. In contrast, the investigators found that naive rats motivated by faradic shock (Justesen et al, 1971b) to the feet under the same contingency in the same apparatus rapidly acquired the escape response (Fig. 3). Carroll et al performed their studies in the wake of earlier reports by Monahan and Ho (1977a, b) that experimentally naive mice, when individually placed in a waveguide and continuously subjected to an intense, 2450-MHz field, exhibited a reliable average decline in rate of energy absorption--from 60 mW/g to 40 mW/g--after initiation of irradiation.

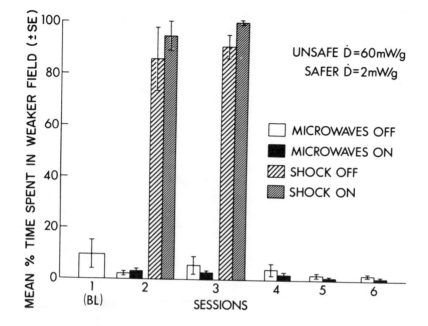

Fig. 2. During each of a series of once-daily sessions, microwave irradiation (918-MHz) was automatically activated five times per session for a 2-min period at 2-min intervals. Entry by a rat into a rectangular area on the floor of a multi-mode cavity (Fig. 3) during periods of irradiation resulted in a reduction of the whole-body-averaged dose rate from 60 to 2 mW/g. Active-control rats escaped from faradic shock by entering the rectangle. Baselines (BL) of the first session were recorded in the absence of motivational stimulation. (From Carroll et al, 1980.)

Monahan and Ho (1977a) interpreted the reduction of dose rate as evidence of "avoidance." Although the field was not avoidable in the continuously excited waveguide, the animals may have been attempting to escape from it. In so doing, they may have learned to reduce the rate of energy absorption by, eg, selective orientation of the body in the field. This interpretation is clouded, however, because the investigators never observed the behavior of their mice. Once installed in the waveguide, a mouse could not be seen. Aversive behavior had been inferred solely from readings of power meters. An alternate interpretation, given the extremely high rates of energy dosing, is thermal collapse.

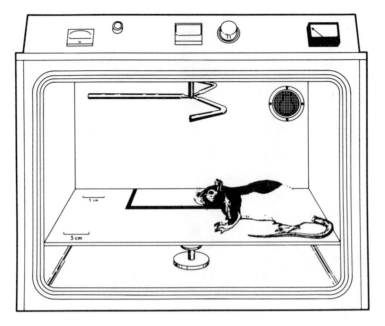

Fig. 3. Artist's rendering of the 918-MHz multi-mode cavity in which the experiments of Carroll et al (1980) and Levinson et al (1982) were performed. When appropriately programmed, entrance by a rat to the area bordered by the rectangle, which encompassed 25-percent of the floor's surface, resulted in reduction or cessation of irradiation, or in cessation of faradic shock to the feet. (From Carroll et al, 1980.)

A mouse prostrate in a waveguide under TE_{10} excitation, which was used by Monahan and Ho, presents a diminished absorptive cross section to the incident field, which would significantly reduce its rate of energy absorption (cf Carroll et al, 1980, with ITT, 1968).

Because a mouse in a waveguide at 2450 Mhz cannot be equated with a rat in a multi-mode cavity at 918 MHz, the question of escape learning vs. thermal collapse by the mice of Monahan et al. was not resolved by the study of Carroll, et al. But a succession of more recent studies of mice and/or rats under motivation by intense 918- and 2450-MHz fields (e.g., Levinson et al, 1982, 1985; Justesen, 1983; Justesen et al, 1985) has revealed that the naive animal usually fails to acquire an escape response under motivation by intense fields, even at lethal intensities. The first of these follow-up studies (Fig. 4), which was

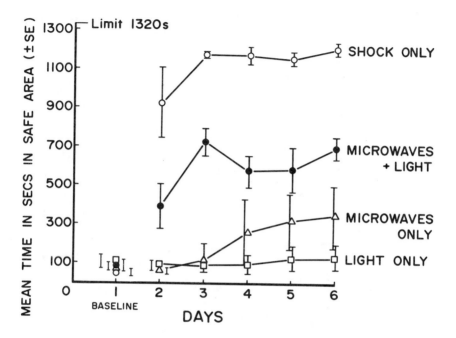

Fig. 4. Means of time per daily session that individual rats of four independent groups spent in the rectangular "safe" area of the multi-mode cavity shown in Fig. 3. (Redrawn from Fig. 3, Levinson et al, 1982.)

reported by Levinson et al (1982), revealed that an absolute reduction of energy dosing in a 918-MHz multipath field (from 60 to 0 mW/g) failed to reinforce an escape response by rats. For another set of rats, cessation of faradic shock was a potent reinforcer. In contrast, rats of yet another group, which were cued by a houselight that illuminated in synchrony with the 918-Mhz field, did learn to escape from the field. Illumination of the lamp in the absence of microwave irradiation failed to result in escape behavior.

The studies of Carroll et al (1980) and of Levinson et al (1982) were based on a series of short, once-daily sessions of 22 minutes per rat; five 2-min. periods of available irradiation alternated with automatic, 2-min. time-

outs. This, to preclude lethality if an animal were continuously irradiated for 10 min. at 60 mW/g.

In a subsequent series of studies of experimentally
naive mice and rats in my laboratory (cf Justesen, 1983;
Justesen et al, 1985), a sink-or-swim protocol was adopted
in which 2450-Mhz irradiation was continuously available at
60 mW/g during a maximum of four, once-daily, 15-min. sessions. Inactivation of the field was contingent on an
animal's entry to a centered circle (Fig. 5) that comprised

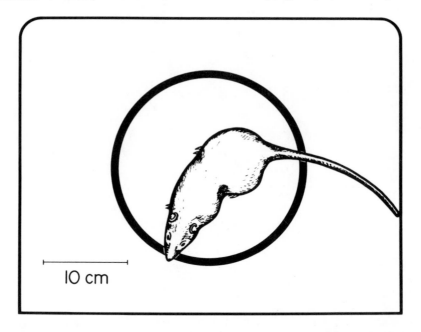

10 cm

Fig. 5. Artist's scale drawing of a rat in the circle of a
false plastic floor that was located in a 2450-MHz multi-
mode cavity. Entry to the circular area inactivated intense
microwave irradiation or faradic shock to the feet. (From
Justesen et al, 1983).

25 percent of the area of the false plastic floor of a 2450-
Mhz multi-mode cavity. None of 10 rats acquired an escape
or avoidance response; all ten expired during the first or
second session of exposure to the 2450-MHz field. Eight of
ten mice survived irradiation at 60 mW/g, but statistical
evaluation of the percentages of time across sessions that

these animals inactivated the field yielded chance differences from baseline values. All ten mice of an additional group expired during sessions in which the available dose rate was 120 mW/g. The escape-to-the-circle response was rapidly acquired by mice and rats under motivation by faradic shock. Most animals eventually avoided the shock by remaining in the circle during all 15 minutes of a daily session.

My colleagues and I assumed that the place response--entry to a large, visually well-demarcated area--to be an extremely easy operant task at time of launching the work on escape-and-avoidance behaviors. Ease of mastery was a preeminent consideration because of the intent to evaluate unaided acquisition of aversive behaviors by the experimentally naive animal. A diversity of false-floor place-response formats was assessed, including the centered circle as well as rectangular and hemicircular areas that bordered a wall of a cavity (Levinson et al, 1985). The data from all assessments supported our assumption of ease-of-mastery when faradic shock was used as the motivating stimulus. But under motivation by microwaves, there was little evidence that cessation of irradiation in the absence of discriminative stimulation would reinforce an escape response. A decision was made therefore to employ an even easier operant task in yet another series of studies on experimentally naive animals (Levinson et al, 1985).

The false, white Plexiglas floors of 918-Mhz and 2450-MHz cavities were divided into equal areas to provide a shuttle-box format. Crossing a black center line to enter one side of the shuttle constituted an escape response; remaining on that side, avoidance. As expected, escape from, then avoidance of, faradic shock by mice and rats was rapidly acquired. When the animals were motivated by microwave irradiation at 60 mW/g, there was a weak but statistically reliable trend of increased time spent on the non-radiated side of the shuttle across four sets of once-daily sessions. There was no evidence of avoidance, and resistance to extinction was nil.

Viewed collectively, the shuttle data are difficult to interpret. Rats of one representative group spent about 25 percent of their time per 15-min. session on the irradiated side of the shuttle. Given the momentary dose rate of 60 mW/g, each animal received session-averaged energy dosing at a rate near 15 mW/g, which is almost double the resting metabolic rate of the species (Hart, 1971; Durney et al, 1978). Conjoined with this high, averaged rate of self-selected energy dosing were signs of thermal stress: frequent urination and defecation, and coating of the pelt with saliva. I think the rats were displaying a thermokinesis quite unrelated to a reinforced escape response. Perhaps an animal moved at random along the 360° perimeter of the cavity's floor, its locomotion simply being more rapid during a 180° excursion under highly thermalizing and motivating radiation than during alternate 180° excursions in the absence of irradiation. On the other hand, the statistically reliable trend toward increased time away from the field may indicate that acquisition of an escape response was slowly developing.

A similar attempt to program cessation of intense microwave irradiation as a reinforcer of escape and avoidance behaviors was reported by Monahan and Henton (1977). These investigators used sonic stimulation (2900 Hz) in synchrony with periods of microwave irradiation (2450-MHz CW) to motivate experimentally naive mice. The mice were individually situated in a special runway within a section of waveguide. Repeatedly during each of eight, once-daily, 30-min. sessions, the sonic stimulus and the microwave field were activated, the latter at ≈45 mW/g. When an animal made an operant escape response by interrupting a beam of light that passed through the waveguide, sonic and microwave stimulation were inactivated for 12 s. Both stimuli were then automatically reactivated--unless an animal again interrupted the light beam within the 12-s time-out, which postponed reactivation for another 12 s. By repeatedly interrupting the beam within the recurring 12-s limit, the mice could have avoided the sonic-microwave stimulation. None of them did. All five mice exhibited both escape and postponement behaviors, some more inclined to escape, others more inclined to postpone, but all animals sustained periods of irradiation and sonic stimulation during all eight sessions. Whether a trend toward avoidance--inactivation of the field during the entirety of a 30-min. session--was developing across sessions was not addressed by the authors.

Complicating interpretation of Monahan and Henton's data is the makeup of their experimental design. The intense microwave irradiation was always presented in synchrony with sonic stimulation, never independently. To conclude, as the authors did, that their mice performed the operant beam-breaking response to escape from or postpone microwave irradiation begs the question of an interaction between the sonic and microwave stimuli. Only observation of escape from microwave irradiation in the absence of sonic stimulation, a condition not included in the authors' study, could justify their conclusion. A control group was included in their study, mice subjected solely to sonic stimulation, which failed to motivate escape or postponement. But data based on their performances are not responsive to the question of negative reinforcement by microwave irradiation as such.

Perhaps the sonic signal served as a discriminative stimulus, a possibility clouded by unreported findings of Richard Lovely, Sheri Mizumori, and Robert Johnson (many personal communications dating from 1977 with Dr. Lovely, who was affiliated with the University of Washington in Seattle). Lovely and colleagues independently programmed both photic and acoustic signals as discriminative stimuli during studies of rats under motivation by an intense, 918-MHz microwave field. A shuttle box was fabricated from a hollow, transparent cylinder of Plexiglas within an open-mesh, circularly polarized waveguide. The centerline of the shuttle box was paralleled by the beam of a light-emitting diode. When an animal left a starting area and crossed the centerline, it interrupted reception of the beam by a photic sensor. Each of a repeated series of trials began with ten seconds of discriminative stimulation; at the end of this period, if an animal had not moved from the starting area to the centerline, the field was activated and was continuously applied (at 30 mW/g) until an animal interrupted the beam of light. On breaking the beam, the microwave field and the discriminative stimulation were inactivated. Avoidance of the field was possible--was contingent on an animal's crossing of the centerline before ten seconds had elapsed.

For rats of one group, Lovely and colleagues illuminated a house light as the discriminative stimulus--to signal the impending activation of the microwave field. For rats of another group, a sonic signal antedated activation of the field. Rats cued by light learned to escape from and, in time, to avoid, the microwave field; not so, the sonically cued rats. Moreover, when rats of yet another group were cued by *inactivation* of an otherwise illuminated house light, they, too, failed to acquire the escape-avoidance response. *Only when the photic stimulus was a posi-*

tive precursor and accompaniment of the intense microwave field was reliable evidence of escape behavior observed. Eventually, the animals cued by the presence of light demonstrated avoidance of microwave irradiation by crossing the centerline of the shuttlebox within the 10-s limit. Five animals each populated the positive-light, the negative-light, and the positively sonically cued groups.

Because the combination of microwave radiation and sonic stimulation was effective in reinforcing escape and postponement behaviors of Monahan and Henton's mice in a shuttle task, the failure of sonic stimulation as a discriminative stimulus in the study of microwave-motivated rats by Lovely et al begs for explanation. The species difference is noted as is the timing of the discriminative stimulus relative to activation of the microwave field: antecedent and conterminous in the studies of Lovely et al, and synchronous in the studies of Monahan and Henton. In one case (Monahan and Henton's), successive trials were continuous during an experimental session; in the other case, a discrete-trial format was used. Also of note is the waveguide that served as a shuttle box in the studies of Monahan and Henton; the only source of illumination within the waveguide was the beam of light that was used to detect escape and postponement responses. In contrast, Lovely et al's rats performed in an illuminated environment that would have masked the weak flux of luminous energy emitted by the photo-diode of their movement detector.

If the beam of light used in photo-detection was readily detected by Monahan and Henton's mice--probable in an otherwise pitch-black surround--it might have served as a collateral discriminative stimulus; i.e., a mouse in passing through and interrupting the beam might have reduced the intensity of light that played on its eyes, which reduction would have been correlated with inactivation of the field. In the absence of specific methodological information--the spectral character and luminance of the beam were not specified--one may only speculate whether the discrepancy in outcomes is more apparent than real. But collateral photic cueing, if critical to the performances of the mice, would reconcile the two sets of findings.

Microwave radiation as a positive reinforcer. To my knowledge, there are no published reports based on the simple contingency in which a brief exposure of an animal to

a microwave field was contingent on a lever-pressing operant. As noted earlier, Stern et al (1979) used microwave
irradiation as a background source of thermal stimulation in
which rats in a cold environment pressed a lever for infrared reinforcers. A similar approach has been taken by Adair
and colleagues (eg, Adair and Adams, 1980, 1982; Adair et
al, 1984) in that microwave irradiation has been applied as
a background stimulus while squirrel monkeys have thermoregulated by controlling the temperature of a draft of air.
The reader may wonder why Stern, et al and Adair and colleagues have not taken the simpler tack of attempting directly to reinforce the operant response by microwave radiation. The answer lies to some extent in their use of free-
field, far-field, 2450-MHz exposure systems; with such systems, relatively high levels of microwave energy from a
relatively distant source are needed to provide even a
modest level of energy dosing.

Bruce-Wolfe and Adair (1985) did make microwave irradiation contingent on an operant response by the experimentally sophisticated squirrel monkey, but their experiments
were based on a complex set of motivational stimuli. Each
of their animals thermoregulated by alternately activating a
draft of cold air and a draft of thermoneutral air by sequential tugs at a cord. Initiation of 2450-MHz irradiation
at a power density of 20, 25, or 30 mW/cm^2 (maximal dose
rate ≈4.5 mW/g) was synchronous with periods of activation of the thermoneutral air. It is highly probable that
the alternately cold and thermoneutral drafts of air that
accompanied successive tugs at the cord served as discriminative stimuli, which factor precludes independent evaluation of the sufficiency of the microwave field as a positive
reinforcer. Noteworthy, however, is that a distinct change
in the performances of the monkeys occurred when the power
density of the field was increased from 25 to 30 mW/cm^2.
That is, the proportion of time per session that the monkeys
selected microwave irradiation and thermoneutral air (≈90
percent) did not differ when the irradiance of the field was
increased from 20 to 25 mW/cm^2. But repeatedly, when the
field was presented at 30 mW/cm^2, that proportion decreased
significantly (to ≈80 percent), a change I attribute to a
perceptual threshold. The reader will recall that the absolute threshold of irradiance in human, part-body detection
of a 2450-MHz CW field averaged 27 mW/cm^2 (see Justesen et
al, 1982, and Fig. 1, this paper). The monkey and human
data were obtained in the same exposure facility.

RECAPITULATION

The behavioral response to microwave and infrared radiations has been unevenly assessed in the operant and psychophysical laboratories. There is a voluminous literature on
the behavioral response to infrared radiations, notwith-
standing the unresolved issue of discriminative cueing by
visible light. The data base on reinforcing potential of
the microwaves is quite meagre by comparison. It follows
that the conclusions I draw from the 1986 data base are
provisional. They are intended as heuristics for a future
agenda of research, not as certainties carved in stone. The
data, such as they are, admit to the following arguments:

1. By introspective report, the sensations imparted
to human observers by microwave and infrared radiations are
indistinguishable (cf, eg, Hendler et al, 1963; Justesen et
al, 1982).

2. Intense, potentially or demonstrably lethal levels
of microwave radiation generally have failed to reinforce an
adaptive escape reaction by the experimentally naive animal
(eg, Carroll et al, 1980).

3. The experimentally naive animal has acquired an
adaptive escape response when visible light has accompanied
the intense microwave field as a discriminative stimulus
(eg, Levinson et al, 1982).

4. Adventitious acquisition ("autoshaping") of an adaptive, operant, heat-seeking response--infrared self-irrad-
iation in a cold environment--has been observed in experimentally naive animals, but visible light accompanied the
infrared radiation, and this light may have served as the
discriminative stimulus that controlled the operant response
(cf Laties and Weiss, 1960, with Satinoff and Hendersen,
1977).

5. Activation of visible light, inactivation of visible light, and activation of sonic stimulation were
independently assessed as discriminative stimuli in studies
of escape and avoidance behaviors of rats under motivation
by intense microwave irradiation. Only when visible light
was *present* as an antecedent-and-conterminous discriminative
stimulus was acquisition of an escape response observed.
(Lovely, Mizumori, and Johnson, unpublished data.)

6. Prolonged training of rats was required to obtain evidence of operant conditioning when the candidate positive reinforcer was infrared radiation in a cold environment. Visible light was eliminated as a discriminative stimulus by quartz filtration, but the initially poor performances of the animals and the need for extensive training comport with the possibility that intense, non-localized, non-visible, infrared radiations, akin to the microwaves, may fail to reinforce an adaptive escape response by the experimentally naive mammal. (See Murgatroyd and Hardy, 1970.)

INTERPRETATION

The large thermal time constants of mammalian tissues, and the relatively great depths of penetration by microwave fields at frequencies below 3 GHz, can give rise to elevations of body temperature that persist long after termination of irradiation. The naive animal that is rendered hyperthermic by an intense field, and that is impelled to increased exploratory activity thereby, may execute fortuitously an adaptive operant response that extinguishes the field. But timely feedback--the sensory-and-affective reinforcement--by which it would "connect" the operant act with respite from excessive heating, is absent. Tens of seconds may pass before a reduction of temperature is detected. The result would be a failure of adaptive escape behavior.

Delay of sensory feedback to explain the absence of an adaptive escape response from intense microwave irradiation was first offered by Carroll et al (1980), and this explanation is consonant with biophysical, psychophysical, and behavioral principles and data (cf, eg, Hendler et al, 1963; Schwan et al, 1966; Bolles, 1967; Justesen et al, 1982, 1983). Acceptance of a delay-of-feedback mechanism does not exclude other explanations, but it does provide a point of departure for inquiry about commonalities and differences in the sensory, motivational, and reinforcing properties of microwave and infrared fields.

Non-localized exposure of the body to infrared radiation may have sharply differentiated effects on behavior when contrasted with the response to microwave radiation. Infrared fields are highly limited in depth of penetration and, at high intensities, can produce rapid elevations of skin temperature and of the skin's superficially situated thermoreceptors. Conversely, termination of infrared ir-

radiation will be associated with a relatively rapid decline
of peripheral temperatures via conduction and circulatory
convection of thermal energy to the much larger bulk of the
body's cooler core. Given the superior kinetics of infrared
heating and dissipation as contrasted with those of the
deeply penetrating microwaves, a good argument can be made
that the sensory dynamics incumbent with infrared irradiation endow it with much the better, positive or negative,
reinforcing properties.

There is a contrary possibility that emerges from the
data: Non-localized infrared irradiation may share with
non-localized microwave irradiation a dependence on visible
light as the discriminative stimulus that controls the *rapid*
behavioral response to external sources of hyperthermalizing
stimulation. During the long course of mammalian evolution,
thermal and visual stimuli have been conjoined in the work-
ings of sun and fire. Perhaps in consequence, as Richard
Lovely speculated in the wake of his work with Mizumori and
Johnson, the photic and thermal sensory modalities of vertebrates are genetically "hardwired."

If Lovely's conception is valid, it has an important
implication for somesthetic taxonomy and functional neuro-
anatomy: The sensory experience associated with an anatom-
ically generalized elevation of body temperature, whether
resulting from internal or external agency, is intrinsically
proprioceptive--is interpreted as "in-the-body." If so,
then only when visible light is covariant with generalized
hyperthermal stimulation can such heating take on the properties of an exteroceptive, "beyond-the-body" experience.

Whether the experience of generalized heating by non-
visible infrared radiation is intrinsically proprioceptive
--is not exteroceptive--is a question that awaits experimental resolution. Whatever the answer, the psychophysical
and operant data on microwave heating are compatible with
the thesis of proprioception, which has an important practical implication with respect to exposure of industrial and
military personnel. Repeatedly in this review, I have
stressed the distinction between the experimentally naive
and the experimentally sophisticated organism. The human
corollary is the experientially naive versus the experientially sophisticated individual. Given the many occupational
and military settings in which exposure to intense shortwave
and microwave fields can occur, what will be the response of

the unsuspecting, technically untrained individual that
unwittingly sustains an accidental overexposure? Will the
sensations of warming from intense, non-localized radiation
be attributed to the external source? or will the individual assume that diffuse sensations of warming are of internal origin?--merely, say, a "hot flash" or a budding fever?
If interpreted as an internal manifestation--if evasive
action is not taken--hyperthermal injury is highly probable.

The available evidence on accidental over-exposure of
human beings to shortwave or microwave radiation is perforce
anecdotal (eg, Harris et al, 1979; Slesin, 1983), but it is
fully compatible with the assumption that the accidentally
hyperthermalized individual does not attribute sensations of
warming to the external source of radiation.

ACKNOWLEDGMENTS

I thank Mary Ellen O'Connor of the University of Tulsa,
who managed the editing of my manuscript and greatly improved it, as did the five anonymous reviewers that provided her
a plenitude of constructive criticisms. Mary Ellen, one-time
protégée, is the most admirable of all good works, persons
or publications, that have issued from my laboratory. The
Battelle Foundation's Richard Lovely, sagacious student of
the behaving rat in the microwave field and co-editor of
this volume, is acknowledged for his creative and quite
possibly correct insights into the role of visible light in
regulation of the mammalian response to highly thermalizing
radiations, whatever their spectral character. I am especially grateful to Eleanor Adair of the John Pierce Foundation and Yale University for keeping me honest, interested,
and informed, and for many years of personal friendship and
scientific comradery. My work, which is largely the expression of untiring, loyal efforts in my laboratory by Daniel
Levinson, Rex Clarke, Robert Smith, and Donald Riffle, is
supported by funds from the Research Service of the U.S.
Veterans Administration and by research grant ESO-2615 from
the National Institute of Environmental Health Sciences.

REFERENCES

Adair ER (1983a): Sensations, subtleties, and standards:
    Synopsis of a panel discussion. In Adair ER (ed):
    "Microwaves and thermoregulation." New York: Aca-
    demic Press, pp 231-238.

Adair ER (1983b): Changes in thermoregulatory behavior during microwave irradiation. In Adair ER (ed): *"Microwaves and thermoregulation."* New York: Academic Press, pp 359-378.

Adair ER, Adams BW (1980): Microwaves modify thermoregulatory behavior in squirrel monkey. *Bioelectromagnetics* *1*:1-20.

Adair ER, Adams BW (1982): Adjustments in metabolic heat production by squirrel monkeys exposed to microwaves. *J Appl Physiol* *52*:1049-1058.

Adair ER, Adams BW, Akel GM (1984): Minimal changes in hypothalamic temperature accompany microwave-induced alteration of thermoregulatory behavior. *Bioelectromagnetics* *5:*13-30.

Baldwin BA, Ingram DL (1967): The effect of heating and cooling the hypothalamus on behavioral thermoregulation in the pig. *J Physiol* *191:*375-392.

Bolles RC (1967): *"Theory of motivation."* New York: Harper & Row, pp 434-451.

Bruce-Wolfe V, Adair ER (1985): Operant control of convective cooling and microwave irradiation by the squirrel monkey. *Bioelectromagnetics* *6:*365-380.

Cabanac M (1983): Thermoregulatory behavioral responses. In Adair ER (ed): *"Microwaves and thermoregulation."* New York: Academic Press, pp 307-357.

Carlisle HJ (1970): Thermal reinforcement and temperature regulation. In Stebbins WC (ed): *"Animal psychophysics: The design and conduct of sensory experiments."* Englewood Cliffs: Prentice-Hall, pp 211-229.

Carlton PL, Marks R (1957): Heat as a reinforcement for operant behavior. *"Technical Report No 229, U.S. Army Medical Research Laboratory."* Fort Knox: Kentucky.

Carroll DR, Levinson DM, Justesen DR (1980): Failure of rats to escape from a potentially lethal microwave field. *Bioelectromagnetics* *1:*101-115.

Cook HF (1952): The pain threshold for microwave and infrared radiations. *J Physiol* *118:*1-11.

Durney CH, Johnson CC, Barber PW, Massoudi H, Iskander MF, Lords JL, Ryser DK, Allen SJ, Mitchell, JC (1978): *"Radiofrequency radiation dosimetry handbook."* 2nd Ed. Report SAM-TR-78-22, U.S. Air Force School of Aerospace Medicine, Brooks Air Force Base, Texas.

Eijkman EG, Vendrik AJH (1961): Dynamic behavior of the warmth sense organ. *J Exp Psychol* *62:*403-408.

Gandhi OP (1974): Polarization and frequency effects on whole-animal absorption of RF energy. *Proc IEEE 62:* 1171-1175.

Gandhi OP (1975): Frequency and orientation effects on whole-animal absorption of electromagnetic waves. *IEEE Trans Biomed Eng BME-22:*536-542.

Guy AW (1971): Analyses of electromagnetic fields induced in biological tissues by thermographic studies on equivalent phantom models. *IEEE Trans Microwave Theory and Tech MTT-19:*205-214.

Guy AW (1983): Quantitation of electromagnetic fields in biological systems. In Osepchuk JM (ed): *"Biological effects of electromagnetic systems."* New York: John Wiley & Sons, pp 1-99.

Guyton AC (1981): *"Textbook of medical physiology,"* 6th ed. Philadelphia: Saunders, p 896.

Hardy JD (1970): Thermal comfort: Skin temperature and physiological thermoregulation. In Hardy JD, Gagge AP, Stolwijk JAJ (eds): *"Physiological and behavioral temperature regulation."* Springfield: Chas C Thomas, pp 856-873.

Hardy JD, Wolff HG, Goodell H (1952): *"Pain sensations and reactions."* Baltimore: Williams & Wilkins, pp 73-79.

Harris EH, Parr WH, Murray WE, Glaser ZR (1979): *"Testimony before U.S. Senate Committee on Commerce, Science, and Transportation: Hearings on irradiation, health, and safety."* Serial No. 95-49. Washington DC: U.S. Government Printing Office, pp 586-587.

Hart JS (1971): Rodents. In Whittow GC (ed): *"Comparative physiology of thermoregulation."* Vol. II. New York: Academic Press, pp 1-149.

Hellon RF, Mitchell D (1975): Characteristics of neurones in the ventral-basal thalamus of the rat which respond to noxious stimulation of the tail. *J Physiol* [London] *50:*29p-30p.

Hendler E, Hardy JD (1960): Infrared and microwave effects on skin heating and temperature sensation. *IRE Trans Med Electron ME-7:*143-152.

Hendler E, Hardy JD, Murgatroyd D (1963): Skin heating and temperature sensation produced by infrared and microwave irradiation. In Herzfeld ME (ed): *"Temperature: Its measurement and control in science and industry."* New York: Reinhold, pp 211-230.

ITT (1968): *"Reference data for radio engineers."* New York: Howard W Sams & Co, p 23.4.

Justesen DR (1975): Toward a prescriptive grammar for the radiobiology of nonionising electromagnetic radiations: Quantities, definitions, and units of absorbed electromagnetic energy. *J Microwave Power 10*:333-356.

Justesen DR (1983): Sensory dynamics of intense microwave irradiation: A comparative study of aversive behaviors by mice and rats. In Adair ER (ed): *"Microwaves and thermoregulation."* New York: Academic Press, pp 203-227.

Justesen DR, King NW (1970): Behavioral effects of low-level microwave irradiation in the closed-space situation. In Cleary SF (ed): *"Biological effects and health implications of microwave radiation."* Publication BRH/DBE 70-2. Washington DC: U.S. Public Health Service, pp 154-179.

Justesen DR, Levinson DM, Clarke RL, and King NW (1971a): A microwave oven for behavioural and biological research: Electrical and structural modifications, calorimetric dosimetry, and functional evaluation. *J Microwave Power 6*:237-258.

Justesen DR, King NW, Clarke RL (1971b): Unavoidable grid shock without scrambling circuitry from a faradic source of low-radio-frequency current. *Behav Res Meth Instrument 3*:131-135.

Justesen DR, Riffle DW, Levinson DM (1985): Sensory, motivational, and reinforcing properties of microwaves: An assay of behavioral thermoregulation by mice and rats. In Monahan JC, D'Andrea JD (eds): *"Behavioral effects of microwave radiation absorption."* Publication FDA 85-8238. Washington DC: Department of Health and Human Services, pp 59-75.

Justesen DR, Adair ER, Stevens JC, Bruce-Wolfe V (1982): A comparative study of human sensory thresholds: 2450-MHz microwaves vs. far-infrared Radiation. *Bioelectromagnetics 3*:117-125.

King NW, Justesen DR, Clarke RL (1971): Behavioral sensitivity to microwave irradiation. *Science 172*:398-401.

Kluger MJ (1979): *"Fever: Its biology, evolution, and function"* Princeton: Princeton University Press, p 8.

Laties VG, Weiss B (1960): Behavior in the cold after acclimation. *Science 131*:1891-1892.

Laudenslager ML, Ryan SM, Drugen RC, Hyson RL, Maier SF (1983): Coping and immunosuppression: Inescapable but not escapable shock suppresses lymphocyte proliferation. *Science 221*:568-570.

Levinson DM, Justesen DR, Riffle DW (1985): Experimental analysis of aversive behavior: Mice and rats in intense microwave fields. In Monahan JC, D'Andrea JD (eds): *"Behavioral effects of microwave radiation absorption."* Publication FDA 85-8238. Washington DC: Department of Health and Human Services, pp 36-58.

Levinson DM, Grove AM, Clarke RL, Justesen DR (1982): Photic cueing of escape by rats from an intense microwave field. *Bioelectromagnetics 3:*105-116.

Lipton JM (1968): Effects of preoptic lesions on heat-escape responding and colonic temperature in the rat. *Physiol Behav 3:*165-169.

Lipton JM (1969): Effects of high-fat diets on caloric intake, body weight and heat-escape responses in normal and hyperphagic rats. *J Comp Physiol Psychol 68:*507-515.

Lipton JM, Marotto DR (1969): Effects of desalivation on behavioral thermoregulation against heat. *Physiol Behav 4:*723-727.

Lipton JM, Avery DD, Marotto DR (1970): Determinants of behavioral thermoregulation against heat: Thermal intensity and skin temperature levels. *Physiol Behav 5:*1083-1088.

Lowenstein E, Dallenback KM (1930): The critical temperatures for heat and burning heat. *Amer J Psychol 42:* 423-429.

Michaelson SM (1972): Cutaneous perception of microwaves. *J Microwave Power 7:*67-73.

Monahan JC, Henton WW (1977): Free-operant avoidance and escape from microwave radiation. In Hazzard DG (ed): *"Symposium on biological effects and measurement of radio-frequency/microwaves"* (Publ. [FDA] 77-8026). Bethesda MD: U.S. Public Health Service, pp 23-33.

Monahan JC, Ho HS (1977a): Microwave-induced avoidance behavior in the mouse. In Johnson CC, Shore ML (eds): *"Biological effects of electromagnetic waves"* (Publ. No. 77-8010). Washington DC: Dept. of Health, Education, and Welfare, pp 274-283.

Monahan JC, Ho, HS (1977b): The effect of ambient temperature on the reduction of microwave-energy absorption by mice. *Radio Science 12/6s:*257-262.

Murgatroyd D, Hardy JD (1970): Central and peripheral temperatures in behavioral thermoregulation of the rat. In Hardy JD, Gagge AP, Stolwijk JAJ (eds): *"Physiological and behavioral temperature regulation."* Springfield: Chas C Thomas, pp 874-891.

Satinoff E (1978): Neural organization and evolution of thermal regulation in mammals. *Science 201:*16-22.

Satinoff E, Hendersen R (1977): Thermoregulatory behavior. In Honig WK, Staddon JER (eds): *"Handbook of operant behavior."* Englewood Cliffs NJ: Prentice-Hall, pp 153-173.

Schwan HP, Anne A, Sher L (1966): *"Heating of living tissues."* Report ACEL-534, Naval Air Electronics Command. Philadelphia: U.S. Naval Air Engineering Center.

Skinner BF (1938): *"The behavior of organisms."* New York: Appleton-Century-Crofts: New York.

Sklar LS, Anisman H (1979): Stress and coping factors influence tumor growth. *Science 205:*513-515.

Slesin L (1983): Radiation accident at Alaska BMEWS radar station. *Microwave News 3:*1-3.

Stern S, Margolin L, Weiss B, Lu S-T, Michaelson SM (1979): Microwaves: Effect on thermoregulatory behavior of rats. *Science 206:*1198-1201.

Stevens JC (1982): Thermal sensation: Infrared and Microwaves. In Adair ER (ed): *"Microwaves and thermoregulation."* New York: Academic Press, pp 191-201.

Stevens JC, Marks LE, Simonson DC (1974): Regional sensitivity and spatial summation in the warmth sense. *Physiol and Behav 13:*825-836.

Vendrik AJH, Voss JJ (1958): Comparison of the stimulation of the warmth-sense organ by microwave and infrared. *J Appl Physiol 13:*435-444.

Visintainer MA, Volpicelli JR, Seligman MEP (1982): Tumor rejection in rat after inescapable or escapable shock. *Science 216:*437-439.

Weiss B (1957): Thermal behavior of the subnourished and pantothenic acid-deprived rat. *J Comp Physiol Psychol 50:*481-485.

Weiss JM (1968): Effects of coping responses on stress. *J Comp Physiol Psychol 65:*151-160.

Weiss JM (1971a): Effects of coping behavior in different warning-signal conditions on stress pathology of rats. *J Comp Physiol Psychol 77:*1-13.

Weiss JM (1971b): Effects of punishing the coping response (conflict) on stress pathology in rats. *J Comp Physiol Psychol 77:*14-21.

Weiss JM (1971c): Effects of coping behavior with and without a feedback signal on stress pathology in rats. *J Comp Physiol Psychol 77:*22-30.

Electromagnetic Fields and Neurobehavioral Function, pages 265–288

PRENATAL MICROWAVE EXPOSURE AND BEHAVIOR

Mary Ellen O'Connor

The University of Tulsa

Tulsa, Oklahoma

INTRODUCTION

Research conducted in the United States on radiofrequency radiation has been guided by attempts to determine safe levels of exposure to this type of radiation, particularly in the microwave range of the spectrum. In evaluating the potential biological impact of any environmental chemical or physical agent one of the most crucial questions is whether the agent can harm developing organisms. The effects from exposure to such agents may not be seen in adult organisms. In fact, they may only be observed in the offspring or, if mutagenic, in future generations. In this regard, previous investigations have been conducted to determine if microwave radiation can induce teratogenic or embryopathic effects in laboratory animals. Most of these studies employed a single, short term exposure to microwave radiation at a power level high enough to result in increased colonic temperature in the maternal subject, and thus her embryonic or fetal contents. Acute studies of this type have not resulted in embryopathic effects unless there was a significant thermal insult to the maternal subject, as documented by measurements of increased colonic temperature. Indeed, the doses at which teratogenesis has been observed are only slightly lower than ones that would result in death to the maternal organism due to hyperthermia (O'Connor, 1980; Berman et al, 1981; Lary et al, 1982).

Few studies have examined the teratogenic potential of multiple exposures to microwave radiation. Over the last several years the research at our laboratory has focused on relatively low-level (from 0 through 30 mW/cm2) exposure of laboratory rodents throughout the gestational period. The results from these studies indicate that exposure at levels as high as 30 mW/cm2 for 6 hours every day throughout the first 18 days of the gestational period does not induce embryopathic or teratogenic effects in either the mouse or the rat. Exposures of maternal guinea pigs to clearly thermal doses also failed to produce deleterious effects in the offspring (O'Connor and Strattan, 1985).

The failure to observe structural abnormalities at relatively low-levels of exposure does not necessarily indicate that there are no potentially harmful effects following long-term exposure to microwave radiation. When the endpoint assessed is structural abnormality, many proven toxic agents (eg, lead and mercury) do not appear to be teratogenic at low levels. Both lead and mercury are neurotoxic but the initial signs of their neurotoxicity are behavioral rather than anatomical. These behavioral symptoms are more subtle and often precede the appearance of more deleterious and life threatening conditions (Weiss, 1983; Fein et al, 1983). It is also true that some behavioral alterations such as poor judgement, loss of motor skills, addiction, etc. can be life threatening in some situations.

The use of the term subtle to describe these behavioral symptoms indicates that behavior can be more sensitive than other responses to some neurotoxic agents. As such, behavioral effects often are observable at low dosage levels where the response is highly variable. The inherent variability of responses at low doses can make the response appear to be elusive. Indeed, behavior is often described in such terms by investigators who are more accustomed to working with dose levels that are capable of inducing anatomical and structural abnormalities. It is the sensitivity of the behavioral response that makes it unique with respect to certain early signs of toxicity, specifically neurotoxicity. Studies that employ sensitive behavioral assays to search for effects at low dosage levels must also include methods to deal with the subtlety or elusiveness that accompanies responsivity in these highly variable ranges. It is the stimulus range or dosage level rather than the fact that the response studied is behavioral that accounts for the variability. When behavior is studied following or during exposure to high dosage levels of proven neurotoxins, the response is no more variable than are other biological indices of damage.

Studies in which postnatal psychophysiological measures were assessed following prenatal microwave exposure at 917-, 2450-, and 6000-MHz (Jensh et al, 1982; 1983; Jensh, 1984) did not produce consistent results. The exposures at 917 MHz apparently did not produce any long term neurophysiologic alterations, while the studies at 2450 MHz resulted in altered activity between the sexes. Some differences were observed at 6000 MHz and Jensh (1984) concluded that prenatal exposure may result in long term neurophysiological changes that are not detectable using standard teratological examination procedures.

The studies reported in this chapter were undertaken to expand our previous teratogenic investigations to include the examination of the potential of microwave radiation to induce behavioral teratogenesis. We chose to study behavior because it can be a sensitive index of neurotoxicity, but also because many of the standards that have been promoted with regard to exposure to microwave radiation have relied on behavioral data as a threshold point for effects. Recommendations for industrial and environmental exposure to radiofrequency radiation have been studied, debated and in some cases adopted by the American National Standards Institute (ANSI), the National Council on Radiation Protection and Measurements (NCRP), as well as the U.S. Environmental Protection Agency (EPA). As part of their effort to arrive at a recommendation, each of these groups attempted to evaluate the currently available behavioral data in the context of potential risk or harm to the human population. How behavioral changes can or should be used in this regard was addressed by all the groups. Apprently, each of the groups independently adopted the position that any effect, including behavioral alterations, should be considered a potential risk or hazard. This is a cautious but questionable position because behavioral symptoms can be, but are not always, early signs of neurotoxicity.

The term behavior refers to a general rather than a unitary process representing many different behaviors that reflect the output from many discrete neurological subsystems. As such, the number of ways in which behavior can be measured is myriad. In designing a behavioral teratology study, the first step is choosing the behavioral parameters that will most likely be effected by exposure to the suspected toxic agent, in this case microwave radiation. In many behavioral teratology studies several parameters are chosen for investigation and comprise a battery of behavioral tests to be made on each subject or on selected subsets of subjects (Norton, 1982). The potential for an effect to elude the investigation is probably increased when low dosages of the agent are employed. In this regard, the use of a battery rather than a single test is particularly important when relatively low dosage levels are being investigated. In determining which behavioral measures to use in the initial investigation, we examined existing reports of effects on laboratory rodents prenatally exposed to microwave radiation. The only consistent effect reported from teratogenic studies is smaller body mass (see O'Connor, 1980). This might indicate retarded growth and development that might be reflected behaviorally in measures of motor development and performance. Also, some preliminary reports had indicated that prenatally exposed rat pups showed signs of neurological changes in the cerebellar cortex (Albert et al, 1984). The battery of tests initially employed in our investigations included some tests for development of motor reflexes and skills, a two-way active avoidance test, and a test for activity and preferred ambient temperature.

GENERAL PROCEDURES

In all the studies reported in this chapter, the subjects were exposed prenatally, delivered naturally, and the pups were tested postnatally for behavioral changes relative to non-exposed control subjects. All of the microwave exposures were performed in a 10 x 10 x 8 ft anechoic chamber lined with absorber material and equipped with a 2450-MHz continuous wave (CW) microwave source. The horn antenna for the microwave power was mounted in the ceiling of the chamber. The maternal subjects were all naive prima-parous Long-Evans sperm-positive rats. During exposure the animals were enclosed in 10.16 cm diameter Plexiglas cylindrical holders and placed on a Styrofoam platform located 154.94 cm beneath the horn. The body of the 16.3 cm long holder sat approximately 2.5 cm off the platform and the cylinders were perforated throughout with 0.95 cm holes to allow for air flow. The temperature and humidity inside the chamber were automatically controlled (22° C, 50%). The subjects were exposed eight at a time for six hours daily from day 1 through day 18 or 19 of gestation. The first investigation exposed for 19 days beginning at 09:00 and the second exposed for 18 days beginning at 10:00. The eight containers were at least one wavelength from one another. Earlier mapping of the chamber with a Narda 8601 Radiation Monitor with an 8621 omnidirection probe indicated that the power density levels to which the rats in these studies were exposed was 27 to 30 mW/cm2.

The rats were born and bred in the colony at The University of Tulsa from stock originally obtained from Charles Rivers Laboratories. In the animal vivarium an ambient temperature of 70° F, relative humidity of 60-75%, and a 12/12 h light/dark cycle was maintained automatically. The animals were housed singly in wire hanging cages and water and laboratory rodent chow specifically formulated for pregnant rodents was available ad lib. Following the final day of exposure, each female was placed in an individual plastic cage with a pine shaving floor covering. The females were observed at least twice per day for birth of the litters.

INVESTIGATION I

In the initial study there were three groups of animals. One group was exposed to microwave radiation while another group was placed in the Plexiglas cylinders where they remained for the entire time that the first group was exposed to microwave radiation. This group is referred to as the holder-control group. The holder- controls were spatially arranged in the same configuration as the microwave-exposed group, but the holder-controls were located on a table in a room adjacent to the animal vivarium. This room was served by the same temperature and humidity control system as the animal vivarium. A third group of animals served as colony-cage controls. Following identification as sperm positive, the colony-cage controls were not handled except for routine maintenance. Of 49 females placed with males for mating, 19 were selected as sperm positive within 5 days of mating and 3 of these females were subsequently determined to be non-gravid. Following delivery 4 litters did not contain enough pups to be used in the study. At 7 days of age, each of the remaining 12 litters was culled to 7 pups. Measurements were thus obtained from 84 pups, 40 females and 44 males from 5 microwave-exposed, 3 holder-control, and 4 cage-control litters.

A number of assessments of ontogeny of behavior and functional development were performed on the offspring. The body mass of the subjects was recorded at birth and each day for the next 25 days. The day on which the subjects had open eyes was also recorded. When the subjects were 9 days of age, testing for accellerated air righting began. The pups were dropped (back downward) from a 30.5 cm height onto cotton bedding. The testing continued until all animals in the litter successfully landed on their feet three trials in a row or until the pups reached 25 days of age. The average for these trials became the righting score reported in Table 1. At least one full day after the pup's eyes were fully open they were tested in a visual cliff apparatus. The pup was placed on a 10.2 cm-wide platform separating the deep from the shallow side of the apparatus. The latency to choose a side was recorded along with the observation as to side chosen. Animals were allowed 180 seconds within which to choose. A trial was complete when the pup had all four feet on the glass. The visual cliff test was repeated when the animals were 28 days of age. The average latency for both trials as well as the average latency for the best of the two trials is presented in Table 1. At 25 days of age the animals were placed on an inclined plane and the time in which they climbed to the horizontal platform located at the top of a 45.7 cm plywood plane was noted. Each pup was given two trials and the average time across both trials as well as the average for the best trial (shortest time) is presented in Table 1. On day 36 the animals were placed in an 76.2 square cm open field apparatus for assessment of activity. The floor of the apparatus was sectioned into 25 , 16.2 square cm grids. The latency to leave the start position, and the number of squares traversed in 180 seconds was recorded along with the number of bolluses in the field and the number of times the animal urinated. This test was repeated on day 66 of age. At 122 days of age the animals were tested in a shuttle box for two-way avoidance. Each pup was given 25 trials per day until it reached the criteria of avoiding shock 22 out of 25 trials, or until a maximum of 200 trials had been attempted. Using analysis of variance, none of these measures of postnatal function and ontogeny of behavior resulted in statistically significant differences between our groups.

Since no single assessment produced a significant difference between groups of exposed and control animals, the ontogenetic measures were combined and a discriminant function analysis was performed to determine if there was a combination of certain tests that indicated differences among the groups. Such a multivariate technique provides a logical procedure for arriving at a relatively compact summary of the sources of the differences amoung the groups on the various dependent (ie, outcome) measures — including descriptions in terms of combinations of these variables that might never have been detected via univariate approaches (Harris, 1985). The results of this discriminant analysis indicated that seven variables were required to predict 91.7% of the cases. The adjusted means for the seven combined variables were 11.18 for the colony cage controls, 8.04 for the microwave exposed group, and − 28.3 for the holder control group. This analysis did not identify a special group of tests that indicated susceptibility to microwave exposure. Even when statistical significance was reached with seven of the variables, the majority of the variance was accounted for by the much lower scores achieved on several of the tests by the holder-control group. The mean litter score per group for each of the above variables is presented in Table 1. Of the 12 variables used in the discriminant analysis, the holder-control group scored lowest on 9 of them.

Table 1. Mean Values Per Litter Per Group For the Variables Included in the Discriminant Analysis

Variable	Control	Cage Holder	Micro-wave
Day of perfect righting	22.0	22.7	22.8
Mean righting score from days 9-25 (# trials)	1.70	1.85	1.61
Day eyes fully open	16.0	16.0	16.2
Mean of both trials for the visual cliff (secs.)	75.2	88.7	80.0
Best of both trials for the visual cliff (secs.)	14.5	12.7	15.4
Mean of both trials for the inclined plane (secs.)	19.3	16.1	17.9
Best of both trials for the inclined plane (secs.)	11.0	7.2	11.3
Activity in open field (# sections crossed)	65.2	57.0	73.2
Bolluses in open field	1.12	1.07	1.15
Urinations in open field	.47	.45	.54
Log of latency to leave start in open field	.73	.91	.74
Mean body mass for days 1 through 25 (grams)	30.3	28.3	28.3

When the subjects were 61 days of age they were given a test that was designed to assess both temperature preference and activity in a temperature gradient. For this study the animals were placed in a Styrofoam and Plexiglas alleyway that was 176 cm long, 24 cm wide, and 44 cm high.

The floor of the alleyway was divided into 12 equal segments. The alleyway was placed inside the anechoic chamber so that ambient air temperature could be varied using the air conditioning system and a series of standard incandescent light bulbs placed under the floor of the alleyway. The air temperature in the anechoic chamber was 16° C. The temperature in the alleyway varied from 17.25° C at one end to 38.29° C at the opposite end. The animals were given a 3-minute habituation trial in the alleybway 4 hours before the actual preference trial. The actual preference trial also lasted for 3 minutes. For data collection, the 3 minute trial was divided into 10 second intervals. The position of the animal in the alleyway as well as the number of times the animal crossed into a different segment of the alleyway was marked on a chart also at 10-second intervals. A small timing light outside the view of the animal aided the experimentor in observing the 10-second intervals. An average position score was calculated for each 10-second interval. This position score was converted to the corresponding temperature score. Individual means for the entire 3-minute trial were determined as were group means. The results showed a significant difference in the temperature choice of the three groups. The microwave-exposed animals spent more time in the coolest part of the alleyway. The average position scores for the microwave, holder-control, and cage-control groups were 6.58, 5.68, and 4.90 respectively. Converted to the corresponding temperatures in these segments, the average for the microwave group was 21.78° C while that for the holder-control group was 23.02° C and the colony cage-control average was 26.66° C.

These same animals were retested in the temperature gradient 4 months later. All of the groups had cooler preference scores but the differences between the groups were not statistically significant. The average for the microwave group was 20.38° C while that for the colony-cage control was 21.53° C and the holder-control average was 17.86° C. When the data from the two testing times was combined the differences were statistically significant.

Of all of the ontogenetic and behavioral measures that we assessed in these animals, the only measure that resulted in significant differences between the groups was temperature preference. One of the differences between this measure and the others is that it is a response to a thermal stimulus.

INVESTIGATION II

Based on the observation that a thermal stimulus produced a differential response in the groups in the first investigation, a second series of studies was designed to further explore prenatal microwave exposure and postnatal responsiveness to thermal cues. The exposure conditions for this second series of studies were the same as reported for the previous studies. Sperm-positive female Long-Evans rats were exposed to 2450-MHz CW microwave radiation for 6 hours daily on days 1 through 18 of gestation. The power density averaged 28 to 31 mW/cm2. The anechoic chamber was maintained at 22° C with 50 % relative humidity. All maternal subjects were born and bred in the laboratory and exposed in the same manner as the earlier study. However, in this study the holder-control group was replaced by a sham-exposure group that was positioned in the anechoic chamber without the microwave exposure. Since the animals were in the chamber 6 hours each day, the sham-exposure group could not be run contiguously with the microwave-exposure group without introducing circadian and other temporal variations. The microwave exposures were conducted each day until the sperm-positive females had completed 18 days of exposure. This same procedure was then repeated for the sham group. A colony-cage-control group was maintained during both the microwave and the sham exposure periods. Pre-exposure and post-exposure rectal temperatures were taken with a Bailey BAT3 thermometer and R3 probes on 2 animals from each of the three groups. Following the 18th exposure the females were placed in the home cage and observed daily for delivery of the litter.

Because of the practical considerations regarding the length of time required to perform these studies and the relatively small number of litters that might constitute the groups at the time of statistical analysis, two considerations guided the choice of the tests to be used in the second investigation.. The first consideration was that the test stimuli would involve a thermal component and the second was that the maximum amount of data would be obtained from each subject without confounding by earlier testing. The three measures chosen were sensitivity to thermally induced seizures, huddle size, and acitivity with and without a prior injection of caffiene.

The test used to assess sensitivity to thermally induced seizures was developed as a potential animal model to study febrile seizures in young mammals (Holtzman et al, 1981). The seizure study was conducted when the pups were 2 and 10 days of age. Selection of pups for this study contributed to the culling of the litters. The first reduction occurred when the litter was 2 days of age and half the number of pups above an n of 8 were chosen randomly from each litter to be subjects in the study. On day 10 the litters were culled to 8 pups each by using the remaining pups above an n of 8 in the seizure study (for example, in a litter of 14 pups, 3 were used in the day 2 test and 3 were used in the day 10 test leaving 8 pups for the other behavioral measures taken after day 11). The n of 8 was chosen based on the smallest litter that had been born when the first day 2 measures were taken. The number of pups used in this study numbered 107 from 23 litters.

The procedure for the seizure study was as follows. An Anchor Hocking glass dish measuring 22.5 x 13.0 x 5.7 cm was placed under a 300 watt

120 volt reflector floodlight. The inside of the dish was heated with the floodlight to 30° C. The pups were removed from their home cages, weighed, and their skin temperature was taken by placing a probe below the back of the head along the spine. A Bailey BAT8 thermometer and R3 probes were used. The animal was placed inside the glass dish which was covered with an aluminum lid so that the floodlight did not shine directly on the pup's skin surface. One probe was taped inside the glass chamber and another was used to measure skin temperature. The experimentor recorded the temperature of the glass chamber as the pup was placed in it, the latency of the pup to seizure, the temperature of the chamber at the time a seizure began, and the skin temperature of the pup following removal from the chamber. The results of the study were analyzed by a 2 x 3 (age x exposure condition) analysis of variance and the Duncan method of post hoc comparisons.

The results for the pre-seizure and the post-seizure skin temperatures showed that all of the measurements taken when the pups were 2 days old differed from all of the day-10 measurements (p's <0.0001). However, for both the 2-day-old and the 10-day-old pups, the pre-seizure skin temperature was not different for the microwave-exposed, sham-exposed or cage-control groups. The post-exposure skin temperatures following seizure did not differ within the day-2 group or within the day-10 group, but as mentioned previously, all the day-2 measures were lower than those taken on day 10.

When chamber temperature was analyzed, there was a significant effect for age at time of testing (p <0.05). The pre-exposure chamber temperature for the cage-controls on day 2 (31.3° C) differed from that of both the microwave-exposure group (30.6° C) and the sham-exposure group (30.5° C). More of the cage-control animals were available on the very first day of testing and the data were collected before a method for cooling the chamber between testings had been adopted. For this reason pre-exposure chamber temperature was covaried out for the latency to seizure, as well as for the pre-seizure and post-seizure skin temperature data. These analyses of covariance produced the same conclusions as the regular analyses of variance. Means of post-exposure chamber temperature did not differ.

Both exposure condition ($\underline{F}$ = 10.152, $\underline{p}$ < 0.0001) and age ($\underline{F}$ = 233.308, $\underline{p}$ <0.0001) were significant sources of variation. The average latencies to seizure were 529 seconds for the cage-control group, 480 seconds for the sham group, and 601 seconds for the microwave group when tested on day 2 of age. The microwave-exposure group's latency to seizure was significantly longer than either the sham- or the cage-control groups but the sham- and cage-control groups did not differ from one another. On day 10 the average latencies were longer for all of the groups. Comparing the day-10 averages showed that the sham-control group (761 seconds) was significantly lower than either the microwave (882 seconds) or cage-control (907 seconds) groups. The microwave-exposed pups exhibited longer latencies on day 2 and their average latency between day 2 and day 10 did not increase as much as the latency for the sham-exposed and cage-control groups.

Microwave radiation has been shown to alter the thermoregulatory behavior of both the squirrel monkey and the rat (Adair and Adams, 1980; Stern et al. 1979). The second assay chosen for inclusion in this series of studies was a non-invasive measure of thermoregulatory behavior. When placed together, young rodents form huddles. Tight huddles are associated with increased body warmth, while loose huddles are associated with cooler temperatures at the skin surface of the young rat (Alberts, 1968). Measuring the size of these huddles does not require any handling of the pups, and thus results in minimal reduction in the pup's experimental naievity that might confound later measures. The size of the huddles was measured at 5, 10, and 15 days of age.

To measure the huddle size, the home cage was removed from the rack and the dam and any more than 8 pups were removed from the cage. The cage was placed under a tripod on which a 35 mm camera was mounted. After a 15 minute adaptation period, 4 photographs were taken at 15 minute intervals. On each of the 3 days, four measurements were taken for 8 cage-control litters, 8 sham-exposed litters, and 13 microwave-exposed litters. Ambient temperature at the time the photograph was taken was also recorded. The slides were developed and projected onto a chalkboard. The projector was positioned 267 cm from the chalkboard and the zoom lens was placed in the most retracted position. The outer perimeter of the huddle was traced with chalk. One tracing was done with the tails included and one tracing excluded the tails of the pups. The length of this chalk line was then traced and measured with a hodometer. The average of the 4 pictures excluding tails for each day was used in the analysis of variance.

The results of this study showed that the average huddle size was significantly different for the 5-day-old sham-exposed and cage control groups. These two measures were statistically different from all other measures. At day 5 the cage-control huddles measured 101.6 cm and the sham-exposed huddles were 101.5 cm. In contrast, the microwave-exposed pup's huddles were 78.7 cm. By day 10 the huddle size for the three groups was 72.4 cm, 74.1 cm, and 82.2 cm respectively. The mean huddle size on day 15 was 84.1 cm, 74.9 cm, and 78.3 cm. The microwave-exposed pups differed only slightly across the 5-, 10-, and 15-day measures. The cage-control and sham-exposed animals formed much larger huddles at 5 days of age than they did at 10 or 15 days.

Another area of considerable interest with regard to the behavioral effects of microwave radiation involves its potential interaction with drugs, particularly with drugs that are commonly

used.   Caffiene is a widely used,   relatively
mild   central   nervous system stimulant   that is
reported to   result   in mild decreases   in body
temperature   as   well   as   increases   in   motor
activity (Greenblat and Osterberg,   1961).   As
such, the third behavioral assay chosen for the
study was activity, measured with and without an
injection of caffeine. This study was conducted
when the pups were 16 days of age. Since this
study   required giving each of the pups an
injection of caffeine or saline, it was the final
study that was performed as part of this series
of investigations.

For   activity measures, first the dam was
separated   from   the   litter by placing her in
another cage.   A pup was selected at random and
injected with saline or 25 mg/kg caffeine and
sodium benzoate in equal parts. Due to the nearly
identical body mass of the pups, each pup was
injected   with approximately 0.08 cc of the
substance.   The   injections were i.p. and were
followed   by   a 15 minute   waiting   period.
Following this period, the pup was placed in the
open field and the number of times that it
crossed a grid line was scored during a 3 minute
period.   The open field apparatus is the same as
described for the first series of studies.   The
pup was removed from the activity chamber and
rectal temperature was taken. The analyses of
variance   indicated   that   no   statistically
significant differences were observed for either
the activity measures or the rectal temperatures.

In the second series of studies, measures
that had not produced significant differences in
earlier studies were not repeated.   Since no
ontogenetic or developmental differences were
observed   in the first investigation,   these
reflexive and motor development measures were not
included in the second investigation.   Removing
these measures also reduced the handling of the
animals to no more than necessary to complete the
three segments of the second investigation. Also
in the first investigation, no differences in the
body mass of pups was observed at birth or on the

25 consecutive days on which body mass was assessed. As such, body mass was only assessed on days in which the pups were scheduled for the seizure or the caffeine and activity study.

In the second investigation the mean litter size of the microwave-exposed litters was 9.64 while the sham-exposed was 10.5 and the cage control was 12.0. It has been reported that exposure to microwave radiation at levels similar to those used in this study results in reduced fetal body mass and increased numbers of resorptions (see O'Connor, 1980). We did not observe postnatal differences in body mass of pups but the smaller litter sizes might be a reflection of an increased resorption rate in the microwave-exposed maternal subjects. After all three parts of the second study were completed, these same maternal subjects were rebred and the number of pups in the second litter was noted. The size of the litters was 11.75, 14.25, and 13.86 for the cage-control, sham-, and microwave-exposed dams. There was a significant difference in litter size between the first and second breeding for the microwave-exposed (t = 2.81, p <0.01) and for the sham-exposed (t = 2.61, p <0.03) groups. The similar litter sizes at second breeding supports the idea that the smaller litter size in the initial breeding was related to a higher rate of resorptions.

Since the number of pups in the litter could have influenced the behavioral measurements, litters with fewer than 8 pups were not used in the studies. An analysis of variance for litter size was conducted for each of the three studies and in no case was there a significant difference in litter size for the litters actually used in the study.

DISCUSSION

Three statistically significant findings emerged from these investigations. Compared with the control groups, the microwave-exposed pups showed a preference for the cooler sections of the temperature-graded alleyway, longer latencies to thermally-induced seizures, and they formed smaller huddles at 5 days of age. In the temperature gradient, the microwave-exposed subjects behaved in a manner that should have resulted in cooler air temperatures at the skin surface, whereas the formation of tighter huddles should have resulted in a warmer skin surface. In the seizure study the longer latencies to seizure were not associated with differences in either pre- or post-seizure skin temperature, nor were differences noted in the temperature of the chamber at the time the seizure began.

This data could be interpreted in several ways and the conclusion to be drawn considering the three findings collectively is not obvious to this author. The apparent lack of clear, consistent, and seemingly logical effects following exposure of laboratory animals to microwave radiation has proven frustrating to investigators in this field. However, such difficulty with regard to interpretation of results from several different studies is not unusual and it is certainly not unique to investigations of non-ionizing radiation. Studies on the response of laboratory rodents to stress contain many examples of experiments for which the results are difficult to interpret. In some cases experimental conditions that are thought to be quite similar produce opposite results. To the contrary, a similar result is sometimes obtained when experimental conditions are very different, eg, overexposure and underexposure to the same class of stimuli (Miller, 1981).

It is sometimes assumed that developmental changes induced by environmental conditions are deliterious to the organism. However, it is possible that rather than retard development, these exposures enhanced fetal development with regard to the control of the response to thermal stress. The levels of microwave radiation to which the subjects in these two investigations were prenatally exposed should not induce extreme temperature changes in either the maternal or the fetal subject. Post-exposure temperatures were not taken on the maternal subjects in the first set of investigations but rectal temperatures from other studies in our laboratory at similar power densities for similar periods of time have demonstrated measureable temperature increments. Also, the post-exposure temperature of the microwave-exposed maternal subjects in the second investigation was 2° C higher than that of the sham-exposed or cage-control maternal subjects. The microwave exposure that these subjects received throughout prenatal development should induce a temperature increase in both the maternal organism and also in the developing embryos and fetuses. The temperature increase in the uterine contents could result from direct heating as well as from heating via the dam's temperature and blood flow. Whether these pups were hotter or cooler than the maternal subject as a result of these processes can not be determined.

In interpreting the results it is important to note that the subjects in the first investigation were 61 days old when they were first tested in the temperature gradient. In contrast the seizure study was performed on 2-day or 10-day old pups and the huddles were measured when the pups were 5, 10, and 15 days of age. Younger pups have fewer mechanisms for maintaining body temperature. As such the performance of the the microwave-exposed pups was similar to what would be expected of slightly older animals in their choice of cooler temperatures in the alleyway and in their formation of tighter huddles. In the seizure study the microwave-exposed pups had longer latencies to seizure. The fact that the latency to seizure was longer while the post-seizure skin temperature did not differ across the groups might be due to the fact that the temperature of the microwave-exposed pups takes longer to rise to the point where a seizure would be induced. It has been well documented that latency to seizure increases with age as does the occurrence and severity of the seizures (Holtzman et al, 1981).

The microwave-exposed pups differed between the 2- and the 10-day measures as did the sham and cage control pups. However, the longer latency to seizure exhibited by the microwave-exposed pups at the 2-day assessment resembled the response expected from an older pup.

It has been reported that rat pups form smaller huddles with increasing age (Alberts, 1968). It might be that in very young pups, the huddle formation is actually maintained by the mother and the younger pups may not have the motor coordination to form the huddle once the mother is removed. This might explain the difference in huddle sizes between the 5-, 10-, and 15-day measurements, but it is not a very likely explanation for the tighter huddles in the microwave exposed pups at 5 days of age. A difference in motor coordination is not likely since the first series of studies included measures of motor development and no indication of enhanced or retarded motor development was observed in any of the groups.

The caffeine study did not result in any differences between the groups. This study was included because some of the most frequently cited studies with regard to behavioral effects following microwave exposure are those of Thomas et al, (1979a; 1979b; and 1980) showing synergistic effects of microwave radiation with several psychoactive drugs. Thomas's studies reported alterations in schedule-controlled (ie, operant behavior) at relatively low-levels of microwave exposure.

When we began our studies, there was a growing literature on behavioral effects during or following microwave exposure. However, in the majority of these studies behavior was examined during or following exposure of a few minutes or hours, and there were only a few studies based on prenatal exposures (Johnson et al, 1977; Jensh et al, 1982, 1983; Jensh, 1984). The apparent reluctance to examine behavioral teratology is probably due in part to practical considerations

in setting up the exposure conditions. Long-term
studies obviously require a lengthy committment
of exposure facilities and other resources. The
exposure facilities impose technical limits on
the number of animals that can be exposed at any
one time. Additionally, in a teratogenic study
the number of sperm-positive females that are
actually gravid is not known until after the
exposures have taken place. These factors place
unavoidable limits on the number of subjects that
may actually be available for postnatal testing
and subsequent statistical analysis.

The results of these studies support but
certainly do not confirm our original hypotheses.
Behavior was chosen as the endpoint in these
studies because it has been shown to be
particularly sensitive to other forms of
neurotoxins. Earlier work indicated that
prenatal exposure to microwave radiation at
levels similar to those used in the present
investigations did not result in skeletal or
physiological abnormalities. However, in the
investigations summarized in this chapter we do
report behavioral changes in the prenatally
exposed groups. The tests chosen for inclusion in
the battery were not expected to be equally
sensitive to microwave radiation and most of the
measures we employed did not differ as a result
of prenatal microwave exposure. Of particular
interest is the fact that the tests that did
result in significant differences all contained
some thermal component.

SUMMARY

The hypotheses for the initial
investigation was based on the idea that failure
to observe structural teratogenesis following
microwave exposure did not preclude the
possibility that such exposure would result in
behavioral changes. We also proposed that such
exposure might specifically alter some aspect of
thermoregulatory behavior. The results of these
studies support both of these hypotheses.
Whether the studies show enhanced thermal

sensitivity or enhanced development, they do support the hypothesis that prenatal exposure to microwave radiation is more likely to alter postnatal sensitivity to thermally related stimuli or conditions as compared to stimuli that are thermally neutral.

ACKNOWLEDGEMENTS

Our laboratory has been generously supported by the United States Environmental Protection Agency, The Office of Naval Research, and The University of Tulsa Faculty and Student Grant Program. The author is indebted to Drs. Robert Strattan, David Bartsch and James Sanza, as well as Mr. Jack Proksa, Mrs. Debra Tremble Limbocker, Mrs. Pam Hons Jones, Ms. Monica Indart, and Mr. James Chrobak for their assistance with these studies.

REFERENCES

Adair ER, Adams BW (1980). Microwaves modify thermoregulatory behavior in squirrel monkey. Bioelectromagnetics 1:1.

Alberts JR (1978). Huddling by rat pups: Group behavioral mechanisms of temperature regulation and energy conservation. J Comp Physio Psych 92:231.

Albert EN, Cohen G, Avelino L, Kornhouser G, Sherif M, Gage M, Monahan J (1984). Effects of microwave exposure on cerebellar purkinje cells and synaptogenesis. Program Abstracts, Gaithersburg, MD: Bioelectromagnetics Society, p 52.

Berman E, Carter HB, House D (1981). Observations of rat fetuses after irradiation with 2450-MHz (CW) microwaves. J Microwave Power 16:9.

Fein GG, Schwartz PM, Jacobson SW, Jacobson JL (1983). Environmental toxins and behavioral development. Amer Psychol 38:1188.

Greenblat EN, Osterberg AC (1961). Correlations of activating and lethal effects of excitory drugs in grouped and isolated mice. J Pharmac Exper Ther 181:115.

Harris RJ, (1985). "A primer of multivariate statistics." New York: Academic Press, Inc.

Hjeresen DL (1984). A microwave hyperthermia model of febrile convulsions. Dissertation Abstracts International 45B:1616.

Holtzman D, Obana K, Olson J (1981). Hyperthermia-induced seizures in the rat pup: A model for febrile convulsions in children. Science 213:1034.

Jensh RP (1984). Studies of the teratogenic potential of exposure of rats to 6000-MHz microwave radiation: II. Postnatal psychophysiologic evaluations. Radiat Res 97:282.

Jensh RP, Vogel WH, Brent RL (1982). Postnatal functional analysis of prenatal exposure of rats to 915 MHz microwave radiation. J Am Coll Toxicol 1:73.

Jensh RP, Vogel WH, Brent RL (1983). An evaluation of the teratogenic potential of protracted exposure of pregnant rats to 2450 MHz microwave radiation: II. postnatal psychophysiologic analysis. J Toxicol Environ Health 11:37.

Johnson RB, Mizumori S, Lovely RH (1977). Adult behavioral deficit in rats exposed prenatally to 918-MHz microwaves. In " Developmental Toxicology of Energy Related Polutants," D.O.E. Symposium Series 47, p 281.

Lary JM, Conover DL, Foley ED, Hanser PL (1982). Teratogenic effects of 27.12 MHz radiofrequency radiation in rats. Teratology 26:299.

Miller NE (1981). An overview of behavioral medicine: Opportunities and Dangers. In Weiss SM, Herd JA, Fox BH (eds): "Perspectives on Behavioral Medicine," New York: Academic Press, p 3.

Norton, S (1982). Methods in behavioral toxicology. In Hayes AW (ed): "Principles and methods of toxicology," New York: Raven Press. p 353.

O'Connor ME (1980). Mammalian teratogenesis and radiofrequency fields. Proc IEEE 68:56.

O'Connor ME, Strattan R (1985): "Teratogenic

effects of microwave radiation." Final Report, available as PB 85-207 462/AS from Springfield VA: National Technical Information Service.

Stern SL, Margolin L, Weiss B, Lu S, Michaelson SM (1979). Microwaves: Effect on thermoregulatory behavior in rats. Science 206:1198.

Thomas JR, Maitland G (1979a). Microwave radiation and dextroamphetamine: Evidence of combined effects on behavior of rats. Radio Sci 14:253.

Thomas JR, Burch LS, Yeandle SS (1979b). Microwave radiation and chlordiazepoxide: Synergistic effects on fixed-interval behavior. Science 203:1357.

Thomas JR, Schrot J, Banvard RA (1980). Behavioral effects of chlorpromazine and diazepam combined with low-level microwaves. Neurobehav Toxicol 2:131

Weiss B (1983) Behavioral toxicology and environmental health science: Opportunity and challenge for psychology. Amer Psychol 38:1174.

Electromagnetic Fields and Neurobehavioral Function, pages 289–308
© 1988 Alan R. Liss, Inc.

REDUCED EXPOSURE TO MICROWAVE RADIATION BY RATS: FREQUENCY SPECIFIC EFFECTS

John A. D'Andrea, Ph.D., John R. DeWitt, Ph.D.
Lupita M. Portuguez, M.S. and Om P. Gandhi, Sc.D.

Departments of Psychology and Electrical Engineering
University of Utah, Salt Lake City, Utah 84112

ABSTRACT

Previous research has shown that SAR "hotspots" are induced within the laboratory rat and that the resulting thermal hotspots are not entirely dissipated by bloodflow. Two experiments were conducted to determine if hotspot formation in the body and tail of the rat, which is radiation frequency specific, would have behavioral consequences. In the first experiment rats were placed in a plexiglas cage one side of which, when occupied by the rat, commenced microwave radiation exposure; occupancy of the other side terminated exposure. Groups of rats were tested during a baseline period to determine the naturally preferred side of the cage. Subsequent exposure to 360-MHz, 700-MHz or 2450-MHz microwave radiation was made contingent on preferred-side occupancy. A significant reduction in occupancy of the preferred side of the cage, and hence, microwaves subsequently occurred. Reduced exposure to 360-MHz and 2450-MHz microwaves at 1, 2, 6 and 10 W/kg were significantly different from 700-MHz microwaves. In the second experiment semichronic exposures revealed the threshold for reduced exposure of 2450-MHz microwaves to be located between whole-body SAR's of 2.1 and 2.8 W/kg.

INTRODUCTION

It is well known that microwave-radiation absorption can vary dramatically with radiation frequency, orientation, body size and shape of the experimental animal (Gandhi, 1974; Durney, et. al. 1978). But most studies of behavioral and physiological effects of microwave-radiation absorption have been conducted at a limited number of radiation frequencies (ie 2450 MHz and 915 MHz), where sufficient power can be generated at low cost. Little is known about behavioral and physiological responses of animals when exposed to microwave radiation at other frequencies, especially for exposures near the whole-body resonant frequency. Since the potential for human exposure can encompass a large portion of the radiofrequency and microwave spectrum, the generation of an animal database for a corresponding portion of the spectrum would be of value in assessment of human exposure hazards. The behavioral experiments reported here comprise one aspect of a research project designed to evaluate the dose-response effects on the behavior of rats at several radiation frequencies at and near the whole-body resonant frequency. In our previously published dosimetry experiments, we have determined both the whole-body averaged specific absorption rate (SAR) as well as the distribution of SAR within the body and tail of the rat for below-resonant, resonant and above-resonant radiation frequencies (D'Andrea et al., 1985). Microwave-induced hotspots occur in the tail and rectum of the rat at 360 MHz and 2450 MHz; these exceed the whole-body averaged SAR by factors of fifty times and eighteen times, respectively. These areas of high energy absorption have generally been thought to be of little consequence when predicting thermal effects of microwave exposure, because it has been presumed that convective heat transfer via the circulatory system redistributes any localized heating. The maximum thermal effect would then be reflected in generalized, rather than localized hyperthermia. However, in a recent experiment by Emmerson et al. (1985) using ketamine-HCL anesthetized rats with circulatory function intact, it was found that localized temperature increases during exposure to 2450-MHz and 360-MHz microwaves remained much greater at hotspot sites than other body sites. The temperature increases at rectum and tail were significantly greater for rats irradiated at 360-MHz and 2450-MHz than those of rats irradiated at 700-MHz. This effect was found for whole-body SAR's as low as 6 W/kg at 360-MHz and 10 W/kg at 2450-MHz. Dosimetry can be used to describe hotspots, but their ultimate significance can only be determined by their influences on alert, behaving animals. This report describes a first attempt to evaluate the effects of microwave radiation frequencies which produce hotspots within the body as indexed by behavioral analyses. Specifically, reduced exposure to microwave fields at three different radiation frequencies with power densities adjusted to give equal whole-body SAR's was measured. Two experiments were performed: in the first avoidance of acute exposure to microwave radiation at 360-MHz, 700-MHz and 2450-MHz was assessed; while in the second, avoidance of semichronic exposure to microwaves at 2450-MHz was measured.

Experiment 1: Behavioral Effects of Acute Microwave Exposure at 360 MHz, 700 MHz and 2450 MHz

METHODS AND MATERIALS

Subjects. The subjects were 48 male Long-Evans rats obtained from Simonsen Laboratories, Gilroy, California, with body masses ranging from 300 to 345 g. The rats were housed individually in hanging rodent cages with free access to tap water and Simonsen No. 7 rodent chow. The lights of the colony room cycled on and off (12 h light-dark), and the room was maintained at an average temperature of 22 degrees celcius (+- 2); relative humidity ranged from 20 to 40 percent as measured by a hygrometric recorder (Rustrak No. 225). All rats were given a 14-day period to acclimate both to the colony room and to daily handling before commencement of the experiment.

APPARATUS

Exposure system 1. This exposure system consisted of an anechoic chamber (7 x 6 x 3.4 m, outside dimension) that was constructed with a metal framework and lined with sheet metal. As illustated in Fig. 1, the interior of the chamber was covered entirely with pyramidal-shaped absorbing material (VHP-24). It contained a suspension floor made of plastic (both Emmerson-Cumming Inc.). The chamber was equipped with a climate-control system (Fedders CKC 060D0B), houselights, and a closed-circuit television monitor. For radiation frequencies of 360 MHz and 700 MHz a dipole antenna mounted within a V-shaped metal reflector was used. Construction of the dipole antenna followed the design of Harris (1972), with removable radiating elements (lamda/4) for each radiation frequency. The dipole was mounted within the metal reflector, which was constructed of aluminum sheet

(90 x 320 cm, 3.18 mm thick). The reflector was supported on a plastic pipe framework 122 cm above the plastic subfloor of the anechoic chamber.

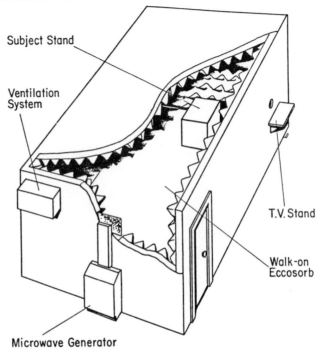

Subject Stand

Ventilation System

T.V. Stand

Walk-on Eccosorb

Microwave Generator

Fig. 1 Schematic representation of the chamber used for exposures to 360-MHz, 700-MHz or 2450 MHz.

For exposures at 2450 MHz, a horn antenna (radiating apeture 34 x 48 cm) was constructed from copper sheet to match a WR-284 waveguide. Microwave power (CW) at 360 MHz and 700 MHz was obtained from 1 kW cavity amplifiers (MCL No. 10110) which were driven by low power oscillators (MCL No. 15222). Power from each source was delivered to the dipole antenna via a coaxial cable (Andrew No. FHJ5). Impedances of the transmission line and antenna were matched by a double-stub tuner. Power delivered to the antenna was measured by a coaxial directional coupler (Bendix No. 538-009) and a digital power meter (Hewlett Packard No. 436A). Microwave power (CW) at 2450 MHz was obtained from a magnetron (Litton 2M53) energized by a variable low-ripple high-voltage power supply and was delivered to the horn antenna via the WR-284 waveguide. A triple-stub waveguide tuner was used to match impedances of the waveguide and horn antenna. Power delivered to the horn antenna was measured by a crossguide directional coupler (Sperry No. 300) and a digital power meter (Hewlett Packard No. 436A). For each antenna, power density was mapped in the area to be occupied by a rat, using omnidirectional field probes (Holaday No. 3002 and Narda No. 8616). The rat, held in a plexiglas cage, was placed 180 cm in front of the irradiating antenna on a styrofoam platform in the E-polarization vector; and was visually monitored via a closed circuit television camera situated 2 m behind and 1 m to the left of the antenna. At 360-MHz and 700-MHz a coaxial switch (Andrew No. 295, 24 V DC operated) which controlled exposure to microwaves was placed between the low power oscillator and the high power amplifier. Exposure of a rat to microwave radiation at either side of the plexiglas cage (see Fig. 2) was programmed using relay circuitry to operate the coaxial switch. For exposures at 2450-MHz the relay circuitry operated a solid state switch which controlled the high voltage output to the magnetron.

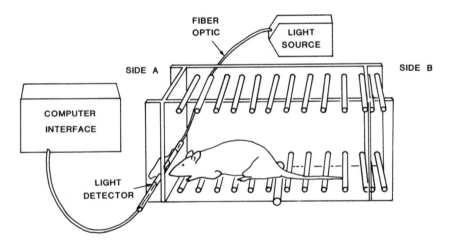

Fig. 2 Schematic representation of the Plexiglas rat cage illustrating the fiberoptic light system to determine the occupied side of the cage by detecting vertical tilt.

Behavioral measurement. The Plexiglas cage (40 x 10 x 9.5 cm interior dimensions) was constructed using Plexiglas sheet (.16 cm thick) for the sides and ends and Plexiglas rods (.31 cm diameter) for the top and floor. The cage, as depicted in Fig. 2, was designed to tilt (4 mm vertical movement at the end) on a Plexiglas rod (.95 cm diameter), which served as a pivot. A fiberoptic light system was used to determine the occupied side of the cage; it detected the vertical tilt at one end of the cage caused by the weight of a rat. White noise was used within the anechoic chamber to mask noise of relay circuitry and microwave power sources and was 70 dBA as measured in the Plexiglas cage with a sound level meter (Quest No. 100).

PROCEDURE

The rats were randomly divided into twelve groups of four each. They were then given twelve one hour sessions (one session per day) in the plastic cage. Sessions 1-4 (baseline) allowed for exploration and adaptation by an animal to the Plexiglas cage and to determine the side of the cage initially preferred by each rat, as evidenced by the side in which the greatest amount of occupancy time occurred. Time spent on each side of the Plexiglas cage and the number of crossovers between the two halves of the cage, were determined by both relay circuitry and pen movements on a stripchart recorder. The preferred side of the plexiglas cage was determined for each rat; this was followed by eight additional one hour sessions during which exposure to microwaves could occur. During sessions 5-8, time that the rat spent on the prefered side of the plexiglas cage resulted in microwave exposure; while during sessions 9-12 time spent on the original nonpreferred side of the cage resulted in microwave exposure. In a 3 x 4 factorial design, each group of rats was subjected to one radiation frequency and one whole-body SAR (360 MHz, 700 MHz or 2450 MHz; 1 W/kg, 2 W/kg, 6 W/kg or 10 W/kg). The field power densities used at each radiation frequency to achieve equal whole-body SAR's are reported in Table 1.

To evaluate time spent on the different sides of the cage during the course of the experiment, a difference score analysis was performed. The average time spent on each side of the Plexiglas cage during sessions 5-8 was subtracted from the average time for sessions 1-4 (Phase-1); while the average scores for sessions 9-12 were subtracted from those of sessions 5-8 (Phase-2). Large positive difference scores reflect less time spent on that side of the cage, and consequently less exposure to microwaves tolerated by the animals. On the contrary, large negative scores reflect more time spent on the side of the cage producing microwave radiation.

TABLE 1

FREQUENCY	WHOLE-BODY AVERAGED SPECIFIC ABSORPTION RATE			
	1 W/kg	2 W/kg	6 W/kg	10 W/kg
	INCIDENT FIELD POWER DENSITY - mW/cm2			
360 MHz -	3.8	7.7	23.1	38.5
700 MHz -	1.4	2.7	8.2	13.7
2450 MHz -	4.2	8.3	25.0	41.7

Whole-body averaged SAR for 1 mW/cm2 incident-

360 MHz - 0.26 W/kg
700 MHz - 0.72 W/kg
2450 MHz - 0.24 W/kg

Table 1. Microwave field power densities used to achive equated whole-body SAR's at each frequency.

RESULTS

The durations of microwave exposures received by the various groups of rats differed significantly as a function of both radiation frequency and whole-body SAR. This finding is reflected in Fig. 3 which presents the difference scores for each radiation frequency and SAR. During 700-MHz exposures at 1 and 2 W/kg, the animals did not leave the preferred side of the cage but actually spent more time on the preferred side during microwave exposure than was measured during the baseline period (as evidenced by the negative difference scores). At whole-body SAR's of 6 and 10 W/kg the rats exposed to 700 MHz spent less time in the microwave fields. However, rats exposed to 360 MHz and 2450 MHz spent considerably less time in the microwave fields than was observed for exposures at 700 MHz (as evidenced by the large positive difference scores). A split-plot analysis of variance for a repeated measures design was used to evaluate the difference scores (Kirk, 1968). There was an

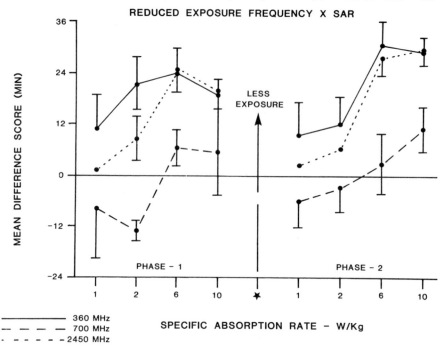

Fig. 3 Experiment-1 mean (+-SEM) difference scores for rats exposed to microwave radiation at 360-MHz, 700-MHz or 2450-MHz. Positive difference scores reflect less exposure to microwaves.

overall significant difference between the exposure frequencies of 360-MHz, 700-MHz, and 2450-MHz [F(2,36)=11.85, P <.001] and between the whole-body SAR's of 1, 2, 6, and 10 W/kg [F(3,36)=7.02, P <.001]. The Tukey HSD multiple comparison of means test (Kirk, 1968) revealed that all means of exposures at 700 MHz were significantly different from means at 360 MHz and 2450 MHz (P <.05). The comparisons between means of 360-MHz and 2450 MHz revealed significant differences only at 1 and 2 W/kg (P < .05).

Finally, a comparison of performance under both exposure contingencies (Phase-1 and Phase-2) showed no differences. This must indicate that the rats were able to determine the side of the cage which produced microwave exposure even after the exposure contingencies were reversed.

The number of crossovers within the Plexiglas cage, as shown in Fig. 4, did not differ for the groups during the

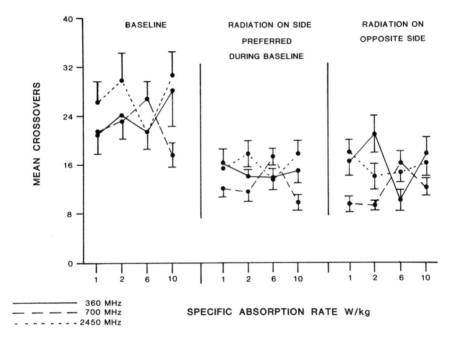

CROSSOVERS X FREQUENCY X SAR

Fig. 4 Experiment 1: Mean crossovers (+-SEM) in the Plexglas cage for rats exposed to microwave radiation at 360-MHz, 700-Mhz or 2450-MHz.

baseline period but did show a significant decrease across the varying conditions of exposure. A split-plot analysis of variance for repeated measures confirmed significance of the decrease [F(11,396)=40.42, P <.001] but did not reveal any significant differences between radiation frequency or whole-body SAR.

CONCLUSIONS

A comparison of the difference scores and crossovers during the course of the experiment indicates that the rats entered and exited the half of the cage which resulted in microwave exposure nearly equally for all frequencies and whole-body SAR's; however, as compared to that for 700-MHz exposures, time on the exposure side of the cage during 360-MHz and 2450-MHz exposures was significantly reduced. This is an interesting outcome since the whole-body SAR's for the varying treatments were made nearly equal. The results of this experiment are, however, in concert with those of our earlier studies on the dosimetry and thermal response of rats exposed to these radiation frequencies (D'Andrea et al., 1985; Emmerson et al., 1985). The actual measurement of whole-body SAR and distributed SAR during behavioral performance of the avoidance task would provide a more direct correlation of microwave induced hotspots and behavioral performance. At the present time, however, this approach is technically impossible since invasive methods must be employed to measure distributed SAR's within the body.

Experiment 2: Behavioral Effects of Semichronic Microwave Exposure at 2450 MHz

METHODS AND MATERIALS

Subjects. The subjects were 80 male Long-Evans rats with body masses ranging from 325 to 350 g. The rats were housed individually as in Experiment-1 and had ad libitum access to food and water, except during periods of sham- and microwave-exposure.

APPARATUS

Exposure system 2. A microwave anechoic chamber (outside dimensions 3.5 x 3.5 x 2.75 m) was constucted of Plywood and divided into two identical subchambers by a partition covered with thin aluminum sheet; it is schematically illustrated in Fig. 5. The partitions formed a ground plane within each chamber. Monopole antennas (0.25-lambda length and 9.53-mm dia.) were mounted at the center

of each ground plane. Other interior surfaces of the
chambers were covered with a pyramidally shaped Eccosorb
(Emmerson and Cumming VHP-12). The end doors are shown open
to illustrate styrofoam supports, which were mounted on the
aluminum ground plane, and were used to hold Plexiglas
cages. Eight styrofoam supports were positioned in a
circular array 90 cm from the monopole antenna of each
chamber. In the configuration shown, the electric field was
parallel to the long axis of the Plexiglas cage and, thus,
of the rat. Each chamber was equipped with one ventilating
fan (0.1m/s averaged lineal velocity air flow) and a

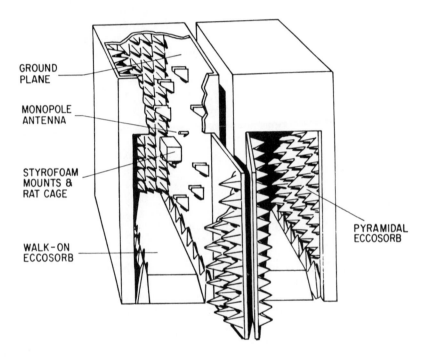

Fig. 5 Schematic representation of the monopole-above-ground
microwave exposure chamber used for 2450-MHz exposures in
Experiment-2.

houselight (40 W). The houselight and fans were mounted on
the wall opposite the monopole antenna. Excrement was
collected on thin paper trays positioned 6 cm below the

floor of the cage and was removed daily. There was no food or water in either chamber. The monopole antenna of one chamber was energized by a 2450-MHz CW magnetron (Amperex No. 2M/107A) with a peak output power of 800 W. The magnetron was coupled to the antenna via a WR-284 waveguide, a coupler (5-db power reduction; MDL No. 284CB336) and a waveguide-to-coaxial-line adaptor. A triple-stub waveguide tuner was used to match the antenna and transmission line impedances. Forward power was monitored by a power meter (Hewlett-Packard No. 436A) and continuously recorded by a stripchart recorder (Soltec No. VP-6232). Panels of pyramidally shaped Eccosorb were positioned so that either half of the Plexiglas cage could be shielded. Consequently, the whole-body SAR (W/kg) of a rat occupying the shielded side of the cage was reduced by 90 percent compared to the unshielded side of the cage. Power densities within each Plexiglas cage were measured by an omnidirectional power monitor (Narda-8616). The output of the magnetron could be adjusted to obtain either 8, 12, or 16 mW/cm2 at each location normally occupied by a rat. These power densities resulted in whole-body SAR's of 1.4, 2.1 and 2.8 W/kg when a rat occupied the unshielded side of the cage and was exposed to microwaves. The whole-body SAR determinations were made using twin-well calorimetry following the procedures outlined by D'Andrea et al. (1985).

Behavioral measurement. Sixteen Plexiglas cages were constructed as described in Experiment-1 and placed on the styrofoam supports in the anechoic chambers. Behind the aluminum ground plane and adjacent to each cage a microswitch was mounted. The microswitch was connected to the cage by nylon cord passed through a hole (0.5 cm diameter) in the ground plane. Vertical tilt of the cage by the weight of a rat on one side of the cage activated the microswitch. A microcomputer located in an adjacent room continuously monitored the microswitches; thus the location of the rat in the cage, and hence the duration of microwave exposure, was directly determined.

PROCEDURE

Experiment 2-A. To investigate a dose-response relationship between SAR and behavioral reduction of microwave exposure three groups of 16 rats (8 sham- and 8 microwave-exposed) were tested. All animals were first given a 4 day period of sham-exposure as a baseline measure, and then 8 days of either sham- or microwave-exposure: 4 days with the shield placed on the side of the cage away from the ground plane, and 4 days with the shield placed on the opposite side of the cage. The daily exposures lasted six hours from 0900 to 1500 hours. Following the daily exposure sessions the rats were returned to their individual cages in the vivarium. Measures of performance included the number of minutes spent per day on the nonshielded side of the cage, and the number of times a rat crossed over from one side of the cage to the other.

Experiment 2-B. Two additional groups of 16 rats were treated identically to those in Experiment-2-A, but exposures were extended to 12 days at 1.4 W/kg and 28 days at 0.7 W/kg. This study was performed to determine if a longer period of access to microwaves, at relatively low power densities, would produce a behavioral reduction in exposure time.

RESULTS

Experiment 2-A. The total time a rat spent on the unshielded side of its Plexiglas cage, during one of the 4-day exposure periods, was analyzed by subtracting it from the total time the rat had spent on the same side during the previous 4 days. Thus, for the first exposure period difference score, the total time spent on the unshielded side was subtracted from the total time spent on that side during the baseline period; and for the second exposure period difference score, the total time spent on the unshielded side was subtracted from the total time spent on the shielded side during the first exposure period. A split-plot factorial analysis of variance was used to evaluate the difference between sham- and microwave-exposed rats. The analyses were performed separately for each exposure condition (1.4, 2.1, and 2.8 W/Kg), because the exposure sessions were conducted at different times.

The difference scores are presented in Figures 6, 7, and 8. No change in occupancy of a preferred side of the cage would result in a difference score of zero. Positive deviations from zero, however, indicate more time spent on the shielded side of the cage, and consequently less exposure to microwave radiation. The sham-exposed rats

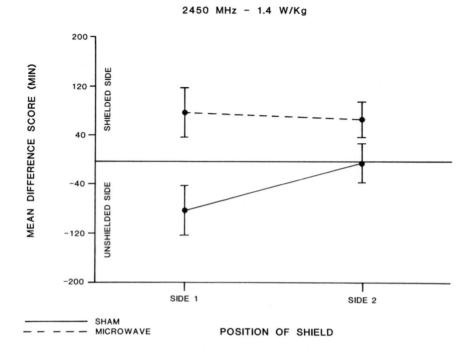

Fig. 6 Experiment-2-A: Mean difference scores (+—SEM) for rats semichronically exposed to 2450-MHz at a whole-body SAR of 1.4 W/kg.

showed an increased preference for the unshielded side of the cage during the course of the experiment subsequently most sham-exposed difference scores are negative values. Rats exposed to microwaves, however, did show more time spent away from the irradiated side of the cage, hence the large positive difference scores. Mean differences scores of rats exposed at a whole-body SAR of 1.4 W/Kg and at 2.8 W/Kg differed significantly from their sham-exposed counterparts [Fs(1,14)=6.98 and 23.87, Ps<.05 and .01, respectively], but rats irradiated at 2.1 W/Kg did not (P>.05). A comparison of both exposure contingencies (shielding side 1 vs side 2) revealed no differences between difference scores of the various groups (P > .05), indicating that the microwave-exposed rats were able to avoid the side of the cage which produced microwave exposure, even after the exposure

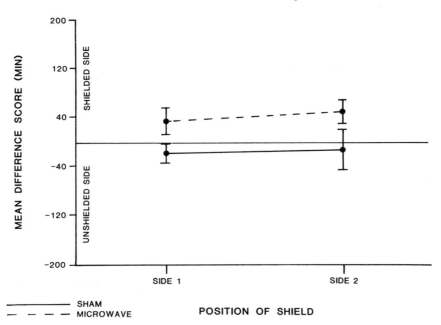

2450 MHZ - 2.1 W/Kg

SHAM
MICROWAVE

POSITION OF SHIELD

Fig. 7 Experiment-2-A: Mean difference scores (+-SEM) for rats semichronically exposed to 2450-MHz microwaves at a whole-body SAR of 2.1 W/kg.

contingencies were reversed. In addition, sham- and microwave-exposed rats did not differ in the number of times they crossed from one side of the Plexiglas cage to the other during exposure sessions (P>.05).

Experiment 2-B. The results of this experiment were analyzed according to the procedures used in Experiment-2-A, except that all difference scores were based on changes only from the baseline period. The diffference scores of the rats exposed for three 4-session blocks at an SAR of 1.4 W/Kg, and of the rats exposed for seven 4-session blocks at an SAR of 0.7 W/Kg are presented in Fig. 9. Difference scores for rats exposed at SAR's of 2.8 and 2.1 W/Kg in Experiment 2-A are included for comparison while sham-exposed groups are omitted for clarity. Rats repeatedly

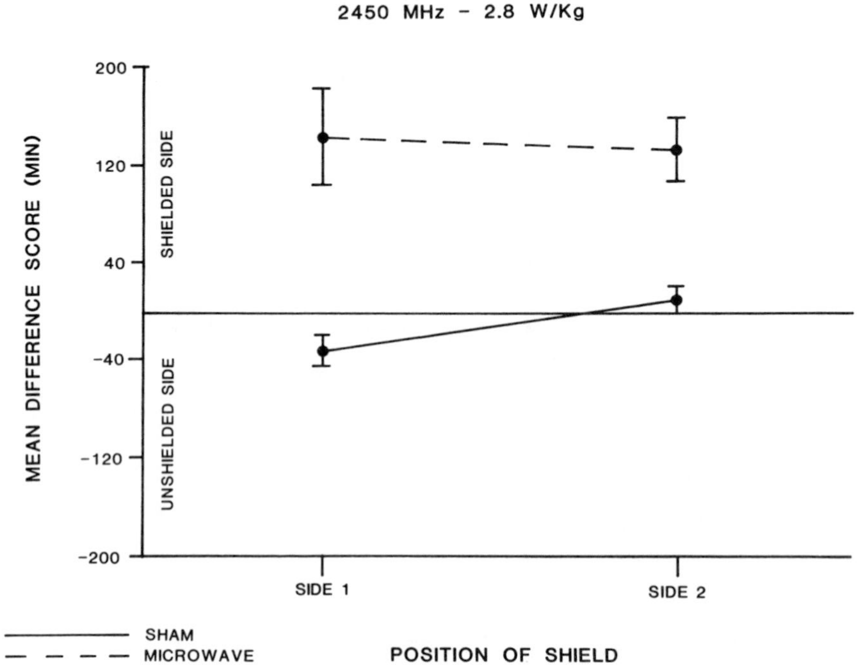

Fig. 8 Experiment-2-A: Mean difference scores (+-SEM) for rats semichronically exposed to 2450-MHz microwaves at a whole-body SAR of 2.8 W/kg.

irradiated at 1.4 W/Kg in this experiment appeared to spend an increasing amount of time on the shielded side of the cage over the three 4-day exposure blocks, however the difference scores of both of the sham- and microwave-irradiated rats were quite variable; consequently the differences between the groups fell short of statistical significance (P >.05). Rats repeatedly exposed at 0.7 W/kg showed little change from their preferred side of the cage over the seven 4-day exposure blocks. Radiation times for rats exposed at 0.7 W/Kg did not statistically differ from those of the sham exposed animals (P >.05).

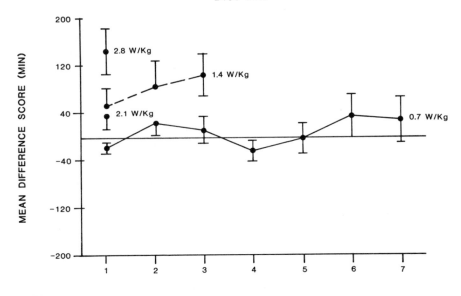

Fig. 9 Experiment-2-B: Mean difference scores (+-SEM) for rats semichronically exposed to 2450-MHz microwaves at a whole-body SAR's of 0.7 and 1.4 W/kg.

CONCLUSIONS

Based on the results of Experiment 2-A, it seems clear that given the opportunity rats will avoid radiation areas at 2450 MHz, which produce relatively high whole-body SAR's. Differences between rats exposed at 2.8 W/Kg and those receiving sham exposure were quite large. Rats exposed at the lower SAR,s also showed some avoidance of microwave exposure but the magnitude of avoidance was reduced, compared to the 2.8 W/kg group. The sham-exposed animals of the 1.4 W/kg group were, for unknown reasons, quite variable across the two conditions of the experiment and this may account for the significant difference from their counterparts exposed to microwaves at 1.4 W/kg. On the contrary, the sham-exposed animals of the 2.1 W/kg group showed little variability during the experiment, and no difference from their exposed counterparts. It is important to notice that there is not a significant difference between the means of animals exposed to 1.4 and 2.1 W/kg (see Fig. 9). If an additional amount of irradiation time is given, animals exposed at 1.4 W/kg (72 hrs total exposure) and at 0.7 W/kg (196 hrs total exposure) do not significantly avoid areas of microwave radiation. Consequently, it is assumed that the threshold for a behavioral reduction of semichronic 2450 MHz microwave exposure must be located between exposures at 2.1 and 2.8 W/kg.

DISCUSSION

The results of this study have shown that rats will prereferentially avoid areas of microwave radiation, and that this effect is highly dependent upon the radiation frequency and whole-body SAR. The reduction of microwave exposure is not simply a passive avoidance since the animals repeatedly enter and exit the radiation exposed half of the Plexiglas cage, as evidenced by a similar number of crossovers at each radiation frequency and whole-body SAR. Rather, this behavior may be best described as an active escape since crossovers in the cage do not differ, but that time spent on the irradiated side of the cage is different depending upon radiation frequency and whole-body SAR.

Rats that were given additional time for irradiation at 2450-MHz in Experiment-2 did not display results different from those observed at the shorter exposure times investigated in Experiment-1. Rats given longer exposures at 0.7, 1.4, and 2.1 W/kg at 2450 MHz did not display significantly reduced irradiation times. The rats exposured at 2.8 W/kg, however, did show significant a reduction in time spent on the irradiated side of the cage, which is similar to the findings at 2450-MHz for Experiment-1.

Since the whole-body SAR's were equated for each radiation frequency in Experiment-1 by adjusting the corresponding field power density, the observed reduction in exposure time by the rats for 360-MHz and 2450-MHz exposures, as compared to 700-MHz exposures, must be based on some other quality of these radiation frequencies than the whole-body SAR. It is known that the distributed SAR in the rat body also depends strongly on the radiation frequency (D'Andrea, et al. 1985), and that significant SAR hotspots exist in the body and tail of the rat at 360-MHz and 2450-MHz but not at 700-MHz. It is very likely that the reduced exposure times observed in Experiment-1 at these frequencies can be explained because of the frequency specific hotspots that are induced. If this were the explanation for the results observed here, then the hotspot phenomena must be effective but subtle stimuli since the rats repeatedly enter and exit the microwave fields. Rats appear to avoid 360-MHz and 2450-MHz microwaves at whole-body SAR's as low as 1 and 2 W/kg, respectively. A similar avoidance is not observed at 700-MHz until a whole-body SAR of 10 W/kg is used. Finally, our rats were tested at ambient temperatures which are below the preferred thermoneutral zone for this species. It is very likely that these thresholds for reduced exposure in rats will depend upon ambient temperature.

REFERENCES

D'andrea JA, Emmerson RY, Bailey CM, Olsen RG, Gandhi OP (1985). Microwave radiation absorption in the rat: frequency dependent SAR distribution in body and tail. Bioelectromagnetics 6 (2):299-206. in press.

Durney CH, Iskander MF, Massoudi H, Allen SJ, Mitchell JC (1978). "Radiofrequency Dosimetry Handbook: Third Edition" Report SAM-TR-80-32 Brooks Air Force Base, Texas, 78235.

Emmerson RY, D'Andrea JA, DeWitt JR, Gandhi OP (1985). Microwave radiation absorption in the anesthetized rat: effect of SAR hotspots in body and tail. Bioelectromagnetics, in press.

Gandhi OP (1974). Polarization and frequency effects on whole animal energy absorption of RF energy. Proceedings of the IEEE 62:1171-1175.

Harris EF (1972). Corner reflector antennas. In Jasik H (ed), "Antenna Engineering Handbook,", San Francisco: McGraw-Hill p. 11(1)-11(8).

Kirk RE (1968). "Experimental Design Procedures for the Behavioral Sciences." Belmont California. Brooks-Cole

This research was supported by a grant to the first author from the National Institute of Environmental Health Sciences No. 1 R01 ES02590 01.

John A. D'Andrea is now at the Naval Aerospace Medical Research Laboratory, Code 42, Naval Air Station, Pensacola, FL. 32508.

Electromagnetic Fields and Neurobehavioral Function, pages 309–326
© 1988 Alan R. Liss, Inc.

MICROWAVE - DRUG INTERACTIONS IN THE CHOLINERGIC NERVOUS
SYSTEM OF THE MOUSE

JOHN C. MONAHAN

FOOD AND DRUG ADMINISTRATION
CENTER FOR DEVICES AND RADIOLOGICAL HEALTH
OFFICE OF SCIENCE AND TECHNOLOGY
ROCKVILLE, MARYLAND 20857

INTRODUCTION

The nervous system is sensitive to a wide range of
chemical and physical agents, and its role in the normal
functioning of the organism including behavior lends itself
to testing for the effects produced by these agents. Some
of these agents produce actual alterations in the nervous
system itself, including morphological, biochemical, and/or
electrical changes that directly affect the ability of the
organism to function. Such changes can sometimes be
detected by changes in behavior. The two studies presented
here were conceived within the framework of this viewpoint
and on the basis of some archival research findings.

Microwave radiation is a physical environmental agent
which has been reported to produce a variety of alterations
in the central nervous system, and also in behavior. For
example, Tolgskaya and Gordon (1973) reported morphological
changes in the brain following exposure to levels of
microwave radiation in excess of 40 mW/cm^2. Albert and
coworkers (1976, 1981a, 1981b) also observed a number of
structural changes following exposure to lower power
densities (10 mW/cm^2) of microwave energy (2.45-GHz). Many
other changes in the central nervous system have been
associated with exposure to microwave radiation (McRee,
1980, Gage and Albert, 1984), including altered EEG
patterns, increased blood-brain barrier permeability, and
alterations in brain metabolism and biochemistry.

Among these reports are some studies in which investigators have attempted to examine whether microwave exposure could result in alteration of the blood-brain barrier permeability. Frey et al (1975) reported increased permeability to fluorescein following exposure to 1200-MHz. They employed both pulsed (0.2 mW/cm^2 average power density) and continuous wave (2.4 mW/cm^2 power density) radiation. Oscar and Hawkins (1977) used radioisotope tracers to investigate the effect of 1300-MHz on blood-brain barrier permeability. They also used both pulsed and continuous wave (CW) exposures and observed increased uptake of labeled inulin and mannitol at power densities as low as 0.3 mW/cm^2. Albert (1977, 1979) and Albert and Kerns (1981) examined the brains of rats and Chinese hamsters following microwave exposure (2450 and 2800-MHz, CW, 10 mW/cm^2). They reported an increased passage of horseradish peroxidase into discrete areas of the brain including thalamus, hypothalamus, medulla, and cerebellum in the exposed subjects indicating that the blood-brain barrier had been breached and permitted the horseradish peroxidase to enter the brain. They also found that two hours following exposure the blood-brain barrier's integrity was again intact.

Merritt and colleagues (1978) attempted to confirm the original findings of Frey et al (1975) and also the work of Oscar and Hawkins (1977). In both of these replicate studies they were unable to demonstrate any increased permeability of the blood-brain barrier attributable to microwave exposure. In addition to these studies, Preston et al (1979) using the same analytical technique employed by Oscar and Hawkins reported no effect of microwave exposure on the passage of labeled mannitol into the brains of rats. In a subsequent study Preston and Prefontaine (1980) exposed rats to 2450-MHz both in an anechoic chamber and also with an applicator applied directly to the head. They did not find any change in permeability associated with either type of exposure situation even at estimated whole body averaged SARs (specific absorption rate) up to 2 W/kg.

Although negative findings do not invalidate positive findings, they do bring into question the robustness and generality of a given effect. The failure of some studies to substantiate alterations of the blood-brain barrier resulting from microwave exposure at best leaves the situation in a state of uncertainty. Interpretation of these discrepant results must include a careful analysis of the procedures and analytical methodologies employed by the various investigators. A review of many of the above studies and an analysis of some of the inherent problems has been provided by Justesen (1980). He cites several possible confounding variables in some of the studies, such as, the use of barbiturate anesthesia and the use of analytical techniques which are sensitive to changes in regional blood flow rates. In an effort to circumvent some of these problem areas we pursued a different approach to assess possible microwave effects on blood–brain barrier permeability. Our rationale was that a psychoactive drug that does not normally cross the blood–brain barrier could be used as an indicator of increased permeability. If microwave exposure increased the passage of this drug into the brain, its behavioral effects would serve as an indicator of increased entry.

The drugs selected for this study were methyl scopolamine, which is normally excluded from the brain, and scopolamine hydrobromide, which readily crosses the blood–brain barrier. Normally methyl scopolamine is prevented from entering the brain and it exerts its pharmacological effects only on the peripheral cholinergic receptors (Seiden and Dykstra, 1977). We reasoned that if a microwave exposure induced an increase in the permeability of the blood–brain barrier to methyl scopolamine then it would bind to cholinergic receptor sites as it does in the peripheral nervous system and interfere with cholinergic transmission. By using scopolamine, which normally passes through the blood–brain barrier and exerts its effect on central cholinergic receptors, we would have a positive control in our behavioral testing situation.

Scopolamine is an anticholinergic drug which exerts its effect by blocking acetylcholine receptors, and thus inhibiting or preventing neural transmission across synaptic functions (Julien 1981). This inhibition of cholinergic transmission results in a broad spectrum of dose-dependent behavioral effects including amnesia, drowsiness, psychological euphoria, confusion, loss of attention, etc. in human beings. In addition, scopolamine produces a number of behavioral changes in experimental animals. The specific change observed is related to dose, route of administration, internal state of the subjects, and, response rates.

EXPERIMENT I - MATERIALS AND METHODS

Adult male ICR mice (35 to 45 g), were individually housed in the vivarium and were maintained on a daily 19-hour food deprivation schedule throughout the study. Food (Purina Lab Chow) was available for 5 hours per day immediately following behavioral sessions, and tap water was continuously available in the home cage. The vivarium has a 24 hour light-dark cycle with light being on between the hours of 0600 and 1800.

The behavioral testing apparatus employed in this study was a clear Plexiglas cubicle (15 x 15 x 21 cm) with a floor made of stainless steel rods for delivery of electrical shock. A glass drinking tube was mounted on the rear wall of the cubicle and protruded 1 cm into the cubicle, at a height of 2 cm above the floor. Drinking (licks) was recorded via a contact relay (BRS/LVE model DR-901-221-05). The equipment for experimental control and data acquisition was located in a room remote from the behavioral testing apparatus, which was located in a sound attenuating room.

Two identical microwave exposure systems (Ho et al, 1973) were employed for irradiation of the mice in this study. Each consists of a 100 W generator producing 2450 MHz (CW) microwaves. The output of the generator was fed through a variable attenuator into the animal exposure chamber. The chamber was a section of WR 430 waveguide (10.9 x 5.5 cm in cross-section) operated in the TE_{10} mode. The waveguide exposure chamber was housed within an environmentally-controlled enclosure that permitted regulation of temperature (24 $+0.5^{\circ}$C), humidity (50 $\pm$ 5%), and airflow (20 l/min) within the waveguide. The forward, reflected, and transmitted powers were measured through coaxial directional couplers and the waveguide was terminated in a resistive load.

The center section of the waveguide was held together with quick-release clamps that permitted rapid insertion and removal of the animal container. This rectangular container was constructed of 2.0 mm black, opaque Plexiglas sheets with holes in either end to permit air flow, and had a sliding top for insertion of the animal. The outside dimensions of the animal container were 26.7 x 5.4 x 3.2 cm; this size permitted the mouse to move about freely during irradiation.

The rate of energy absorption varied during the course of irradiation due to the subject's movement within the animal container. Therefore, we integrated the readings from the power meters over time to arrive at an integral dose rate for an irradiation session. This approach permits calculation of the whole-body averaged SAR (specific absorption rate) (Ho et al, 1973).

The drugs employed in the study were scopolamine methyl bromide and scopolamine hydrobromide obtained from Sigma Chemical Company (St. Louis, Missouri). Drugs were prepared for intraperitoneal injection by dissolving the respective compounds in physiological saline to yield an injection volume of 1 ml/100 g body mass. Drug doses were based on the mass of the salt of the specific compound. The dose of scopolamine hydrobromide was chosen following preliminary dose-response determinations in ICR mice using our behavioral procedure. A weight equivalent dose of scopolamine methylbromide was used.

The behavioral procedure which we employed in this study was a modification of the one-trial conditioned suppression paradigm of Leaf and Muller (1965) consisting of three separate stages i.e., training (day 1-7), shock conditioning (day 8), and retention testing (day 9). Preliminary training consisted of the mice learning to drink a milk solution (one part Borden's Eagle Brand sweetened condensed milk to two parts tap water) during seven daily training sessions. Each session consisted of 10 minutes or 100 licks of milk solution, whichever occurred first. Mice whose latency was more than 50 seconds on the last three days of training were dropped from the study. The remaining subjects were assigned to one of eighteen treatment groups in a 3 x 3 x 2 factorial design (N > 10 mice/cell). The three factors of the design were drug (saline, methyl scopolamine, or scopolamine), microwave exposure (SARs of 0, 1, or 10 mW/g), and conditioning (shock or no shock).

On the shock conditioning day (day 8) mice were injected intraperitoneally with either saline, methyl scopolamine 1 mg/kg, or scopolamine 1 mg/kg and then were immediately placed in the microwave exposure apparatus and were exposed for 30 minutes to 2450-MHz CW radiation at whole body averaged SARs of 0, 1, or 10 mW/g. Immediately following irradiation mice were placed in the drinking cubicle for 5 minutes. They were permitted unlimited access to the drinking tube during this period. However, 0.6 mA of shock was delivered to one half of the subjects in each group thru the milk by a programmable shocker (Coulbourn Instruments Inc., Lehigh Valley, Pa.). Thus each time a mouse licked the milk from the drinking tube they received a shock to the tongue. During the 5 minute conditioning session mice were observed via closed circuit TV. Most mice received about 6 shocks. The remaining one half of the subjects did not receive any shock during this conditioning session.

On the following day (test day) mice were again placed in the drinking cubicle and their latency to complete 100 licks of milk solution was determined. No shock was present during this session. This test session was terminated at the end of 10 minutes if they had not completed the requisite number of licks. The test day latencies of groups were compared using an analysis of variance for an unbalanced design due to the unequal number of mice per cell.

EXPERIMENT I - RESULTS

All nine treatment groups that received drug and microwave exposure on day eight, but no shock during the conditioning session, had test day mean latencies of 35 seconds or less. These latencies are not statistically different from the preconditioning mean latencies of day 7 and indicate that on the test day there were no residual effects on latencies of drug and microwave treatments given on the previous day.

The subjects that received shock conditioning, saline injection and 0 mW/g (sham) microwave exposure had mean test day latencies of 335 seconds (Fig. 1). Shock conditioning produced a significant (P <0.01) increase in the latency on subsequent testing when compared to subjects that received no shock during the conditioning session. Animals that received saline and either 1 or 10 mW/g microwave exposure in conjunction with shock conditioning had mean test day latencies of 373 and 461 seconds, respectively. There were no significant differences between these groups and the group that received sham microwave exposure (Fig. 1).

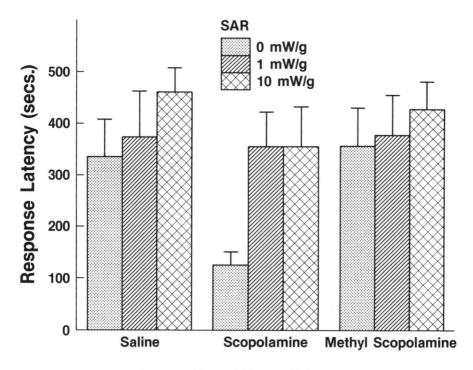

Figure 1. Mean test day latencies plus SEM. Latency of
   mice to complete 100 licks of milk solution twenty four
   hours following shock conditioning in which they
   received 0.6 mA of shock to the tongue each time they
   licked the milk tube.

Animals that received scopolamine and 0 mW/g (sham)
microwave exposure in conjunction with shock conditioning
had a mean drinking latency of 125 seconds (Fig. 1). This
is a statistically significant difference (P <0.01), when
compared to the saline-sham exposed mice. Although this
shorter mean latency is not as low as that observed in the
unshocked control group, it does demonstrate that the
administration of scopolamine prior to shock conditioning
resulted in a poorer association between shock and milk
(i.e. scopolamine reduced the effect of the shock
conditioning).

In the shock conditioned subjects that received either 1 or 10 mW/g microwave exposure plus scopolamine (Fig. 1) their test day mean latencies were comparable to those of the saline-microwave groups. The difference between the scopolamine-sham exposure group and the scopolaminemicrowave groups was significant (P<0.01). The data show that microwave irradiation at either 1 or 10 mW/g abolished the scopolamine-induced reduction in latencies associated with shock conditioning.

EXPERIMENT I - DISCUSSION

Our original intent in this study was to examine via behavior the effect of microwave irradiation on the permeability of the blood-brain barrier. We attempted to do this by using the passage of methyl scopolamine into the brain and then measuring the behavioral effect produced by this drug.

An unexpected finding in the present study was that, when scopolamine was combined with microwave irradiation the anticipated effect of scopolamine on retention of shock conditioning (i.e. reduced latency) was partially abolished. At SARs of both 1 and 10 mW/g a diminished effectiveness of scopolamine on associative processes was observed during subsequent testing. These subjects responded in nearly the same way as subjects given only saline and microwave exposure. It appears that microwave exposure decreased the potency of a 1 mg/kg dose of scopolamine.

If microwave exposure did not produce an increase in permeability of the barrier, then methyl scopolamine would be prevented from entering the brain and no effect of this drug would be observed in our test procedure. On the other hand, if microwave exposure did increase the permeability and permitted the methyl scopolamine to enter the brain its effect may have been abolished by the microwaves and again no effect would have been observed. No difference was observed between the scopolamine-microwave and the methyl scopolamine-microwave groups on their test day latencies but this does not mean that no alteration in blood-brain barrier permeability occurred. Since microwave exposure appears to abolish the effect of scopolamine on the central nervous system no conclusions can be made regarding permeability changes in the blood-brain barrier.

The finding that microwave exposure can decrease at least one of the behavioral effects of scopolamine has some rather interesting implications when considered in the context of some previous research. Other investigators have reported microwave-drug interactions for other drugs which have totally different pharmacological activity. For example, Servantie et al (1974) found a decreased effectiveness of curare-like drugs in both rats and in vitro neuromuscular preparations exposed to microwaves. Exposure produced a decreased susceptibility to the paralyzing effects of the compounds. Cleary and Wangemann (1976) reported a decreased effectiveness of pentobarbital on sleeping time in rabbits produced by microwave exposure. Subsequently Thomas et al (1979) and Thomas and Maitland (1979) found a potentiation of behavioral effects by both dextroamphetamine and chlordiazepoxide when the rats were also exposed to microwave radiation. In addition to these studies, which demonstrate a microwave-drug interaction, other research on the central nervous system has examined the levels of neurotransmitters following irradiation.

Snyder (1971) found reductions in serotonin and 5-HIAA levels following repeated exposures at 10 mW/cm^2. Merritt et al (1976) also observed regional decreases in brain norepinephrine, dopamine, and serotonin levels following brief exposure to high power densities (80 mW/cm^2). They attributed these changes to induced localized temperature elevations in the brain. In a subsequent study Merritt et al (1977) observed decreased hypothalmic norepinephrine following a brief exposure to a 1600-MHz field at 20 mW/cm^2. Although the results on microwave-drug interactions and neurotransmitter levels are amenable to different interpretations, one possibility is that microwave radiation can produce biochemical changes that impact on neural transmission and behavior.

The aim of the second study was to extend the unexpected scopolamine results of Experiment I using another behavioral testing situation, and to attempt through additional manipulation of the cholinergic transmitter system to clarify the microwave-induced changes which were observed. There are no known specific compounds to deplete or replace acetylcholine in the central nervous system. Thus it is difficult to directly alter acetylcholine levels; however, the function of the cholinergic system can be altered indirectly by the administration of compounds which block cholinergic transmission, by cholinergic agonists, and by cholinesterase inhibitors. This indirect manipulation of the cholinergic system is the approach utilized in the second study. We chose scopolamine, an anticholinergic which blocks cholinergic receptors in order to inhibit cholinergic transmission in the experimental subjects. The other drug which we employed in Experiment II, physostigmine, is a cholinesterase inhibitor. This compound exerts its effect by inhibiting acetylcholinesterase, which breaks down acetylcholine in the synaptic cleft. This drug therefore increases acetylcholine concentrations in those areas of the nervous system where it is released.

EXPERIMENT II - MATERIALS and METHODS

Adult male ICR mice (40 to 50g) were used in this study and maintenance conditions were the same as described in Experiment I except that food (Purina Lab Chow) was continuously available. The behavioral testing apparatus employed in this study was a residential maze (figure-8 maze) manufactured by Scientific and Professional Support Group (La Jolla, California). This apparatus is designed to detect locomotor activity as the subject moves from one portion of the maze to another. Locomotion in each area of the maze is automatically detected by a photodiode sensing system, and is recorded as frequency counts on a remote data acquisition unit.

The microwave exposure apparatus and the environmental conditions employed in this study were the same as those used in Experiment I.

The drugs employed in the study were scopolamine hydrobromide and physostigmine salicylate which were obtained from Sigma Chemical Company (St. Louis, Missouri). Drugs were prepared for injection by dissolving the respective compounds in physiological saline. All drug concentrations were based on the salt mass of the specific compound, and the drug solutions were prepared so that the desired dose would be administered in a volume of 1 ml/100 g of body mass. Doses of scopolamine and physostigmine were selected on the basis of preliminary dose-response work using activity in ICR mice. The dose of scopolamine was selected to yield an increase in activity and a subthreshold dose of physostigmine which did not decrease activity was chosen.

All mice were habituated in the residential maze for 4 sessions over 4 consecutive days and their activity counts were recorded. Each session consisted of 30 minutes in the maze, which was located in a dark sound attenuating room. Examination of the data from these 4 sessions permitted us to select for testing those subjects with relatively stable locomotor activity as indicated by the cumulative counts of activity for 30 minute periods. Subjects whose activity deviated from their mean 4 day locomotor score by more than +20 percent on days 3 or 4 were discarded.

Mice with "stable" locomotor activity were randomly assigned to one of the treatment groups. A 2 X 3 factorial design was used with an N of 10 subjects per cell. The first factor was drug treatment (saline, scopolamine 2.0 mg/kg, or physostigmine 0.2 mg/kg) and the second factor was microwave irradiation (SARs of 0, 1, or 10 mW/g). On day 5, each subject was injected intraperitoneally with either saline, scopolamine, or physostigmine solution. Following the injection, the mice were immediately placed in the microwave exposure apparatus for 30 minutes where they were exposed to 2450-MHz (CW) radiation at SARs of 0, 1, or 10 mW/g. Immediately following termination of exposure, each subject was placed in the residential maze and its cumulative locomotor activity counts for 30 minutes were determined. Individual subjects were habituated and tested at the same time of day during the course of the study and treatment conditions were balanced out over time.

EXPERIMENT II - RESULTS

For each treatment group, the total locomotor activity counts for day 5 (test day) were compared with the mean activity counts of the previous 4 days, to determine treatment effects. The activity counts were evaluated by a 3 way analysis of variance and class variables were day, microwave exposure, and drug treatment. The activity of mice that received saline and sham (0 mW/g) exposure was not significantly different during the test session when compared with their baseline activity. Although they showed a 14 percent decrease in activity (Fig. 2) this is not

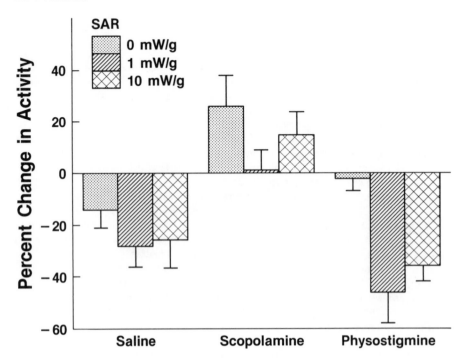

Figure 2. Mean percent change plus SEM in locomotor act-ivity of mice compared to mean baseline activity (0 percent line) of the previous four days. Activity is defined as the total number of counts registered during the 30 minute test session in the residential maze.

significantly below baseline and it may reflect a sampling error or an effect due to the stress of injection and/or the 30 minute sham exposure. The two groups that received saline and 1 or 10 mW/g microwave exposure showed a 28 and 26 percent decrease, respectively, in locomotor activity, when compared with baselines (Fig. 2). These differences are statistically significant (P<0.01), and indicate that SARs of these magnitudes can result in a reduction of locomotor activity immediately following cessation of microwave irradiation.

Mice that received scopolamine and sham irradiation exhibited a significant increase (P<0.01) in locomotor activity when compared with their baseline levels (Fig. 2). Scopolamine has been demonstrated to increase locomotor activity (Meyers et al, 1964), thus the increased activity we observed was the anticipated finding. Mice that received a combination of scopolamine and microwave exposure at 1 mW/g showed a 1 percent increase in activity. Scopolamine in combination with exposure at 10 mW/g resulted in a 14 percent increase. Neither increase is statistically significant when compared to baseline. Thus, it appears that microwave irradiation at 1 or 10 mW/g at least partially abolishes the behavioral increase in locomotor activity normally induced by the administration of 2 mg/kg scopolamine.

The activity of mice that received physostigmine and sham irradiation (0 mW/g) was not significantly different than their baseline (Fig. 2). Although, physostigmine has been shown to decrease locomotor activity (Pradhan and Mhatre, 1970), a sub-threshold dose for producing locomotor changes was utilized in this study. Mice that received physostigmine and irradiation at 1 or 10 mW/g showed a 46 and 36 percent decrease in activity respectively (Fig. 2). These differences are statistically significant (P<0.01) when compared with baseline locomotor activity. It should be noted that these decreases are 18 and 10 percent greater than those produced by saline plus microwave exposure at comparable dose rates but are not significantly different when compared with these groups. Although these differences are not significant the data suggest that the simultaneous administration of physostigmine (0.02 mg/kg) may enhance the reduction in locomotor activity induced by microwave exposure alone.

EXPERIMENT II - DISCUSSION

Under the conditions of Experiment II, a significant increase in locomotor activity was observed in subjects under the influence of scopolamine. This is consistent with the results of other investigators. For example, Meyers (1965) found an increase in activity in two different types of avoidance testing. Meyers et al (1964) also observed scopolamine-induced increases in locomotor activity in a study specifically designed to examine this endpoint. Thus it appears that a decrease in cholinergically mediated transmission produces increased activity.

In both studies reported here, in those subjects administered scopolamine and exposed to microwaves, we observed a diminution of the scopolamine effect.

Pradhan and Mhatre (1970) demonstrated that increasing acetylcholine concentrations by administration of physostigmine produces a decrease in locomotor activity. Under the conditions of our experiments and the subthreshold dose of physostigmine (0.02 mg/kg) used, no effect on locomotor activity was observed. However, when the drug was administered in conjunction with microwave irradiation, significant decreases in activity were noted in comparison to baseline. These decreases were greater then observed with microwaves alone, but these differences do not reach statistical significance. Physostigmine may enhance the decrease in activity induced by microwave irradiation but the present data are only suggestive.

Two explanations that have been postulated to explain the results of previous studies involving microwaves and drugs in combination are: increases in metabolism, and/or increases in blood flow. These explanations are based on the assumption that regional or localized increases of temperature are produced by microwave energy deposition. Although such explanations cannot be completely excluded for the present results, they appear to be unlikely, since an inhibition of activity was observed for one drug and a potentiation of activity for the other drug. In addition to the differential direction of the drug effects we observed one would expect only minimal if any compensatory thermoregulatory mechanisms such as increases in local brain blood flow at an SAR of 1 mW/g. Because our subjects were free to move about during irradiation, localized energy deposition in the brain and the resultant need to increase blood flow is extremely remote.

Although several hypotheses can be postulated to account for our findings, one possible explanation for our observations is that microwave irradiation enhances cholinergic transmission. This would account for the decrease in activity observed with no drug present because increased acetylcholine transmission with physostigmine has been shown to decrease locomotor activity (Pradhan and

Mhatre, 1970). In Experiment I, testing was conducted 24 hours after exposure. With this time interval between exposure and test it is unlikely that any increase in cholinergic transmission associated with microwave exposure would manifest itself and no saline-microwave effect was noted in Experiment I. An increased cholinergic transmission would account for the inhibition of scopolamine (a cholinergic blocker) because presumably, more acetylcholine would be present to bind to the available receptors and counteract the effect of the drug during conditioning. We observed this inhibition of scopolamine in both experiments at comparable microwave dose rates, but in two very different behavioral paradigms. And finally, administration of physostigmine (a cholinesterase inhibitor) in conjunction with microwave exposure would produce a greater enhancement of cholinergic transmission than either treatment given alone. In Experiment II we observed a tendency in this direction although the data did not reach statistical significance.

Based on the present results, it is impossible to determine the actual mechanisms underlying our observations. Certainly a membrane effect (enhanced receptor activity), an enzymatic effect (cholinesterase inhibition), or perhaps enhanced release of acetylcholine cannot be ruled out, and they offer some possible directions for future investigation.

CONCLUSIONS

1. Microwave absorption of 1 or 10 mW/g at a frequency of 2.45-GHz (CW) inhibits the scopolamine induced reduction in latencies associated with shock conditioning during subsequent testing.

2. Microwave absorption of 1 or 10 mW/g at a frequency of 2.45-GHz (CW) results in decreased locomotor actitity immediately following exposure in mice.

3. Microwave absorption at these SARs inhibit the locomotor activity increases which are produced by administration of scopolamine (a cholinergic blocker).

4. The effect of microwave absorption at these SARs which results in decreased locomotor activity appears to be

enhanced by the simultaneous administration of physostigmine (a cholinesterase inhibitor).

REFERENCES

Albert EN (1977). Light and electron microscopic observations on the blood-brain barrier after microwave irradiation. In Hazard DG (ed): "Symposium on Biological Effects and Measurement of Radio Frequency/Microwaves," Rockville, Maryland: HEW Publication (FDA) 77-8026, p 294.

Albert EN (1979). Reversibility of microwave induced blood-brain barrier permeability. Radio Sci 14:323.

Albert EN, DeSantis M (1976). Histological observations on Central Nervous System. In Johnson CC, Shore ML (eds): "Biological Effects of Electromagnetic Waves, Vol 1," Rockville, Maryland: HEW Publication (FDA) 77-8010, p 299.

Albert EN, Kerns JM (1981). Reversible microwave effects on the blood-brain barrier. Brain Res 230:153.

Albert EN, Sherif MF, Papadopoulos NJ (1981a). Effects of nonionizing radiation on the purkinje cells of the uvula in squirrel monkey cerebellum. Bioelectromagnetics 2:241.

Albert EN, Sherif MF, Papadopoulos NJ, Slaby FJ, Monahan J. (1981b). Effect of nonionizing radiation on the purkinje cells of the rat cerebellum. Bioelectromagnetics 2:247.

Cleary SF, Wangemann RT (1976). Effect of microwave radiation on pentobarbitol-induced sleeping time. In Johnson CC, Shore ML (eds): "Biological Effects of Electromagnetic Waves, Vol 1," Rockville, Maryland: HEW Publication (FDA) 77-8010, p 311.

Frey AH, Feld SR, Frey B (1975). Neural function and behavior: Defining the relationship. Ann NY Acad Sci 247:433.

Gage MI, Albert EN (1984). Nervous system. In Elder JA, Cahill DF (eds): "Biological Effects of Radiofrequency Radiation," Environmental Protection Agency Publication EPA-600/8-83-026F, p 5-43.

Ho HS, Ginns EI, Christman CL (1973). Environmentally controlled waveguide irradiation facility. IEEE Trans MTT 21:837.

Julien RM (1981). "A Primer of Drug Action." San Francisco, California: WH Freeman and Company, p 138.

Justesen DR (1980). Microwave irradiation and the blood-brain barrier. Proceed IEEE 68:60.

Leaf RC, Muller SA, (1965). Simple method for CER conditioning and measurement. Psychol Rpts 17:211.

McRee DI (1980). Soviet and Eastern European research on biological effects of microwave radiation. Proceedings of the IEEE 68:84.

Merritt JH, Hartzell RH, Frazer JW (1976). The effect of 1.6 GHz radiation on neurotransmitters in discrete areas of the rat brain. In Johnson CC, Shore ML (eds): "Biological Effects of Electromagnetic Waves, Vol 1," Rockville, Maryland: HEW Publication (FDA) 77-8010, p 290.

Merritt JH, Chamness AF, Hartzell RH, Allen SJ (1977). Orientation effects on microwave-induced hyperthermia and neurochemical correlates. J Microwave Power 12:167.

Merritt JH, Chamness AF, Allen SJ (1978). Studies on blood-brain barrier permeability after microwave radiation. Radiat Environ Biophys 15:367.

Meyers B (1965). Some effects of scopolamine on a passive avoidance response in rats. Psychoparmacologica 8:111.

Meyers B, Roberts KH, Riciputi RH, Domino EF (1964). Some effects of muscarinic cholinergic blocking drugs on behavior and the electrocorticogram. Psychopharmacologia 5:289.

Oscar KJ, Hawkins TD (1977). Microwave alteration of the blood-brain barrier system of rats. Brain Res 126:281.

Pradhan SN, Mhatre RM (1970). Effects of two anticholinesterases on behavior and cholinesterase activity in the rat. Res Comm Chem Path Pharmacol 1:682.

Preston E, Vavasour EJ, Assenheim HM (1979). Permeability of the blood-brain barrier to mannitol in the rat following 2450 MHz microwave irradiation. Brain Res 174:109.

Preston E, Prefontaine G (1980). Cerebrovascular permeability to sucrose in the rat exposed to 2450 MHz microwaves. J Appl Physiol 49:218.

Seiden LS and LS Dykstra (1977). "Psychopharmacology a Biochemical and Behavioral Approach." New York, New York: Van Nostrand Reinhold Company, p 213.

Servantie B, Bertharion G, Joly R, Servantie A, Etienne J, Dreyfus P, Escoubet P (1974). Pharmacologic effects of a pulsed microwave field. In Czerski P, Ostrowski K,

Shore ML, Silverman C, Suess MJ, Waldeskog B (eds): "Biological Effects and Health Hazards of Microwave Radiation," Warsaw, Poland: Polish Medical Publishers, p 36.

Snyder SH (1971). The effect of microwave irradiation on the turnover rate of serotonin and norepinephrine and the effect of monamine metabolizing enzymes. Final Report, Contract No DADA 17-69-C-9144, US Army Medical Research and Development Command, Washington, DC.

Thomas JR Maitland G (1979). Microwave radiation and dextroamphetamine: Evidence of combined effects on behavior of rats. Radio Sci 14:253.

Thomas JR, Burch LS, Yeadle SS (1979). Microwave radiation and chlordiazepoxide: Synergistic effects on fixed-interval behavior. Science 203:1357.

Tolgskaya MS Gordon ZV (1973). Pathological effects of radio waves (translated from Russian by Haigh B) Library of Congress Cat Card 72-94825.

Electromagnetic Fields and Neurobehavioral Function, pages 327–347
© 1988 Alan R. Liss, Inc.

RECENT STUDIES IN THE BEHAVIORAL TOXICOLOGY OF ELF ELECTRIC
AND MAGNETIC FIELDS

Richard H. Lovely

Neurosciences Group
Battelle, Pacific Northwest Laboratories
Richland, WA 99352

INTRODUCTION

This review summarizes and evaluates the recent scientific literature on the behavioral effects of exposure to
electric and magnetic fields ranging in frequency from 1-
300 Hz extremely low frequency (ELF). Most of this work
has been carried out at 60 Hz.

Much of what is known about the behavioral effects of
exposure to ELF fields is summarized by a National Academy
of Sciences (NAS) report (1977). Since the time of that
report, considerable research has been carried out to assess specifically the "health effects" of exposure to ELF
fields. The impetus for this work comes from the U.S. Department of Energy (DOE) and the public power industry,
both here and abroad, because of their interest in identifying possible deleterious effects that might result from
exposure to power-frequency (50- and 60-Hz) electric and
magnetic fields. Because of their goals, much of the research emanating from these and other programs has been
toxicological in nature--at least more so than in past researches. In other words, because of the implicit risk-
benefit analysis that will eventuate from these studies,
the researches are often cast in toxicologic context.
Among other things this means most (but not all) of the
work is well conceived and designed, correctly analyzed,
establishes dose-dependence when an effect is obtained,
attempts to replicate initial effects, attempts to general-
ize the existence of significant effects to more than one
species, and attempts to evaluate established effects with

regard to their being placed under the rubrics of "effect" or "hazard." Thus, a number of behavioral effects of expo- sure to ELF fields that have been identified since 1977, can be considered well-established effects. These consti- tute the majority of material reviewed in this paper. How- ever, effects that are less well established are reviewed, and, where relevant, their implications for our understand- ing of the behavioral toxicology of exposure to ELF fields are considered.

The principal behavioral effects reviewed in the fol- lowing pages appear under the following ordered headings:

- Perception and Behavioral Detection
- Arousal Response and Activity
- Aversive Behaviors
- Neurobehavioral Teratology
- Behavioral Effects in Humans.

BEHAVIORAL EFFECTS

Perception and Behavioral Detection

A number of vertebrate species are able to detect the presence of ELF electric and magnetic fields and they do so by a variety of means.

By far and away the most sensitive of these detection abilities is that termed "electroreception." Because this is such a large body of literature and because it is treated elsewhere in this volume, I will not review it in any detail here. The major developments in this area since the report by NAS (1977) have dealt with identifying and differentiating the various forms of electroreception that appear in a number of fish. Bullock (1982) suggests that evolution "invented" electroreception at least three dif- ferent times.

For our purposes, it will suffice to indicate that there are two broad classes of receptors that respond, at least in part, to ELF electric fields. The low-frequency receptors, known as Ampullary organs, have a frequency re- sponse of from 0.1 to 50 Hz. The high-frequency receptors respond from 50 to 2,000 Hz, and are classed as Tuberous organs. The absolute threshold for behavioral detection in different species can range from as high as 10 mV/cm to as low as about 5 nV/cm. The latter sensitivity is for the Ampulae of Lorenzini of the Elasmobranchs such as sharks, rays, and skates (Bullock, 1982).

How such weak electric fields are transduced into classical neural firing patterns is not yet known. It seems unlikely that local currents directly depolarize receptors because the fields to which these fish respond are several orders of magnitude below the voltage required for classical neuronal firing. Patch-clamp techniques should help unravel the biophysics of transduction in the near future.

Other species are also able to detect electric fields, although this occurs at much higher field strengths. Cooper et al. (1981) trained pigeons to respond on a variable-interval 90-second reinforcement schedule. Once stable behavioral baselines were obtained, the pigeons underwent classical conditioning trials that paired 60-Hz electric fields (25 or 50 kV/m; 10.5 or 21 kV/m at the pigeon's head) with an impending shock. Following sufficient training, the pigeons could then be probed with the electric field alone. Had they been able to detect the electric field during conditioning, then, when probed later, the pigeons would show conditioned suppression, i.e., they would suppress responding for food relative to their baseline behavior on the interval schedule of reinforcement. Cooper's pigeons suppressed at the higher field strength, but not at the lesser one. A second report from this laboratory (Graves, 1981) assessed the pigeons with and without shielding by a Faraday cage. If the pigeons had suppressed responding because of cueing by stimuli other than the fields (e.g., noise, vibration) then they should suppress inside or outside of the Faraday cage. The results made it clear that the pigeons' suppression was under electric-field control. This is a well-done study that recognizes and tests for possible sources of artifact.

Stern et al. (1983) have similarly evaluated behavioral detection of 60-Hz electric fields in male rats. Their rats were trained to make a nose-poke operant on a parallel-plate exposure system. Using a rigorous signal-detection paradigm, Stern et al. found that the range of values bracketing the absolute threshold for detection of the electric field ranged from 3 to 8 kV/m. In a second study (Stern and Laties, 1985), female rats were similarly evaluated in a signal-detection paradigm. The thresholds of female rats were not different from those of male rats. Sagan (unpublished data) has obtained very similar thresholds in male rats. Sagan also used a signal-detection approach, although there are significant procedural differences in the two studies. Both of these detection studies using rats are well done; the Stern et al. study was especially thorough in testing the possibility that their rats might be responding to some cue other than the electric field. The data made it clear that they were not.

What these studies do not tell us is _how_ these animals detect the electric fields to which they were exposed. Certainly, they do not have electroreceptors. What, then, is the "site of action"? The answer is, "we do not know," although there are at least three possible sites of action. One is that the animals are affected by and may perceive the external fields; this would include such secondary effects as piloerection induced by the oscillating field forces. A second possibility is that the internal fields (i.e., fields in tissues) are somehow detectable. A third, and related possibility is that the current flow produced by the internal fields is somehow detectable.

If we allow the human detection of electric fields to serve as a guide (Reilly, 1978), pigeons and rats probably detect the fields because of their effects on the surface of the body, e.g., piloerection. There are a number of studies in progress attempting to address the site-of-action question. However, for now, we can only guess that it is the external field forces to which rats perceive and respond. Internal fields, and the related current flow that occurs, could possibly induce phosphenes. However, the currents demanded for this to happen would have to be larger than those induced by the low fields employed in these detection studies. For example, in man, the minimal current flow for phosphene induction is about 150 μA, _if_ it is applied near the eyes; applied elsewhere on the head, it would take well over 200 μA to induce phosphenes (Adrian, 1977).

Arousal Response and Activity

Another index of field perception/detection is the arousal response an animal shows to a stimulus. It is not as precise, nor is it as quantifiable, an index of perception/detection as those indices obtained from detection studies. But it does suggest some form of perception (e.g., an orienting response), given one rules out direct neural stimulation by ELF fields (e.g., of the reticular formation).

Hackman and Graves (1981) exposed an outbred strain of mice to 25- or 50-kV/m, 60-Hz electric fields and determined plasma corticosterone levels at various time intervals after exposure. In the first experiment, these intervals were on the order of minutes; the second experiment was on the order of hours; the third experiment was on the order of days. Positive controls were included that measured plasma corticosterone responses to social and auditory stressors. While the positive controls showed significant increases in plasma steroid levels (stress), the two groups exposed to electric fields were not different from one another nor from the sham-exposed/unhandled controls. The field-exposed groups did show a transient rise at 5 minutes after field onset, but were nearly normal by 15 minutes after field onset. The authors, appropriately, interpreted these transient changes as an orienting (arousal) response and not as indicative of stress.

A similar transient response was reported by Rosenberg et al. (1981). They exposed mice (Peromyscus leucopus) to 100-kV/m, 60-Hz electric fields. The animals were exposed for 1 hour four times with 1-hour intervals between each exposure. Gross motor activity, and a number of metabolic indexes were monitored throughout the 1-hour exposures. These investigators found an immediate, but transient, increase in activity and an increase in the use/production of O_2/CO_2. These responses were not elevated following the second 1-hour exposure (i.e., habituation). In a subsequent study, Rosenberg et al. (1983) were able to show that the threshold for the arousal response in their mice ranged between 35 and 50 kV/m, values reasonably consistent with the Hackman and Graves' index of arousal, as is the transient nature of the response.

Other investigators have reported ELF field-induced changes in activity and where there have been transient elevations, one is inclined to interpret them as reflections of arousal given the preceding findings. For example, Hjeresen et al. (1980) exposed rats to an intense 60-Hz electric field in a study of "perception" and avoidance. At field strengths greater than 75 kV/m, rats tested in a lucite alley took residence on the side covered with a Faraday cage. However, rats tested at all field strengths (25 to 100 kV/m) showed increased activity in the first hour of the 23.5-hour test, but not thereafter, when compared with sham-exposed controls.

In all of the foregoing studies, animals rapidly habituated to the novel electric fields to which they were exposed. Such was not the finding when Smith and Justesen (1977) exposed two strains of mice to a 60-Hz field with a dominant magnetic component at 1.7 mT. The exposures were recurrent 120-second presentations of the field. Both strains (DBA/J and CD-1) showed significant increments in activity over all test sessions (i.e., they did not habituate from day to day over the 48 hours of exposure). Of the two strains tested, the DBAs showed greater reactivity to the magnetic field's presence.

A number of studies that have exposed animals for longer durations have reported mixed findings--but these differences are related to procedure. For example, some investigators have found changes in adult activity as a result of prenatal exposure to ELF fields. Such studies are discussed later in the section on "Neurobehavioral Teratology." Other studies have exposed adult animals to ELF fields for longer durations and found minimal effects of exposure. Lovely et al. (1984b) exposed rats for 30 to 37 days and, in two different studies (one at 1.9 kV/m and another at 40 kV/m), found no remarkable effects of exposure on postexposure exploration, activity or its circadian distribution. The first study at 1.9 kV/m tested rats for only 1 hour following a month of exposure to a 60-Hz electric field. Half the rats were observed in the morning and half were observed in the afternoon in a residential or figure-8 maze. The exposed rats appeared to show a reversal of the early morning to late afternoon activity differences typically seen in this environment and as was evident in the sham-exposed rats. In the second study, at 40 kV/m, rats were tested in the same maze for 23-hour periods following 30 to 37 days of exposure. The data showed no significant perturbation of the normal circadian distribution of activity despite the fact that the findings at the lower-field strength had shown a difference. One is inclined to dismiss the initial finding as a false positive, unless there is an intensity "window" at 1.9 kV/m.

Aversive Behaviors

Exposure of rodents to 50- or 60-Hz, primarily electric, fields will lead to aversive behavior if the fields are strong enough.

Bayer et al. (1977) observed that female rats, given a choice between two living environments connected by a runway, would traverse the runway to avoid exposure to a 50-Hz, 100-kV/m electric field. However, the female rats would re-enter the field during the nocturnal portion of the day/night cycle on which they were maintained. While this observation was made on only a handful of animals, the effect was later observed by Hjeresen et al. (1980) for 60-Hz electric fields at, or above, field strengths of 75 kV/m. Hjeresen et al. also observed the nocturnal reversal seen by Bayer et al. Hjeresen et al. employed much larger sample sizes of male Sprague-Dawley rats and found that the aversive behavior: 1) develops within 45 to 60 minutes, 2) is unaffected by up to 1 month of prior exposure to intense (100-kV/m) electric fields, and 3) occurs independent of possible electric shock, corona discharge, ozone, audible noise or vibration of the exposure system as a source of "artifact." The statistical analyses were appropriate for the data collected, and in a subsequent study, Hjeresen et al. (1982) demonstrated similar phenomenon in Hanford Miniature swine (HMS) that had already been on exposure (20 hours/day for up to 3,600 hours) to a 30-kV/m, 60-Hz electric field. The data also made it clear that the diurnal swine show the opposite effect of the nocturnal rat with regard to day/night dependence of field aversions. Thus, the pigs tended to remain in the field during the daylight hours and avoid field exposure at night.

Despite the fact that this aversive behavior appears to be robust and generalizes across species, test parameters, and laboratories, it would be premature to conclude that intense electric fields are an adverse stimulus that easily motivates aversive behavior in the species tested. Creim et al. (1982) employed the same test apparatus used by Hjeresen et al. (1980) and found that rats that experience electric-field exposure in a slowly ascending sequence of field strengths (0, 25, 50, 75, and 100 kV/m, with each 1-hour test carried out every 15 days) fail to avoid electric fields at field strengths up to 100 kV/m in the later tests. The study appears to be free from artifact, is well-designed (other groups with random or descending sequences of field strengths do show the typical field aversion), and is properly analyzed statistically. Thus, the nature of an animal's prior experience with the electric field may serve to completely attenuate the typically observed aversion.

Another study by Creim et al. (1984b) paired saccharin-flavored water with a 3-hour exposure to 60-Hz electric fields at intensities up to 130 kV/m in an attempt to obtain taste-aversion (TA) learning. When novel tastes, such as saccharin-flavored water, are paired with stimuli producing illness or malaise, generally (Garcia and Koelling, 1967), or gastrointestinal (GI) distress, specifically (Pelchat et al., 1983), the adversive agent is a sufficient condition for TA learning to occur in rats (and most other species). In a series of three experiments, Creim et al. failed to find evidence for TA learning as a result of electric-field exposure up to 5 hours in duration. They also failed to find any synergistic (additive) effect of combining clyclophosphamide (an agent that does produce GI distress) and electric-field exposure for 5 hours after consumption of saccharin-flavored water. They did find TA learning with cyclophosphamide alone, thus validating their procedures and experimental design. So, here is more evidence that allows one to narrow the possible interpretations of the aversive behavior induced by exposure to electric fields.

Although rats may fail to show TA learning, they will avoid saccharin-flavored food when its consumption necessitates traversing an alley from the Faraday-shielded half of an alley to the half exposed to a 100-kV/m, 60-Hz electric field (Creim et al., 1983). The effect is large, easily replicable (in the same laboratory), and is strictly contingent on the presence of the electric field. Indeed, the rats develop a preference for saccharin prior to any electric-field exposure. Nevertheless, the preference is abandoned when consumption requires exposure (i.e., entry) to the electric field. This series of studies is well-designed and is based on large sample sizes (original effect based on 18 rats/group). A rather tortuous series of subsequent experiments (Creim et al., 1984a) finally revealed that this apparently robust effect depended on as subtle a variable as whether the container holding the saccharin-flavored food was above, or below, the ground plane on which the animal was exposed to the 60-Hz electric fields. Finally, the most recent study of this series (Lovely et al., 1985) has revealed that the saccharin-flavored food aversion is largely eliminated if the rats' vibrissae and eyebrows are shaved prior to testing. Of greater interest is the finding that the field aversion typically seen in this laboratory (Hjeresen et al., 1980) was also greatly attenuated when the rats' vibrissae and eyebrows were shaved prior to testing. One is inclined to conclude that the behavioral aversions are based on no more than stimulation of facial hair in the rat. If this intepretation is correct, then the extensive series of studies documenting behavioral aversions that result from exposure to 60-Hz electric fields may be unique to the rat, and some other species, that find stimulation of their facial hair an "adversive" experience.

Neurobehavioral Teratology

Neurobehavioral teratology refers to the early ontogenetic and adult neural and behavioral changes that occur due to perinatal exposure to a putative toxic agent or substance. It is one of the most sensitive "preparations" that can be employed by the behavioral toxicologist because subtle events happening in utero leave not-so-subtle markers on adult nervous system function, including behavior. The primary reason for this, if exposures are appropriately timed, is that differentiation and migration of neural cell types are not complete until well after birth. Perturbation of these processes will often manifest themselves as changes in the development of neural responses or in their adult expression or in both. More often than not, the adult changes are permanent.

It is another issue as to whether one decides to interpret adult behavioral change due to perinatal influences as an "effect" or a "hazard." In other words, one cannot assume that all perinatal manipulations that produce neural changes are necessarily bad. Greenough (Turner and Greenough, 1983) is one of a number of researchers who manipulate the quality and quantity of environmental stimulation that a rodent receives during rearing. Over the years, profound effects have been shown to occur at all levels of neural organization--morphological, chemical, and behavioral. But these effects are not hazards; they merely reflect the plasticity of the developing nervous system.

When we turn to studies evaluating the neurobehavioral effects of perinatal exposure to ELF fields, the safest generalization we can make is that there is an insufficient data base at this time to come to any sound conclusions regarding the putative toxicity of perinatal exposure to ELF fields.

Frey (1982) exposed pregnant Sprague-Dawley rats to a 60-Hz electric field at 3.5 kV/m from the first to the nineteenth day of gestation. The experimental design allowed for cross-fostering within a day after parturition to eliminate postnatal mothering effects. The author claims a number of postnatal alterations in behavior, including open-field activity, but the methods and statistics are reported in insufficient detail to evaluate this report fairly.

Lovely et al. (1984c) also exposed gravid Sprague-Dawley rats to a 60-Hz electric field at 60 kV/m. Exposures were for 20 hours/day from conception to 21 days of postnatal age. There were no attempts to eliminate mothering effects. At 90 days of age, male/female littermates were tested in three tasks: shuttlebox avoidance, a residential maze, and the preference/aversion task described by Hjeresen et al. (1980). They found that the perinatal exposure to a 60-Hz electric field versus sham-exposure failed to statistically differentiate groups in any of the tasks employed. There are two shortcomings of this study. First, the sample sizes (n = 10 subjects/subgroup) is small for a behavioral teratology study. This is especially unfortunate because a number of consistent trends in the data are suggestive of an effect of exposure on activity measures of female progeny. Second, the range of behaviors examined is not a very complete assessment for postnatal neural alteration (e.g., no sensory or motor tests, no memory tests, no analgesia tests, etc.).

In another study (Lovely et al., 1982, 1984a), post-natal behavioral tests were carried out on F_2 generation HMS that had been exposed prenatally to a 60-Hz, 30-kV/m electric field. The assessments included a test for neuro-muscular development at 3 days of age (righting and nega-tive geotaxis), a test for open-field activity, vocaliza-tions, orienting response/habituation at 1, 3, and 5 weeks of age; and learning/memory in a multi-choice T-maze at 8, 12, and 16 weeks of age. There were no statistically sig-nificant differences between exposed and sham-exposed swine in the neuromuscular tests (although there were some ani-mals failing to respond in the exposed group). Similarly, there were no significant differences in the T-maze tests for learning and memory (parameters assessed included startbox latency, goalbox speed, errors made, trials to criterion or completed/30-minute test). However, in the open field, the exposed females made significantly less vocalizations, both within and across all 15-minute test sessions. The same females were also less active in the test at 1 week of age. The nature of the overall design precluded cross-fostering at parturition, so it is not pos-sible to determine if the effect is the result of prenatal exposure, postnatal exposure, or altered mothering. It is known that the mothers of these swine showed anomalous re-productive behavior prior to conception and farrowing (Si-kov et al., 1984).

Neural functions other than behavior have been evalu-ated following prenatal exposure to ELF fields. Jaffe et al. (1983) monitored the ontogeny of the visual-evoked re-sponse in rats prenatally exposed to 60-Hz electric fields at 65 kV/m, and found no significant effects of exposure. The study is well-designed and the evoked-potential data appear to be appropriately analyzed.

Hansson (1981) exposed rabbits to a 50-Hz, 14-kV/m electric field throughout gestation and through 7.5 weeks postnatally. He found a number of histological changes in the cerebellar Purkinje cells of his exposed rabbits. These included a reduction in the size and number of Nissl bodies, a reduction in the rough endoplasmic reticulum, and the appearance of lamellar bodies. There were also signif-icant reductions in the body weights of his exposed rab-bits, suggesting more general deleterious effects of expo-sure or possibly other stressers in the exposure environ-ment. However, in subsequent experiments where the exposed

subjects appeared to be generally healthy and better maintained (Hansson, this volume), similar findings were reported as a result of perinatal exposure to electric
fields. In a different laboratory, Albert et al. (1984)
has observed similar effects in rats; the appearance of
lamellar bodies both in cerebellar Purkinje cells and hippocampal pyramidal cells was the result of prenatal exposure to a 60-Hz electric field at 60 kV/m. So, despite
reservations about the exposure environment in Hansson's
initial study (1981), there may be genuine neurohistologi-
cal changes due to perinatal exposure to ELF fields.
Whether these alterations portend pathology is not yet
clear.

Behavioral Effects in Humans

Although Russian investigators have reported that
switchyard workers exposed to 50-Hz electric fields suffer
from a number of neurovegetative disorders (e.g., Asanova
and Rakov, 1966; Filipov, 1972; Korobkova et al., 1972), it
is difficult to evaluate these reports because there is no
real measurement of the fields to which the workers were
exposed; nor is there a meaningful estimate of the duration
of exposure. Had a rigorous dosimetric investigation been
conducted, it might just as well turn out that these effects result from mini-shocks and not from exposure to ELF
fields per se. Changes in neurovegetative function might
be more understandable if they had come from mini-shocks.

More recently however, a series of studies (Norris,
Male, and Bonnell, this volume) have been reported that
document, in detail, the fields or currents experienced by
human subjects and relate these values to the subjects'
physical and psychological well-being. In the first of two
study types, nearly 400 occupationally exposed personnel
completed a widely used health-questionnaire interview
(Broadbent and Gath, 1979; Crown and Crisp, 1966, 1979).
Estimates of exposure to 50-Hz electric and magnetic fields
were obtained, and, on nearly 300 of the 400 workers, actual measurements over a 2-week period were also obtained.
The results were unequivocal. First, estimates of exposure
tended to exceed actual measured exposure (measured mean of
30.5 kV/m-hours twice/week). Second, no significant correlations between either estimated exposure or actual expo-

sure and health status was found. The study is statistically sound and was conducted blind.

In a second type of study, 76 healthy human volunteer subjects had electrodes placed over 10 locations on the upper body, whereby a total of 500 μA at 50 Hz could be injected into the subjects. The decision to inject current was in deference to possible effects of hair stimulation (and resulting perception) that would occur if subjects were actually exposed to 50-Hz electric fields. The authors estimated that the summed-current injected was equivalent to that which might result from a grounded man standing in a 35-kV/m field. The subjects were tested over two sessions with half the subjects receiving injected current the first session, and half receiving it in the second session. The four major tests the subjects took under both conditions were: syntactic reasoning, semantic reasoning, visual search, and serial reaction time. Stress/arousal levels were also determined using a mood-adjective checklist at the start and end of each session. The study was conducted double-blind. Two significant differences were found. The first was a significant shift in the ability to determine truth of sentences. However, the results make it impossible to determine if the effect of injected current is to improve learning in the first session or impair performance in the second session (or impair performance generally). The second and similarly ordered effect relates to the self-report of arousal; it emerged as a significant interaction effect: arousal falls from the start to the end of a session; but it falls less for the current-off group only in the second session. Even though these are rather minimal effects, it is unfortunate that other "dose" groups were not included (i.e., 500 μA, albeit distributed, is a fair amount of current). One would be more concerned with such findings at 50-μA summed current injected.

DISCUSSION

If we exclude the specialized response systems that have evolved in some species (e.g., electroreception, homing, and navigation), it is tempting to conclude that remarkably little, if any, behavior is radically altered by exposure to ELF fields. What then are we to make of Hansson's findings (1981), that prenatal exposure to 50-Hz electric fields leads to a number of histologic anomalies in the rabbit cerebellum, and the Albert et al. observations (1984) of similar exposure-dependent changes in the rat's cerebellum and hippocampus? What are we to make of Wilson et al. (1981), who reports that 1 month of exposure to 60-Hz electric fields at 65 kV/m suppresses nocturnal melatonin levels and serotonin-N-acetyltransferase (SNAT) activity in the pineal gland of rats? The pineal observations have been subsequently obtained at field strengths as low as 1.9 kV/m (Anderson, personal communication). And what are we to make of the efflux of calcium ions that occur in chick, cat, and rat cortices when tissues are exposed in vitro to electromagnetic fields modulated at particular ELF frequencies (e.g., Bawin and Adey, 1976; Blackman et al., 1985)? If these neural alterations occur in the same animals tested in behavioral experiments, then why has so remarkedly little been found? Are these neural effects just "noise" to a behaving organism? Or, are there other possible explanations for the lack of concordance? One possible answer to this question relates to the very substance of behavioral neuroscience and physiological psychology.

The primary objective of the physiological psychologist is to identify the rules of correspondence that are the linkages between the simple elements in the nervous system (neurons, glia, transmitters, receptor types, etc., and their general organization) and behavior. These rules of correspondence are not yet well understood, and as a result it is difficult for behavioral scientists to know whether they are asking the right question of the animal or even using the right species and behavioral preparation. In a few cases, some of the rules of correspondence are being worked out, and the astute behavioral scientists should apply these to evaluate the putative toxicity of ELF fields. An example or two should suffice to make the point. Thompson (1983) has provided evidence that the dentate and interpositus nuclei of the cerebellum are the substrate of memory for a simple learned motor habit in the rabbit. With this in mind, and in light of Hansson's observations (1981) of histological change in the rat cerebellum (which include the dentate and interpositus nuclei), an appropriate experiment to evaluate the functional/behavioral significance of Hansson's finding would be to prenatally expose rabbits to ELF fields as Hansson has done and then, when the progeny are adults, test them for classically conditioned leg flexion or the nictitating membrane response as Thompson has done. To date, no one has done this experiment nor have they proposed to do it.

One of the most frequent questions asked of Bawin and Adey (1976) and of Blackman et al. (1985) is, "what is the functional significance of your observations of efflux of calcium ions from cortices exposed invitro"? To answer that question, behaviorally, we need to again establish what linkages exist between subtle changes in neuronal calcium pools in cortex and behavior. One answer to that question is elegantly detailed by Lynch and Beaudry (1984). Calcium-ion infusion into the subsynaptic space is requisite for cortical memories to be formed. Events, other than exposure to ELF fields, which perturb the normal calcium-ion influx into the subsynaptic space disrupt behavioral indices of memory (e.g., rodent memory in a radial-arm maze), as well as electrophysiological events that are taken as reflecting the substrate of memory, e.g., long-term potentiation (LTP) in the hippocampus. So, here again, because some rules of correspondence appear to be in place, the physiological psychologist has some idea of what questions to ask under ELF exposure conditions approximating those in which Bawin and Adey (1976) and Blackman et al. (1985) obtained their calcium-ion effects. But, what behavioral scientist has studied radial-arm maze performance during exposure to an ELF field; similarly who has evaluated LTP under ELF exposure conditions that approximate those of Bawin and Adey or Blackman et al.?

Beyond the approaches detailed above, there are a number of other behavioral researches that need to be carried out before one can conclude that exposure to ELF fields is without effect on behavior. The data base for neurobehavioral teratology is inadequate. It is especially inadequate given suggestions in the literature that ELF electric and magnetic fields may be potent teratogens (Sikov et al., 1984). There are a number of postnatal parameters that have yet to be assessed following prenatal exposure to ELF fields. Among these are learning and memory, sensory and motor function and analgesia. The activity assessments reported by Lovely, Creim, and Phillips (1984a, 1984c) and Frey (1982) should be repeated with larger sample sizes, and, as indicated above, someone should specifically address whether rabbits exposed prenatally show learning deficits in the acquisition of a classically conditioned motor response.

Finally, there is a need to evaluate populations at risk or populations already compromised by exposure to other agents. In the real world, there are subsets of the general population that are "at risk." They tend to be more susceptible to secondary stressers. But few, if any, synergy-type studies have been conducted employing ELF fields. There are other research needs, but the above are essential.

SUMMARY

Behavioral responses to ELF electric and magnetic fields are reviewed starting with the simple sensory awareness or detection by an animal and moving on through more-complicated behavioral responses such as behavior that averts exposure. The literature selected in this review is taken primarily from the area of behavioral toxicology. As such, it does not review work on specialized response systems to ELF fields. The most notable of these omitted specialized response systems are electroreception, (see Kalmijn, this volume), which occurs in a number of fish species, and homing/navigation and communication of the location of food that occurs in several species of birds and in honeybees, respectively.

The toxicologic orientation of most researches that evaluate the effects of exposure to ELF electric and magnetic fields has been influenced primarily by the "missions" of DOE and the power industry programs to determine the health effects of power frequency (50- and 60-Hz) electric and magnetic fields. Because of these large programmatic efforts, most of the recent research has in fact been done at 50 or 60 Hz.

In the context of the above limitations, remarkably few robust behavioral effects have been reported. Those that have been reported probably relate to an animal's perception of the electric field, although there are some exceptions to this generalization.

The apparent lack of deleterious effects in animals is consistent with recent studies on humans that have been conducted in the UK. With this in mind, it is tempting to conclude that exposure to an ELF field is a rather innocuous event and, other than possible mini-shocks, is without hazard. However, if this is the case, then what sense are we to make of reports of altered neural function (other than behavior) that result from exposure to ELF fields (e.g., suppressed melatonin and SNAT activity in the rat pineal; efflux of calcium ions from brain cortices; histological change in the cerebellum and hippocampus following perinatal exposure, etc.)? Are these neural effects no more than "noise" to the behaving organism? Possible reasons form the disparity between cell biology, neurochemistry, and behavior have been presented in this chapter, and based on the hypothesized reasons for the existing disparity, a number of experiments were suggested.

ACKNOWLEDGMENTS

The research reviewed in this paper, which was conducted in the authors' laboratory, was presented at the Conference on Electromagnetic Waves and Neurobehavioral Function, Corsendonk, Belgium, August 19-23, 1984. Major portions of this paper were published by the American Institute of Biological Sciences (AIBS) in May 1985, under the title "Assessments and Viewpoints on the Biological and Human Health Effects of Extremely Low Frequency (ELF) Electromagnetic Fields," and I am indebted to the AIBS for their permission to reproduce that material here. Preparation of this review was supported, in part, by the U.S. Department of Energy under Contracts DE-AC06-76RLO-1830 and DE-AC06-76RLO-1831.

REFERENCES

Adrian DJ (1977). Auditory and visual sensation stimulated by low frequency electric currents. Radio Sci 12(6S): 243-250.

Albert E, Cohen G, Avellino L, Kornhouser G, Yoshida A (1984). Electron microscopic observation on rat cerebellum and hippocampus after exposure to 60 Hz electric fields. In "Sixth Annual Scientific Session of the Bioelectromagnetics Society, July 15-19, 1984, Atlanta, GA (abstrast), p 4.

Asanova TP, Rakov AN (1966). The state of health of persons working in the electric field of outdoor 400-kV and 500-kV switchyards. Leningrad: Institute of Labor Hygiene and Professional Diseases. Reprint. 1974.

Specical Publication No. 10. Piscataway, NJ: IEEE Power Engineering Society.

Bawin SM and Adey WR (1976). Sensitivity of calcium binding in cerebral tissue to weak environmental electric fields oscillating at low frequency. Proc Natl Acad Sci USA 73:1999-2003.

Bayer A, Brinkman J, Wittke G (1977). Experimentelle untersuchungen an ratten zur frage der wirkung elektrischer wechselfelder auf lebewesen. Elektrizitaetswirtschaft 4:77-81.

Blackman CF, Benane SG, House DE, Jocines WT (1985). Effects of ELF (1-120 Hz) and modulated (50 Hz) RF fields on the effect of calcium ions from brain tissue in vitro. Bioelectromagnetics 6:1-19.

Broadbent DE, Gath D (1979). Chronic effects of repetitive and nonrepetitive work. In Mackay C and Cox T (eds): "Response to Stress," London: IPC, pp 120-128.

Bullock TH (1982). Electroreception. Annu Rev Neurosci 5:121-170.

Cooper LJ, Graves HB, Smith JC, Poznaniak D, Madjid AH (1981). Behavioral responses of pigeons to 60-Hz electric fields. Behav Neural Biol 32:214-228.

Creim JA, Hilton DI, Lovely RH, Phillips RD (1983). Motivational aspect of electric-field avoidance in rats. In "Fifth Annual Scientific Session of the Bioelectromagnetics Society," June 12-17, 1983, Boulder, CO (abstract), p 113.

Creim JA, Lovely RH, Hilton DI, Phillips RD, Kaune WT (1984a). Rats preference for saccharin-flavored chow depends on feeder location in a 60-Hz electric field. In "Sixth Annual Scientific Session of the Bioelectromagnetics Society," July 15-19, 1984, Atlanta, GA (abstract), p 67.

Creim JA, Lovely RH, Kaune WT, Phillips RD (1984b). Attempts to produce taste-aversion learning in rats exposed to 60-Hz electric fields. Bioelectromagnetics 5:271-282.

Creim JA, Lovely RH, Phillips RD (1982). Role of previous exposure history on preference to minimize exposure to 60-Hz electric fields in rats. In "Fourth Annual Scientific Session of the Bioelectromagnetics Society," June 23-July 2, 1982, Los Angeles, CA (abstract), p 47.

Crown S, Crisp AH (1966). A short clinical diagnostic self-rating scale for psycho-neurotic patients. Br J Psychiatry 112:917-923.

Crown S, Crisp AH (1979). "Manual of the Crown-Crisp Experimental Index." London: Hodder and Stoughton.

Filipov V (1972). Effect of alternating electric field on man. Chapter 2. In "Second International Colloquiam on Prevention of Occupational Risk due to Electricity," November 30-December 1, 1972, Köln.

Frey AH (1982). Neural and behavioral consequences of prenatal exposure to 3.5 kV/m 60 Hz fields. In "Fourth Annual Scientific Session of the Bioelectromagnetics Society," June 28-July 2, 1982, Los Angeles, CA (abstract), p 6.

Garcia J, Koelling RA (1967). A comparison of aversions induced by X-rays, toxins, and drugs in the rat. Radiat Res 7:439-450.

Graves HB (1981). Detection of a 60-Hz electric field by pigeons. Behav Neural Biol 32:229-234.

Hackman RM, Graves HB (1981). Corticosterone levels in mice exposed to high-intensity electric fields. Behav Neural Biol 32:201-213.

Hansson HA (1981). Lamellar bodies in Purkinje cells experimentally induced by electric fields. Brain Res 216:1-10.

Hjeresen DL, Kaune WT, Decker JR, Phillips RD (1980). Effects of 60-Hz electric fields on avoidance behavior and activity of rats. Bioelectromagnetics 1:299-321.

Hjeresen DL, Miller MC, Kaune WT, Phillips RD (1982). A behavioral response of swine to a 60-Hz electric field. Bioelectromagnetics 3:443-451.

Jaffe RA, Lopresti CA, Carr DB, Phillips RD (1983). Prenatal exposure to 60-Hz electric fields: Effects on the development of the visual-evoked response in rats. Bioelectromagnetics 4:327-339.

Korobkova RP, Morozov Yu A, Stolarov MS, Yakub Yu A (1972). Influence of the electric field in 500 and 750 kV switchyards on maintenance staff and means for it protection. Conf Int Grand Res Elec (CIGRE, Paris), paper 22-06.

Lovely RH, Creim JA, Anderson LE (1985). The role of ears, vibrissae and other body hair in the rats aversions to intense 60-Hz electric fields. In "Abstracts, Seventh Annual Meeting of the Bioelectromagnetics Society, June 16-20, 1985, San Francisco, CA, p 58.

Lovely RH, Creim JA, Phillips RD (1982). Early neuromuscular development in three-day-old F-2 generation miniature swine is unaffected by prenatal exposure to 60-Hz electric fields. In "Fourth Annual Scientific Session of the Bioelectromagnetics Society," June 28-July 2, 1982, Los Angeles, CA (abstract), p 7.

Lovely RH, Creim JA, Phillips RD (1984a). Adult behavioral effects of prenatal and early postnatal exposure to 60-Hz electric fields in rats. In "Interaction of Electromagnetic Fields with Biological System," 21st General Assembly of the International URSI, August 27-30, 1984, Florence, Italy (abstract).

Lovely RH, Creim JA, Phillips RD (1984b). Effects of prenatal exposure to 60-Hz electric fields on open field and maze performance of F-2 generation Hanford Miniature swine. In "Sixth Annual Scientific Session of the Bioelectromagnetics Society," July 15-19, 1984, Atlanta, GA (abstract), p 10.

Lovely RH, Creim JA, Phillips RD (1984c). 60-Hz electric field effects on exploration and circadian distribution of activity in the rat. In "Sixth Annual Scientific Session of the Bioelectromagnetics Society," July 15-19, 1984, Atlanta, GA (abstract), p 11.

Lynch G Beaudry M (1984). The biochemistry of memory: A new and specific hypothesis. Science 224:1057-1063.

National Academy of Sciences (1977). Biologic effects of electric and magnetic fields associated with proposed Project Seafarer. In "Report of the Committee on Biosphere Effects of Extremely-Low Frequency Radiation," NAS: Washington, DC.

Pelchat ML, Grill JG, Rozin P, Jacobs J (1983). Quality of acquired responses to tastes by Rattus norvegicus depends on the type of associated discomfort. J Comp Psychol 97:140-153.

Reilly JP (1978). Electric and magnetic field coupling from high voltage AC power transmission lines -- Classification of short term effects on people. IEEE Power Engineering Meeting, New York, January 29-30, 1978, Piscataway, NJ. IEEE Report No. F78 167-9, 1-10.

Rosenberg RS, Duffy PH, Sacher GA (1981). Effects of intermittent 60-Hz high voltage electric fields on metabolism, activity and temperature in mice. Bioelectromagnetics 2:291-304.

Rosenberg RS, Duffy PH, Sacher GA, Ehret CF (1983). Relationship between field strength and arousal response in mice exposed to 60-Hz electric fields. Bioelectromagnetics 4:181-191.

Sikov MR, Buschbom RL, Kaune WT, Rommereim DN, Beamer JL, Phillips RD (1984). Evaluation of reproduction and development in Hanford Miniature Swine exposed to 60-Hz electric fields. In "Interaction of Biological Systems with Static and ELF Electric and Magnetic Fields," 23rd Hanford Life Sciences Symposium, October 2-4, 1984, Richland, WA (abstract), p 58.

Smith RF, Justesen DR (1977). Effects of a 60-Hz magnetic field on activity levels of mice. Radio Sci 12(6S):- 279-286.

Stern S, Laties VG (1985). 60-Hz electric fields: Detection by female rats. Bioelectromagnetics 6:99-103.

Stern S, Laties VG, Stancampiano CV, Cox C, DeLorge JO (1983). Behavioral detection of 60-Hz electric fields by rats. Bioelectromagnetics 4:215-248.

Thompson RF (1983). Neural substrates of simple associate learning: Classical conditioning. Trends Neurosci 7:270-274.

Turner M, Greenough WT (1983). Numerical density of synapses in neuropil of occipital cortex of rats reared in complex, social, or isolated environments. In "Thirteenth Annual Meeting of the Society for Neuroscience," November 6-11, 1983, Boston, MA (abstract), p 55.

Wilson BW, Anderson LE, Hilton, Phillips RD (1981). Chronic exposure to 60-Hz electric fields: Effects on pineal function in rats. Bioelectromagnetics 2:371- 380.

Electromagnetic Fields and Neurobehavioral Function, pages 349–365
© 1988 Alan R. Liss, Inc.

PEOPLE IN 50 Hz ELECTRIC AND MAGNETIC FIELDS: STUDIES
IN THE UNITED KINGDOM

W.T. Norris and J.A. Bonnell

Central Electricity Generating Board

   This paper discusses a programme designed to provide
information to help in deciding whether or not the health of
people living and working near electric power transmission
equipment is substantially affected by the 50-Hz electric or
magnetic fields it produces in its vicinity. The main work
was concerned with electric fields; it is only these that
produce directly discernible responses in people and attention
had been directed to them by earlier publications (e.g.
Korobkova et al., 1972; see also Bridges and Preache, 1981 for
a full discussion).

   Electric fields at ground level under the highest voltage
electric power transmission lines in the UK - those at 400 kV -
rise to about 11 kV m^{-1}; in 400 kV substations (American;
switchyards) they rise to about 22 kV m^{-1}. Because of
topographical constraints on tower siting the spans with the
lowest design clearance to ground are rarely found. Objects
such as buildings and trees also reduce ground level fields
in their vicinity. The average value under the conductors
of 400 kV lines is lower than 5 kV m^{-1} and the average value
is lower yet under lower voltage lines. For cognate reasons
fields in substations are for the most part less than 5 kV m^{-1}.

   There is no specified width of right-of-way in the UK.
Land is not usually bought by the electricity supply authorities
for transmission lines; an easement to erect and use a line
is obtained and payments are made for the disturbance caused
and for loss of facility. Provided that safety clearances to
prevent heavy current flashover are maintained, buildings and
houses are erected beneath lines.

At least since the 1930s electricity supply engineers have had experience in dealing with directly perceived effects of electric induction under a.c. transmission lines (e.g. Barber et al, 1972). Practical difficulties are few and are readily overcome by screening or earthing.

Magnetic fields near lines fluctuate widely during the day and the seasons as the power flow rises and falls; an average value beneath a 400 kV line is below 20 A m^{-1} but at peak load 80 A m^{-1} may be found. Magnetic fields in houses due to distribution cables are rarely more than 100 mA m^{-1}. Near domestic equipment one may find greater field strengths. These magnetic fields are not directly perceived by people.

With regard to these electric and magnetic fields a question we saw as needing resolution was, were there surreptitious effects on health which were provoked during exposure but with the people being unaware that they were being affected especially when they could perceive nothing. Physically this means, is the current flow induced inside the body by the electric or magnetic field physiologically active at the field strengths concerned? For completeness one might also consider direct magnetic interactions at the cellular or molecular levels but we know of no good biological or medical grounds for introducing such a consideration.

Basis of the Work

We took the view that we needed to study people. We came to this view partly because we were aware of the extensive and high quality work being done on animals and on tissue in vitro in Europe and the United States from which we hoped to learn and upon which we could not expect to improve without inordinate effort.

The Central Electricity Generating Board (CEGB) in collaboration with others therefore has supported:

-   an epidemiological study of people occupationally exposed to electric fields

-   a laboratory study of mood, memory, vigilance, concentration and verbal reasoning skills when 50-Hz currents were passed through people

- a survey of the incidence of childhood cancer and its relation to environmental magnetic fields

- a study of the performance of pacemakers when the wearer encounters strong electric fields.

We wished to do a survey of the general health of public living near overhead lines but saw no way in which general morbidity data could be collected so as to account plausibly and usefully for confounding factors, and thus show influences of electric and magnetic fields. The cancer survey was facilitated by the existence of a well maintained set of records about the incidence of that particular group of diseases in a large geographical area.

This programme is now largely completed apart from the cancer survey. The remainder of this paper outlines the results of the work done and discusses their implications in the light of work done elsewhere.

Epidemiology of Occupationally Exposed People; South West Britain Survey

Broadbent, Broadbent, Male and Jones (1985) describe the survey in detail. The results cover 390 electric power transmission and distribution staff. A health questionnaire was administered by nurses specially trained for a standard interview of about 150 questions and which lasted about an hour. Exposure to electric fields was (a) measured over the fortnight before the interview and (b) estimated by supervisory engineers for time spent exposed to low (1.5-5.5 kV m^{-1}), medium (5.5-9.5 kV m^{-1}) and high (>9.5 kV m^{-1}) strength fields over the previous six months and the previous fifteen years.

Perhaps because of inexperience in making such estimates (and with no exposure measurements to guide them) the average of the engineers estimations was about ten times the average of the measured values. This sort of discrepancy has been noted by others and is due partly to there being more screening of electric fields by objects near people at work than had been supposed and partly to underestimation of time spent travelling and doing preparatory work outside high voltage areas.

Measurements were made of the time integral of unperturbed field strength using the electrochemical meter devised by Deno (1977). The meter was worn in an armband sleeve and so held facing outwards on the upper arm. This is not a sensitive position. Errors were estimated to be about 50%. Random zero drift of the meters meant that detection of low levels was unreliable: a threshold of 6.6 kV m^{-1}hr was eventually adopted and only 28 subjects received exposure above this threshold during the fortnight of measurement. There was some correlation between the short term exposure measurement and the estimates of longer term exposure. It seems that the scale of the estimates was wrong but there is no special reason to say the ranking of individuals was incorrect.

Health measures included numbers of visits to the doctor, use of medicines (both prescribed and unprescribed), incidence of headaches and cognitive failure. A modified version of the Middlesex Hospital Questionnaire (MHQ) (Crown and Crisp, 1966, 1979) was used to estimate anxiety, depression and somatic and obsessional symptoms. Job factors were also included: e.g. amount of physical work, shift changes, time spent travelling, overtime, discretion exercised on the job, and variety of things to be remembered.

The results were analysed in several ways. For example, the fortnight measurements of exposure were taken at face value in one analysis; those for whom the fortnight exposure was above the threshold were studied in a companion analysis.

In the first analysis of the sixty correlations tested only 6 were of statistical significance, all with longer term estimates of exposure.

Five of these, concerned with visits to the doctor and the taking of unprescribed medicines suggested that more exposed people had fewer symptoms. The sixth factor suggested that those more exposed in the previous six months to medium fields took fewer prescribed medicines. When only those people who had had significant exposure in the fortnight before the interview were considered there were no fresh findings apart from a single correlation between frequency of visits to the doctor and 15-year exposure to high fields. These rather paradoxical relationships appear to result from the exposure being different in different jobs but it is other features of the jobs that

tend to produce health effects and this was borne out by
further analysis. Factors such as overtime, working alone
or having changed shift several times in the past three
days were correlated with the total MHQ score, depression
and somatic symptoms.

However, after allowing for these effects no
significant correlations of health either with measures
or with estimated exposure to electric fields was found.

Laboratory Study of Mood, Memory, Vigilance and Verbal-Reasoning Skills

This study is reported in detail by Stollery (1984
and 1985 to be published). We believed it was important
to eliminate perception of the electric field. Instead
of placing subjects beneath high voltage electrodes which
would lead to hair and skin stimulation, 500 µA at 50 Hz
was passed through ten electrodes attached to the upper
body (including four on the head) to the feet. As we
shall see we were not entirely successful in suppressing
perception . This total current is equivalent to that
induced in a person standing in an electric field of about
35 kV m^{-1} (Deno, 1977), If however one regards the current
to the head (200 µA) as critical the equivalent field is
47 kV m^{-1} (Deno, 1977). These equivalent fields assume
the person is well earthed; if this is not the case the
equivalent fields are higher. We had originally intended
to use three current levels up to the traditional minimum
perception current of 500 µA with a view to establishing
a biological gradient. However, in a pilot study of 20
people we saw no effects at 500 µA and so decided to devote
all the main study to one current level thereby improving
sensitivity.

The electrodes concentrate the current beneath them
and to the extent they do this the current flow pattern
in the body departs from the spatial variation of current
in-flow through the surface from the external
displacement currents that typify being beneath an overhead
line. This discrepancy does not seem important.

No specific illness had been suspected to result from
exposure to electric fields near transmission plants but
some studies (see Male and Norris, 1981 and Bonnell, 1982,
for references) had suggested that non-specific responses

might be consequent on or expressed as changes in the action of the central nervous system.

We did not do tests on blood because the work of Hauf (1974) showed only small efects in broadly comparable work and the changes were within the normal physiological range. Animal work (e.g. Phillips 1985) had provided no indications of biochemical parameters that showed enough promise of being useful to justify the considerable technical effort needed to measure them in our proposed experiment. The measures of central nervous function we chose as most useful were psychometric tests.

Subjects were male volunteers aged between 18 and 65. Each of the 76 subjects undertook a sequence of four such tests, the sequence being undertaken four times during each of two 5.5 hr days. The tests were of syntactic reasoning, semantic reasoning , visual search and serial reaction time. Stress and arousal were self reported using a mood adjective check list at the start and end of each day.

For one group of subjects, Group A, current was passed only on the first day; for the remainder, Group B, current was passed only on the second day.

Double blind procedures were adopted. Subjects had been asked to note down when they felt current flow during the day. Before the main test period each day current was raised through one electrode until the subject 'perceived' current flow. They thus had an idea of what current flow felt like. The values of current used in this test were always substantially higher than the 50 µA per electrode of the main test.

Some subjects did report sensations of current flow. Some reports were on both days (i.e. both when current was flowing and when it was not); some in group B reported sensations only when no current was flowing. Sensations occurred at electrodes, mainly those on the arm. The electrode arrangment had been modified because of much more extensive reports of sensation during the pilot study. We surmise that reports of sensations when no current was flowing were due to electrodes moving across the skin.

The durations of sensation were of a few minutes. The duration during exposure (8.4 minutes on average) was (significantly) longer than during sham exposure (2.6 minutes). Thus the double blind nature of the study was compromised to some extent. We judge this to be minor.

Of all the interactions covered by the analysis of variation of the parameters of the psychometric tests and the arousal and stress responses two main factors emerged implying an effect of current (see papers by Stollery for other matters).

The first factor concerned the ability to determine the truth of sentences. A television screen displayed to subjects a sentence describing the order of two letters A and B (not to be confused with the test groups) and the pair of letters in random order. E.g.

A follows B   AB
B is not followed by A   BA.

Subjects had to press one of two keys to indicate whether the sentence did or did not correctly describe the final letter order. The first example is 'false' and the second is 'false' too. Many trials were made in each ten minute session. Overall accuracy was 98.5%. Co-variates were examined and subjects who had slept longer on the previous night verified statements more quickly. The only effect that appeared to be related to current was in the time to correctly respond to sentences in the passive voice (p=0.03).

Figure 1 shows the mean reaction times for the two groups on the two days. Both groups improve from day 1 to day 2 but group A improves more than group B. The performances of the groups are indistinguishable on the first day.

The results do not allow one to distinguish whether current flow improved the learning acquired on the first day, impaired performance on the second day or impaired performance generally. The third possibility requires that the groups although picked at random were actually of different ability: the rest of the data do not support that assumption.

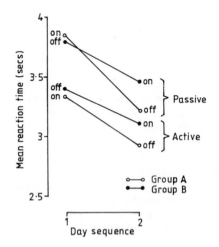

Fig.1. Correct-response reaction times to determine the
truth of sentences. Only responses to passive sentences
show a day - group interaction implying a possible effect
of current.

Figure 2 shows the averaged reaction times for each
individual and is presented to illustrate the scatter in
the measurements. The reaction time on the second day
is plotted against the reaction time on the first day.
The tendency of the points to fall to the lower right part
of the plot illustrates how performance improves from day
1 to day 2. The average points repeat the information
given in figure 1.

The second effect was in self reported arousal
(p = 0.01). At the beginning and end of each day subjects
were presented with a list of adjectives and were asked
to pick those which they felt applied to them. The
adjectives are listed in table 1. One group applies to
feelings of stressfulness, one group to degree of arousal.

Subjects were asked to say which applied to them.
In the list presented to subjects the order was jumbled
from that given here.

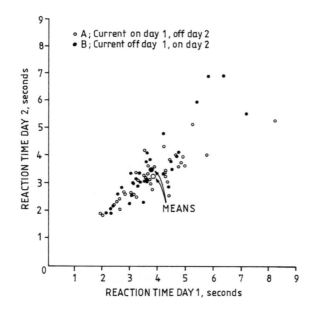

Fig. 2. Individual average correct response reaction times
to passive statements. This plot is to illustrate the
scatter. The difference in mean scores between Group A
and Group B is significant (p = 0.03).

There were no effects of current on stress as assessed
in this way. However, in those subjects who reported
sensations on days when current was flowing those sensations
tended to last longer in those who reported feeling more
stressed. This association suggests that psychological
and biochemical stress responses reported in earlier studies
of electric field exposure may relate to perceived effects
rather than to unfelt flow of electric current.

Figure 3 illustrates the average measures of arousal.
The effect appears to be localised to group A who were
less aroused at the end of the first (exposure) day than
at the end of the second (non exposure) day. Post session
scores for group B did not differ significantly on the
two days.

Table 1 Mood Adjectives. At the start and end of each day

Stress	Arousal
Tense	Active
Worried	Energetic
Apprehensive	Vigorous
Bothered	Alert
Uneasy	Lively
Dejected	Activated
Jittery	Stimulated
Nervous	Drowsy
Distressed	Tired
Peaceful	Idle
Relaxed	Sluggish
Cheerful	Sleepy
Contented	
Pleasant	
Comfortable	
Calm	
Restful	

Figure 4 illustrates the scatter on the individual results. It is a complicated diagram and should either be taken at a glance or examined carefully to see what is being portrayed.

These two results in which no differences are discernable between the groups on the first day allow no clear interpretation. If the two groups were intriniscally different then the results could be interpreted as a simple effect of current. But there is no evidence to say the groups were different. One is then left with transfer effects in which a first experience, with or without current, affects the second experience, without or with current. From these results one can bring forward only a selection of alternative explanations. Amongst these explanations is one that there is no effect at all.

It is perplexing trying to see how best to proceed in further investigation. One might note that the currents used here are much higher than those encountered in present practice near overhead lines and in substations. The effects

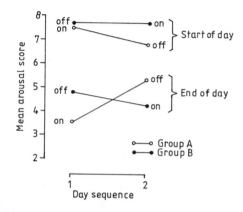

Fig. 3. Average arousal scores for the two exposure groups. The significant aspect is the change in arousal at the end of the day for group A between the first and second day.

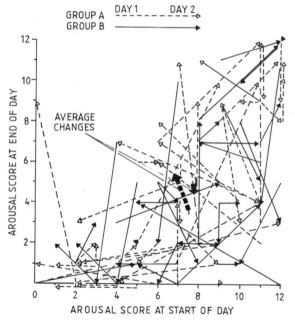

Fig. 4. Scatter of arousal scores. Each arrow represents an individual. The tail of the arrow corresponds to the first day and the point to the second day. The broad arrows are the averages for the two groups.

reported are mild. It does not seem unreasonable to take the view that for practical purposes these results give no cause for disquiet and to allow the case to rest for the time being.

If one determines to continue investigations none of the apparent alternative courses is particularly attractive. A straight forward replication is the orthodox approach but it would be expensive and, even if the effects were confirmed, would leave many questions open. Thus one turns to looking for a scheme which would not only confirm (or not confirm) the present findings but would also give additional information of the kind that one might wish if simple replication had confirmed the original result. Possibilities for future work include

a)   use of more delicate psychological tests which invoke higher mental functions .
b)   use of lower currents (to seek thresholds) or higher currents (to get clearer effects) or a multilevel experiment.
c)   concurrent measurements of other factors such as evoked potentials .
d)   use of shorter timescales of testing. The effects on syntactic reasoning were apparent from the results of the first hour of testing on the second day suggesting that any response is within an hour.
e)   trying to identify susceptible individuals .

The current to the head in these experiments was 200 μA. This current is on the low side of the border line for producing electrical phosphenes or electrosleep: 150 μA flowing into the head near the eyes (Adrian, 1977) produces phosphenes; 500 μA to the head is reported to induce electrosleep.

There is no recorded information to show adequately the extent of variation in individual susceptibility. However, in our experiments no one fell asleep, and no one reported phosphenes. It seems one may discount both phosphenes and electrosleep as contributory factors to the observations though one might consider whether some less marked phenomena related to them may be at play at these lower currents.

Overhead Power Lines and Childhood Cancer

This work is not yet complete but is to be published in due course. Myers et al (1985) provide more detail on the work described here. Registers of childhood cancers diagnosed between 1970 and 1979 were used covering the Yorkshire Health Region. The coverage was not complete but deficiencies appeared small enough to be insignificant. Controls had been established from birth registers choosing children born as near as possible in time to the case child and with a nearby birth address. Some sets of records had two controls per case. Account was taken of moves in and out of the district. In all there were 376 cases and 590 controls.

A survey of magnetic fields in and near houses suggested that the cables in the street or nearly overhead lines were responsible for most of background magnetic field inside a house. Values of such background field due to distribution were estimated to range from 0.01 mG to 0.45 mG. Higher fields are found within a metre or so of some pieces of electrical equipment when it is energised. Higher background fields (up to 4 mG) were also found in apartments especially on the ground floor and are presumably due to cables inside the building. The houses studied were not those of cases or controls from the registers. We had no ready means of finding the historic distribution cable loadings near the houses of cases and controls at the time of diagnoses and no way of discriminating residences on account of magnetic fields produced by distrubution cables. We are taking steps with a view to overcoming this feature.

However, overhead lines produce higher magnetic fields than distribution cables and we estimated (using for the work done so far the maximum recorded current over the period 1974 to 1984) the magnetic field in houses due to nearby overhead lines. 'Nearby' covered a distance up to 100m away but more remote lines will be included in further analysis.

Both lines and cables were identified using maps and the addresses of controls and cases. This identification and assessment of magnetic field exposure was done blind by people not knowing whether an address referred to a case or control.

Only a small proportion of cases and controls lived near overhead lines. Table 2 gives the number of cases and controls living in various estimated range of magnetic field strength.

Table 2   Cases and Controls Living in Various Bands of Estimated Magnetic Field

Field Strength range, mG	No. of cases	No. of controls	Risk ratio
0.1 - 0.99	9	15	1.0
1 - 9.99	4	5	1.3
>10	2	3	1.1

The analysis so far shows no apparent relationship between overhead power lines and childhood cancer.

A comparable study of adult cancers is planned and we seek improved methods of assessing the ambient magnetic field at a residence. It would be an advantage to be able to account for distribution cables since more cases and controls can then be included.

Cardiac Pacemaker Performance

Bridges, Frazier and Hauser (1978) had reported electronic tests on cardiac pacemakers both on the bench and in pacemakers fitted in baboons.

This work has been followed up recently by testing a variety of cardiac pacemakers which had been fitted in people suffering from various cardiac disorders. In the first experiments (Butrous et al., 1983) people stood on the ground beneath a high voltage electrode whose potential could be varied, thus changing the electric field strength to which the people were exposed. Pacemaker performance was observed by measuring heart performance in an instrument attached to the person. The signal from this instrument was telemetered a few meters at radio frequency to a receiver and recorder. This arrangment avoided additional uncontrolled 50-Hz currents that might have flowed to the body in any solid connection between heart monitor and recorder. The arrangements allowed the imposed electric field to be removed in the event of unusual cardiac behaviour.

In other experiments (Camm et al., 1984), electric
currents were fed to the shoulders and taken from the feet
by electrodes attached to the skin. This simulates the
current induced by exposure to a strong electric field.
It is a much more convenient procedure, and it can be done
in a hospital with the patient in bed. Precautions are
needed in designing and making the current source so as
to avoid accidental electric shock.

Some designs of pacemaker are insenstive to
interference induced by fields even as high as 20 kV m^{-1}
which is about the highest field likely to be experienced
in practice. The most sensitive pacemaker was affected
by a field of only about 2 kV m^{-1}. All pacemakers recovered
as soon as the electrical interference was removed.

In some cases the interference resulted in the
pacemaker providing sustained regular stimulation to the
heart even when not needed. This is not believed to be
harmful but did in one case cause discomfort. Some
sensitive pacemakers may either stimulate irregularly or
fail to stimulate at all. We know of no experience of
this last kind of interference in practice either in a
member of the public or in a person exposed occupationally.

Exposure to strong electric fields is not the only
source of electrical interference that may affect an
implanted pacemaker. Leakage currents from electrical
equipment can in some circumstances be sufficiently strong
to alter the mode of operation even when the leakage
currents are below levels specified in National Standards
for new equipment.

For these reasons cardiologists should use pacemakers
which are insensitive to electrical interference and advise
patients already fitted with sensitive pacemakers to
approach unfamiliar electrical equipment cautiously.

Concluding Remarks

The work undertaken in this programme has confirmed
that the function of some types of cardiac pacemaker is
susceptible to electrical interference. The work has also
served to put limits on possible changes in health and
physiological function in people in 50 Hz electric and

magnetic fields. The degree of delimitation is not
quantifiable since the range of effects that can be
concerned is wide and covers different qualities of possible
response. Nonetheless the investigations were penetrating
and do not point to any effect on health identifiable
in those living or working near electric power plants.

Acknowledgements

It is a pleasure to acknowledge the collaboration
of many colleagues in the CEGB, especially Dr. P.F. Chester
and Dr. John Male, and of Dr. Donald Broadbent at Oxford
University, of Professor Tim Lee and Dr. Brian Stollery
at Manchester, Professor John Camm and Dr. Ghazwan Butrous
at St. Bartholomew's Hospital, London, Dr. R.A. Cartwright
at Cookridge Hospital, Leeds and Dr. A. Myers at Leeds
University.

This paper is published by permission of the Central
Electricity Generating Board.

References

Adrian, D.J., 1977, Auditory and visual sensations
  stimulated by low frequency electric current, Radio
  Science, 12(6(S)), 243-250
Barber, P.B., Looms, J.S.T., Oakeshott, D.F., Prest,J.,
  Stringfellow, G.C., Stevens, D.R. and Watson, R.P.E.,
  1974, Transmission lines in the environment of England
  and Wales, CIGRE Paper 22-01, Paris
Bridges, J.E., Frazier, M.J. and Hauser, R.G., 1978, The
  effect of 60 Hz electric fields and currents on implanted
  cardiac pacemakers, IEEE Int. Sym. Elec. Comp., p 258
  own, S. and Crisp, A.H., 1966, A short clinical
  diagnostic self-rating scale for psycho-neurotic patients,
  Brit. J. Psychiatry, 112, 917-923
Butrous,G.S., Male, J.C., Webber, R.S., Barton, D.G.,
  Meldrum, S.J., Bonnel, J.A. and Camm, A.J., 1983. The
  effect of power frequency high intensity electric fields
  on implanted cardiac pacemakers, PACE, 6. 1282 - 1292.
Camm, A.J., Butrous, G.S., Kaye, G., Maltz, M.B., Meldrum,
  S.J. and Male, J, 1984. The responses of implanted
  cardiac pacemakers to 50 Hz electric interference, 5th
  Asian Congress of Cardiology, Bangkok, November. Also
  presented at Cardiostim '84 Meeting, Monte Carlo.

Crown, S. and Crisp, A.M., 1966, A short clinical
diagnostic self-rating scale for psycho-neurotic patients,
Brit. J. Psychiatry, 112, 917 - 923.
Crown, S. and Crisp, A.H., 1979, Manual of the Crown-Crisp
Experiential Index, Stodder and Houghton, London
Deno, D.W., 1977, Currents induced in the human body by
high voltage transmission line electric fields -
measurement and calculation of distribution and dose,
IEEE Trans. Pow. App. Syst., PAS-96(S), 1517-1527
Fulton, J.P., Cobb, S., Preble, L., Leone, L. and Forman,E.,
1980, Electrical wiring configurations and childhood
leukaemia in Rhode Island, Am. J. Epidemiology, 111,
292-296
Hauf, R., 1974, Effect of 50 Hz alternating fields on man,
Electrotechnische Zeitschrift, 26, 12
Korobkova, V.P., Morozov, Yu.A., Stolarov, M.S. and
Yakub, Yu.A., 1972, Influence of the electric field in
500 and 750 kV switchyards on maintenance staff and means
for its protection, Conf. Int. Grand. Res. Elec, (CIGRE,
Paris), paper 22-06.
Male, J.C. and Norris, W.T., 1982, The nature of exposure
to low frequency electric fields near electric power
plant, Institution of Electrical Engineers Colloquium
on Some Biological Effects of Electric and Magnetic
Fields, 26 May, London
Male, J.C., Norris, W.T. and Watts, M.W., 1984, Exposure
of people to power-frequency electric and magnetic fields,
23rd Hanford Life Sciences Symposium, Richland,
Washington
Myers, A., Cartwright, R.A., Bonnell, J.A., Male, J.C.
and Cartwright, S.C., 1985, Overhead power lines and
childhood cancer, IEE Conference on Electric and Magnetic
Fields in Medicine and Biology, London, November.
Phillips, R.D., 1985, Neurophysiological response to
extremely low frequency electric fields,
Stollery, B. T., 1984, Human exposure to 50 Hz electric
currents, 23rd Hanford Life Sciences Symposium, Richland,
Washington
Stollery, B.T., 1985, Effects of 50 Hz electric currents
psychological functioning. I Mood and Verbal - Reasoning
skills, Brit. J. Indust. Med., to be published.
Wertheimer, N. and Leeper, E., 1979, Electrical wiring
configurations and childhood cancer, Am. J. of
Epidemiology, 109, 273-284

Electromagnetic Fields and Neurobehavioral Function, pages 367–376
© 1988 Alan R. Liss, Inc.

POSSIBLE PHYSIOLOGICAL MECHANISMS FOR NEUROBEHAVIORAL EFFECTS OF ELECTROMAGNETIC EXPOSURE

M. G. Shandala

A. N. Marzeev Research Institute of General and Communal Hygiene

Kiev, USSR

EDITORS' NOTE

The following chapter represents abbreviated, edited exerpts from the presentation given by Dr. Shandala.

INTRODUCTION

Changes in the nervous system as well as overt behavioral changes have been produced by radiofrequency (RF) electromagnetic fields (EMF). These changes have been described by a number of Soviet and foreign authors both at high (thermal) and low (non-thermal) exposure levels. We believe that there are different physiological mechanisms underlying these behavioral effects at the lower versus higher levels and, therefore, they should be given separate consideration. Intermediate levels resulting from power densities (PD) less than 10- but more than 1-mW/cm^2 may present an exception.

On the basis of her laboratory investigations, Gordon (1964, 1966) has suggested a two phase response to SHF radiation exposure. The first phase is characterized by central nervous system (CNS) excitation, increase in blood cholinesterase activity, hypertension and stimulation of development. According to Gordon, this phase cannot be interpreted as a positive shift due to active inhibition. During the second phase, referred to as protective inhibition, there is a weakening of CNS excitation, a decrease in cholinesterase activity, hypotension and developmental suppression. These effects are considered harmful to the organism.

Unlike the two phase theory suggested by Gordon,
Subbotin (1957, 1958) divided the types of responses to SHF
irradiation into adaptation and accumulation. The first
reaction phase was identified by Subbotin in his tests
using the classical conditioning method and 10 cm radiation
at 5 to 10 mW/cm^2 with 16 - 18 trials given in 2 hours. At
the beginning of the exposure, the response latency
decreased and the conditioned-salivation response
increased. These parameters returned to normal levels by
the end of the exposure period. The authors suggest that
this is due to adaptation. However, we suggest that it was
the result of prolongation of the second, i.e. protective
inhibition, phase.

Interesting investigations have been conducted in our
institute by Professor Dumansky. Rats were exposed to
continuous (12.6 cm, 0.5- 5-, and 10-mW/cm^2) and pulsed
(3cm, 1pps, f = 1000 Hz) waves with antenna rotation and
ray apperture of 2° and a rotation frequency of 1 rot/min
at 20, 10, 5, and 1 mW/cm^2 for 8-10 hours during 3-4
months. Changes in CNS activity were observed. There was
an increase in cortical excitation as demonstrated by
decreases in latency and increases in conditioned
responses. After 3 - 10 days there was an increase in
inhibition as shown by such changes as an increase in
latency and decreased food intake. Inhibition was strongest
during the 1st and 2nd months of exposure (Dumansky et al.,
1975).

Considerable experimental data on behavioral changes
have been obtained at both high (thermal) and low (non-
thermal) levels. However, there is no generally accepted
explanation of the observed changes. Behavioral changes
have been observed in studies of CNS activity at power
densities corresponding to those that might be encountered
in industrial situations. The studies reported at levels
corresponding to those that might be encountered by the
general population have not provided consistent results and
the number of such investigations is more limited. The
questions regarding the behavioral dynamics of changes seen
during and ,particularly, after the field exposure are not
resolved. The studies need to be replicated in order to
substantiate decision-making with regard to exposure
levels. Further investigation of CNS activity is needed at
low exposure levels. The question of whether these effects

might appear after, not during, the exposure period needs
to be identified. Most important, studies need to approach
the question of the theoretical mechanisms for
understanding the observed effects.

Neurobehavioral effects at low levels following
chronic exposure are the most interesting with regard to
environmental health and establishing safety standards for
the general population. Such studies are presented in this
report.

INVESTIGATIVE METHODS

For evaluation of CNS activity we employed several
behavioral indices including both conditioned response (CR)
methods and a number of non-conditioned approaches
including open field tests and electric shock threshold
measures.

A modified shuttle-box consisting of three chambers
was used to study conditioned avoidance. The device could
deliver electric shock via metal bars which constituted the
floor of the chambers. During conditioning, a signal (CS)
was given for 6 seconds (a sound at 75db and a 500 Hz light
at 10V). The electric shock was turned on in the
"dangerous" chamber and in all the passages between the
chambers 3 seconds after the CS. A successful CR was
recorded when the rat avoided the shock by running to a
"safe" chamber. In each daily session trials were
continued until the rat performed 5 successive CRs, or to
90 trials. The procedure was repeated for 1 or 2 days
until the criterion of 5 successive CRs was obtained.

The open field test was used as a measure of non-
conditioned responses such as exploratory behavior and
emotional tension reflecting the level of CNS excitability.
The open field test consisted of 3 trials each lasting 1
min with a 15-20 sec intertrial interval. At the beginning
of each trial the rat was placed in an opaque container in
the center of the field. During a trial the total number
of squares crossed, the number of center squares (the
middle nine squares) crossed after initially leaving this
area, and the number of vertical rearings were recorded.
In general, the rat would run into a corner following the
removal of the opaque container and subsequently begin to

explore the field. Therefore, the crossing of the nine
central squares was measured independently.

A test for electroshock threshold was also included.
A pulsed current device YEI-I with stabilization on shock
intensity was used as a source. The shock persisted until
the rat withdrew the front paws from metal bars
constituting the floor of the chamber. The intensity of
current required for withdrawal (100 Hz, lpps) and the
latency to withdraw the front paws from the metal bar floor
were recorded.

Studies of chronic exposure to 2450 MHz fields upon
behavior were carried out using white, random bred male and
female rats who were 4 to 5 months of age at the beginning
of the exposure. In the first set of tests the animals
were exposed 7 hours daily for a month at a power density
of 500 mW/cm^2. In the second set of tests the power
density was 50 mW/cm^2 or 10 mW/cm^2 for 3 months for 7 hours
daily. The animals were monitored for 3 months following
the exposure periods (post-exposure period) with recordings
made every 10-30 days. Conditioned responses in the
shuttle box used male rats while the other tests used
females. Initial, baseline measures were recorded for all
the tests and then the animals were divided into
homogeneous exposure and control groups. Behavioral
changes observed in the exposure groups were compared with
the corresponding control group.

For the third set of tests using pulsed EM fields, 80
random bred albino rats were divided into 3 experimental
and 1 control group containing 20 rats each. The animals
received 0, 100, 500, or 2500 mW/cm^2 for 4 months, 16 hours
per day. Behavioral measurements included investigative
and motor activity, electroshock threshold, and conditioned
avoidance. The open field test as well as the electroshock
thresholds and conditioned avoidance apparatus and
measurements were as indicated for the previous
experiments. A maze was used to evaluate motor activity.
The maze had 5 compartments with openings in opposing
corners for adjacent compartments. The path through the
maze required crossing from side to side through the
adjacent compartments. Ten aluminum plates were fixed on
the compartment floor in two lines parallel to the long

side of the maze. The animal was placed in the first maze compartment and an automatic timer was set for 2 and 4 minutes. The counters registered the closing of the circuits between 2 adjacent aluminum plates by movement of the rat's body. The current is 0.01 mA which is not considered stressful to the animal.

EXPOSURE SYSTEM AND CONDITIONS

The animal exposure system was designed to model the natural exposure conditions of the general population. The chamber floor, ceiling and walls were covered with special absorbing plates "Luch-50". During normal EM exposure the incident energy is fully absorbed by the plate surface creating optimal conditions for the biological experiments.

The 2450+50 MHz generator fed the energy through an attenuating cable to the horn which emitted the power parallel to the long axis of the chamber. Fluctuations of the E-field vector occurred in the vertical plane perpendicular to the floor surface of the chamber.

The homogeneous nature of the exposure conditions was measured using the 500 mW/cm^2 test set conditions. Nine cages were irradiated simultaneously. The cages were placed on three floors, three cages on each floor. To minimize cage interference the long axis of the cages was oriented to the horn emitter center. Optimal distance between the exposure zone and the horn emitter was determined empirically. Power density was measured with a PO-1 type thermistor power device that has an accuracy of $\pm$ 30%. The power density was measured at 18 points evenly located on the exposure zone surface. At each point the measuring antenna horn was directed to the center of the EM waves. For the 500 mW/cm^2 test, the deviation in the 18 points varied from 6- to 22.4%. The average deviation of the entire exposure volume was 71.2 mW/cm^2. Periodical measurement of power density at a single point showed that fluctuations did not exceed $\pm$ 3.5% of the originally observed value. Thus, there was no need to correct the power during the experiments. The power density measurements were taken without animals in the cages.

The third set of experiments studied behavior during exposure to pulsed EM. The frequency was 2750-MHz with a

400 Hz pulse frequency. Pulse duration simulated radar antenna rotation at 3 rotations per min, 40 msec per 20 sec, 16 pulses at a pulse burst. EM energy was conducted via a waveguide to an emitting antenna fixed to the ceiling of the anechoic chamber. Experimental animals were placed in plexiglas cages 2.7m under the emitting antennae. The distribution of the EM energy inside the chamber did not vary by more than 10%.

RESULTS

The non-conditioned reflex tests at 500 mW/cm^2 seemed to be the most sensitive. A statistically significant decrease in exploratory activity was identified by the 20th day of exposure. This inhibition was present till the 30th day but was progressively less evident. The inhibition changed into excitation (increased exploratory activity) during the post-exposure period. Significantly higher exploratory activity was recorded on the 30th day and the 90th day of the post-exposure period. The other measures recorded in the open field test produced the same pattern of results. The activity in the central area decreased on day 30 of the exposure period and increased by day 30 of the post-exposure period. Rearing did not show any significant changes.

The electroshock threshold tests also appeared to be sensitive indices of the CNS state. There was a significant increase in the threshold in the exposed group on the 20th day of exposure. The threshold decreased on the 30th day of exposure. The threshold also decreased on the 30th and 60th day of the post-exposure period. The conditioned avoidance response measures remained unchanged under the 500 mW/cm^2 level.

There were many similarities to the 500 mW/cm^2 data in the responses at the 50 and 10 mW/cm^2 levels. The electroshock threshold decreased on the 10th day of exposure. By day 90 the threshold in the experimental group was higher than the control. In the open field test there was a decrease in exploratory activity in general and in the central area on the 30th day of exposure. This decrease was maintained through the 60 days of exposure. Vertical rearing decreased on day 30 of exposure. During the post-exposure period all of the average values for the measures were higher for the experimental as compared to the control group.

At the 50mW/cm^2 level there were CR changes both during and after exposure. The number of trials to reach criterion was checked on day 60 and 90 of exposure as well as day 30 and 90 of the post-exposure period. The sharpest increase was observed on the 90th day of exposure. These changes suggest CNS inhibition. At 10 mW/cm^2 it took longer for the excitation phase at the beginning of exposure to develop. There were significant decreases of electroshock threshold on the 10th and 30th days of exposure. No further changes in the thresholds were observed.

CNS inhibition was suggested by decreases in exploratory activity in the open field test. All types of activity including vertical rearing, total exploration and exploration in the central area were decreased on the 30th day of exposure. All three types of exploratory measures were also decreased on the 60th day. The CNS activation phase observed at the end of the 50 mW/cm^2 exposure was suggested by significant increases in central exploratory activity on the 30th and 90th days.

In the third set of tests in pulsed fields, no changes in central exploratory activity or vertical rearing were seen. At 100 mW/cm^2 there was some inhibition during the 3rd and 4th month of exposure. At the same time, power densities of 500 and 2500 mW/cm^2 showed decreases in exploratory behavior without the activation phase. No activation or inhibition of central exploratory activity or vertical rearing were observed. The dynamics of motor activity changes assessed from the total number of circuit closures in the maze reflected the same pattern of exploratory activity as obtained in the open field.

Statistically significant decreases in the number of maze compartments investigated was seen at 100 mW/cm^2 but not at 500 and 2500 mW/cm^2.

Electroshock thresholds (EST) were statistically different in experimental animals. At 100 mW/cm^2 the EST decreased during the first two months of exposure suggesting CNS activation. Following the decrease there

was an increase that was statistically significant at the
end of the 4th month of exposure. At power densities of
500 mW/cm^2 there was a significant EST decrease during the
entire exposure period. Exposure at 2500 mW/cm^2 resulted
in decreased EST at the third month with further increase
at the fourth month. These results suggest inhibition of
non-conditioned reactions in animals.

Other investigators have suggested that the
conditioned avoidance method fails to show significance in
experiments that are terminated in less than 2 or 3
months. Therefore, CNS conditioned avoidance activity was
taken at the end of the 4th month of exposure. The CRs of
experimental animals at all three power densities were
statistically different. At 2500 mW/cm^2 the was a
significant increase in the number of non-conditioned
reactions during the training process. At this level, the
response latency was significantly increased. The changes
suggest inhibition of the CNS. A power density level of
500 mW/cm^2 failed to produce changes in these indices. The
100 mW/cm^2 level produced some CNS activation. There was a
decrease in both the non-conditioned defensive response
fall out and the total number of trials to criterion.

At exposures to different non-heating SHF energy
levels there were many common observation in the dynamics
of the behavioral responses. Inhibition of CNS was
observed at all levels. A CNS excitation phase was
recorded at the beginning of exposure. After exposure the
inhibition phase is replaced by another CNS activation
phase. This is observed most clearly in the non-
conditioned response measures, especially at 500 mW/cm^2.
However in animal groups with developed CR, inhibition
during the exposures at 50 and 10 mW/cm^2 increased. The
inhibited state remained for 3 months in the 50 mW/cm^2
group.

CONCLUSIONS

At exposures to different non-heating SHF energy
levels there were many common observation in the dynamics
of the behavioral responses. Inhibition of CNS was
observed at all levels. A CNS excitation phase was
recorded at the beginning of exposure. After exposure the
inhibition phase is replaced by another CNS activation

phase. This is observed most clearly in the non-conditioned response measures, especially at 500 mW/cm^2. However in animal groups with developed CR, inhibition during the exposures at 50 and 10 mW/cm^2 increased. The inhibited state remained for 3 months in the 50 mW/cm^2 group.

As the results of the three sets of studies were compared, many similarities in the dynamics of the behavioral responses under study became evident. In general the initial inhibition or activation was followed by a reversal that persisted not only through the latter exposure periods but also for some months following the exposures.

USSR HUMAN EXPOSURE STANDARD

On the basis of these and previous studies the USSR has proposed the following standard for exposure of the general population to EM.

Frequency Range	Old Values	New Values
Long Waves (30 - 300 kHz)	20 V/m	25 V/m
Middle Waves (0.3 - 3 MHz)	10 V/m	15 V/m
Short Waves (3 - 30 MHz)	4 V/m	10 V/m
Ultrashort Waves (30 - 300 MHz)	2 V/m	3 V/m
Microwaves (300 MHz - 300 GHz)	5 $microW/cm^2$	10 $microW/cm^2$

REFERENCES

Gordon S, (1964). The outcome of a complex study of biolo-
    gical effects of radiofrequency waves and future out-
    look on further research. In "On the biological effects
    of radiofrequency waves," pp 3-9.

Gordon S, (1966). Problems in industrial hygiene and biolo-
    gical effects of very high frequency electromagnetic
    fields. 163 pages.

Subbotin A, (1957). On the effect of very high frequency
    electromagnetic fields on the higher nervous activity
    of dogs. In "On the biological effect of very high
    frequency electromagnetic fields," Leningrad, pp35-57.

Subbotin A, (1958). On the effect of pulsed very high
    frequency electromagnetic fields on the higher nervous
    activity of dogs. Bulletin of Experimental Biology
    and Medicine 46:55.

Dumansky Y, Serdyuk AM, Los' IP, (1975) The effect of radio-
    frequency electromagnetic fields on humans. Kiev,
    159 pages.

Electromagnetic Fields and Neurobehavioral Function, pages 377–388
© 1988 Alan R. Liss, Inc.

ELECTROMAGNETIC WAVES AND NEUROBEHAVIORAL FUNCTION
Comments from Clinical Medicine

Paul J. Rosch, M.D., F.A.C.P.

I too wish to add my thanks to the organizers and
sponsors of this stimulating and delightful conference.
One of the previous speakers in commenting on the wide
variety of interesting presentations in allied fields that
had relevance for his own research noted that he felt
somewhat like Alice in Wonderland. As the conference
developed, I could readily appreciate the analogy for those
of you engaged in the varied, fascinating, broad subject of
electromagnetic energy and neurobehavioral function. I
must confess, however, that my initial reaction was more
akin to feeling like a fish out of water, since I did not
have adequate background in mathematics or physics to
appreciate Dr. Van Bladel's detailed, eloquent equations.
My experience is primarily that of having been a practicing
physician for 35 years with a particular research interest
in relationships between stress and illness. Fortunately,
in my early training, I spent some time in Selye's animal
laboratory. During post graduate training at Johns Hopkins
where I worked in the Endocrine Clinic and subsequently at
the Walter Reed Army Institute of Research as Director of
the Endocrine Laboratories, I was able to gain some
experience in basic research, conducting experiments, and
writing scientific reports. Consequently, I was able to
appreciate, if not marvel at, the very meticulous and
superb scientific logic and methodology that characterized
the presentations we heard during this workshop.
Furthermore, I was readily able to see the clinical
implications and relevance of many of the topics to my own
interests.

This was particularly apparent in Dr. Adey's very lucid paper and those that followed dealing with the role of calcium in cell biology which brought into focus the current flurry of interest in the use of calcium channel blocking agents in heart disease, hypertension, migraine, Raynaud's and other stress related disorders. Similarly, Dr. Ehret's discussion of circadian rhythms and the influence of zeitgebers provided additional insight into the growing discipline of chronopharmacology which deals with variation in drug effect according to time of administration. I was also intrigued by the role of various stressors as zeitgebers, and the possible correlation of emotional states and altered ultradian rhythms, etc. Dr. Norris' attempts to study the effects of magnetic fields on human performance in the workplace again vividly demonstrated the numerous difficulties associated with attempting to evaluate the important components of job stress.

In reflecting on the events of the past three days and attempting to correlate them with my own clinical and research experience over the past three and one half decades, there are certain conclusions or at least impressions that have crossed my mind, some half dozen of which I would like to share with you.

(1) Life on earth and the biologic phenomena associated with it generally exhibit an often unappreciated or unrecognized wisdom, shaped by hundreds of thousands of years of evolutionary adaptational responses to a variety of external stimuli and stressors that ultimately appear to result in the survival of the fittest, or as Jonas Salk might say "the wisest." This is quite apparent in the studies presented on the magnetic detection systems of pigeons by Dr. Semm and the navigational abilities of sharks by Dr. Baker.

(2) Our concept of the human brain as a complicated electronic switchboard (which is what I learned in medical school) has now been superceded by an acknowledgement of its role as a vast endocrine organ with awesome power and potential. With that, perhaps, comes an important caveat, namely that, because of man's highly developed cerebral cortex, it may become increasingly difficult to apply the

results of certain psychological experiments in laboratory animals dealing with perception of stress to meaningful conclusions in humans.

(3) Our ability to recognize or comprehend the full significance of research findings is entirely dependent on being able to identify and measure all the potential components that contribute to adaptive responses. Very often our hypotheses are correct based on existing evidence. However, when subsequent observations conflict, there may be a tendency to try to bend the data to fit in with some preconceived framework rather than abandon a pet theory. When all you have is a hammer at your disposal, you tend to view everything as a nail.

(5) While many adaptive responses appear to be useless or even harmful, they most likely can ultimately be shown to have had some teleologic purpose during the course of evolution. We were talking at breakfast the other morning about "goose flesh" and the bristling of the hairs on the back of the neck in response to acute fear. While that reaction appears purposeless in humans, you will recall that the bristling of the fur on the arched back of an aroused cat makes it appear more ferocious to a potential assailant and that the stimulation of those same arrectores pilorum muscles provides a very effective means of defense for the porcupine. As we shall see, other adaptive responses of man to acute stress which involve intense stimulation of the sympathetic nervous system and the release of catecholamines to facilitate lifesaving "fight or flight" activities also undoubtedly had survival value for primitive man. However, they have now become not only inappropriate but dangerous responses to modern stressors and a major contributor to heart attacks, hypertension, and a host of other "Diseases of Civilization."

(6) The truth is not that which is demonstrable but rather that which is inescapable or as St. Exupery noted "ineluctable." Evidence is not the same as proof, and it is ultimately proof that the scientific community demands.

Now, what has all of this to do with stress and the influence of electromagnetic waves on neurobehavioral function? At first, you may properly ask "what is stress?" For the pure scientist, it is a useless term simply because it means different things to different people and it is different things for each one of us. A good example of

this is afforded by observing individuals on a roller
coaster ride. Some sit in the back seats cringing, eyes
shut, and teeth clenched, white knuckled as they grasp the
retaining bar, praying for the ordeal to end so that they
can get out of the torture chamber and back to terra firma.
Up front are the wide-eyed thrill seekers, shrieking and
relishing every steep plunge, who quickly scurry to get on
the very next ride. In between are those seemingly
unaffected by the experience with an air of insouciance
that almost borders on boredom. So, was the roller coaster
ride stressful? Obviously, for some it was very
distressful and for others, it provided an exhilarating
experience. Thus, stress cannot be defined satisfactorily
from an objective point of view. For our purposes, I shall
define it merely as "the response of the body to any demand
for change." Despite the fact that we can't satisfactorily
define stress, one thing seems clear from most laboratory
and clinical research, namely that a sense or feeling of
"being out of control" is very distressful. Similarly,
another lesson afforded by the example of the roller
coaster ride is that it is not necessarily the <u>nature</u> of
the stressor, but rather our <u>perception</u> of it that is
really important. It is necessary to keep such
observations in mind when attempting to transpose the
results of animal studies in clinical situations dealing
with apparently stressful states that have such a strong
subjective component.

I emphasize this simply because many of the research
reports deal in rather general terms with the effects of
"non-specific stress" in referring to the nature of certain
interventions as well as the significance of their
consequences. The term has tended to become a wastebasket
and source of confusion since it can be interpreted in so
many different ways. Despite such drawbacks, "stress"
provides an attractive rubric to describe the variegated
aspects and phenomena associated with the mind-body
relationship. Consequently, it attracts investigators from
otherwise disparate disciplines having concerns that are
surprisingly common. Therefore, it might be instructive
for us to review the origins of the concept of "stress."

Certainly, the notion that the mind can affect the
body or that emotions could play an important role in
health and illness is not a novel idea. It is present in
our earliest medical writings and is evident in most great

philosophies and religions dating back to ancient Hindu Scriptures.

The scientific study of stress probably had its origins in the investigations of the great 19th century physiologist, Claude Bernard, who developed the concept of good health and survival as being dependent upon the ability to maintain the constancy or stability of the internal environment (milieu interne). Thus, man and homeothermic animals exposed to the subzero temperatures of the Arctic or the blistering heat of the desert tend to maintain a body temperature of 98.6^0F by virtue of a series of integrated adaptive responses that produce shivering or vasoconstriction to generate or retain heat or vasodilation and perspiration in an effort to dissipate it. Similarly, ingestion of excessive amounts of sugar which cause a rise in blood glucose evoke a series of hormonal responses such as insulin to lower it. If the drop is too great, adrenalin and cortisol bring it back to normal range. If too much salt or other elements are ingested, increased excretion through renal and other mechanisms come into play to maintain the status quo. In a very general sense, Bernard taught that good health was essentially dependent upon good and effective communication between the internal constituent components of the organism and the external environment. That same philosophy would appear to be applicable to all the hierarchial components of living systems ranging from a single cell to a tissue, organ, individual, family, nation, society, etc. where effective internal and external communications also appear to be essential for good health and survival.

In the early part of this century, Walter Cannon, the great Harvard physiologist, extended Bernard's concept of the "milieu interne" which he termed the "steady state," and for which he coined the term "homeostasis." Cannon was probably the first to employ the term stress in its present context and it was clear that his appreciation of the term included both psychological and physical stimuli. His classical studies of the effects of life threatening fear in dogs demonstrated that there was a marked stimulation of the sympathetic nervous system with an outpouring of adrenalin-like hormones which appeared to assist the animal in life saving "fight or flight." Thus, the pupils dilated to promote better vision, there was an increased flow of blood to the brain to improve decision making, glycogen

stores were quickly broken down to provide an elevated
blood sugar for more energy, blood clotted more quickly to
minimize loss from henorrhage and blood flow was shunted
away from the gut where it was no longer needed for
processes of digestion to the large muscles of the arms and
legs to assist in this vital "fight or flight" response.
While such adaptive responses would undoubtedly have had
survival value for primitive man suddenly confronted with a
sabre-toothed tiger, the nature of stress for modern man is
more apt to be getting stuck in a traffic jam on the way to
the airport, or fights with the boss, customers, wife,
children, girlfriend, etc. Unfortunately, our bodies still
respond in that same old archaic fashion but now the
outpouring of such stress related hormones no longer serves
any useful purpose. In fact, there is increasing evidence
that such repetitive responses occurring many times a day
rather than once a fortnight contributes significantly to
cardiovascular diseases, peptic ulcer, diabetes, as well as
suppression of immune system defenses against cancer and a
host of infections ranging from herpes to tuberculosis.

Our current concept and preoccupation with stress,
however, stems almost entirely from the work of Hans Selye,
who essentially coined the term, borrowing it from physics
where it had long been employed to describe the elastic
properties of solids exposed to external loads (Hooke's
Law). Selye was impressed with the fact that in thousands
of laboratory experiments where experimental animals were
exposed to a variety of different and even opposite noxious
stimuli (severe heat, freezing, bright lights, loud noises,
psychological frustration, muscular exercise to the point
of exhausation), identical pathological changes could be
demonstrated at autopsy. Regardless of the nature of the
offending agency, the acute response to stress which Selye
termed the "Alarm Reaction" was always accompanied by
hemorrhages and ulceration in the gastric mucosa, a
dissolution or atrophy of the thymus gland and lymphatic
tissues, and hypertrophy of the adrenal cortex. If the
offending stimulus persisted, the animal appeared to enter
a second phase or "Stage of Resistance" during which body
defenses appeared to be maximized and finally a persistent
third or final "Stage of Exhaustion" and ultimately death
ensued. Selye named this triparte response the "General
Adaptation Syndrome." Autopsy studies conducted during
various phases of this "General Adaptation Syndrome"
revealed microscopic changes indistinguishable from those

seen in humans with hypertension, coronary heart disease, rheumatoid arthritis, peptic ulcer, nephrosclerosis, etc. Selye reasoned that if such "non-specific" stress could cause these changes in his laboratory animals, perhaps it played a similar important role in such human illnesses which he labelled "Diseases of Adaptation."

As a consequence, he ran into all sorts of other semantic problems and when invited to give a lecture at The College de France, the officials there who had custody of maintaining the purity of the French language had great difficulty in finding a word or expression that could be used to translate "stress" accurately. After much deliberation, a new French word, "stress," was born and after an equally spirited discussion concerning the appropriate gender, the male chauvinists apparently won out and le stress was quickly followed by el stress, lo stress, der stress, etc. in other languages.

Cannon's appreciation of the pathophysiology of stress was limited to the sympathetic adrenal medullary system because that was all he could measure. Similarly, Selye's belief in the "non-specificity" of stress was also a function of the parameters of pituitary-adrenal activity available to him. However, as new refinements in biochemical techniques became available, it became quite obvious that stress involved a whole repertoire of humoral secretion including a host of newly discovered small brain peptides such as melatonin and the endorphins. Far from being non-specific, it was increasingly apparent that the overall response to stress was highly personalized, and varied considerably from individual to individual or even in the same subject at different times. In addition, in humans, the harmful effects of stress were produced not only by the types of noxious stimuli studied in Selye's rats, but a host of other more subtle and less quantifiable psychosocial threats such as bereavement, isolation, retirement, poverty, etc. They could also be invoked by any number of seemingly insignificant minor hassles ranging from a broken shoelace to a traffic ticket. In some, it apparently could be self-generated as in the individual with the Type A coronary prone behavior pattern. Today, all these situations have come to be included under the broad heading of "stress" in humans and all may have adverse health consequences.

Thus, our theories concerning the role of stress in illness have had to be constantly revised as new advances and discoveries required changes in the overall framework. Our current appreciation of stress and its health effects are far different than could have been possibly anticipated thirty-five years ago when the concept was born.

As I listened to the various presentations, I could not help but feel that this field is also in its infancy if not gestation. If we were to return 5 or 10 years hence, Dr. Ehret would probably have the blackboard filled with new definitions. We would likely have discovered zeitgebers that could not only influence the hour hand but perhaps the minute or even second hand as we learn more about a host of as yet unsuspected circadian, ultradian, and infradian rhythms. The apparent recent discovery of the elusive magnetic monopole, a bizarre theoretical particle with only one magnetic pole, has vast implications for understanding fundamental forces of nature such as magnetism and gravity. Similarly, I have no doubt that future experiments in man and laboratory animals that can be performed in outer space, divorced from the effects of the earth's gravity, may likely yield other important information about homeostatic functions and adaptive strategies that are as yet unsuspected or not clearly understood. The development of newer imaging techniques such as nuclear magnetic resonance and positive emission tomography will likely provide still further unsuspected data about the interface between emotions, behavior, neuroendocrine, and other metabolic changes in the brain.

I have been asked by some of you in the past few days to discuss our current concept of the significance and dimensions of the role of stress in illness. Obviously, that is not possible in the time allotted but let me offer the following observations. It is estimated that up to 90% of visits to primary care practitioners are for stress related disorders or complaints. Stress in the workplace is thought by many to be the number 1 health problem in the United States today in the adult population with costs to industry estimated at 100 billion dollars annually - more than 10 times the cost of all strikes combined. There is increasing recognition that stress and coronary prone behavior are the most significant risk factor for coronary heart disease. Attempts to reduce the incidence of recurrent heart attacks by modifying such standard risk factors as cigarette smoking, cholesterol, and hypertension have generally proved unsuccessful as evidenced by the recent Multiple Risk Factor Intervention Trial (MRFIT). The only successful strategies in preventing heart attacks have been the administration of beta blockers or techniques used to reduce coronary prone behavior. In both instances, the beneficial effects appear to be a consequence of reducing or blunting the effects of stress related catecholamines known to cause direct myocardial damage. The link between cigarette smoking, hypertension, cholesterol, and coronary heart disease may, to a large extent, be due to the fact that these also may be manifestations of coronary prone behavior.

Currently, there is a great deal of interest in the effects of psychosocial stress on immune system dysfunction. In most scales that attempt to quantify or "rate" stress, loss of a spouse heads the list. In connection with this, it is of interest to note that widowed individuals die at rates 3 to 13 times higher than their married counterparts in the 12 to 24 months following bereavement for all the 10 leading causes of death. Why? How? Recent studies in Australia and New York provide some helpful clues as they demonstrate that immediately following bereavement, there is a prompt and impressive decline in components of the immune system known to be responsible for defenses against malignancy and infection.

However, it is not all bad news. All the great adaptive and integrating mechanisms that have been developed in the course of evolution operate on a system of checks and balances. The autonomic nervous system has complementary and antagonistic sympathetic and parasympathetic influences. Similarly, the endocrine system operates on a self-regulating feedback mechanism whereby target gland hormones are stimulated by pituitary trophic influences or levels of peripheral metabolites which they in turn control. Consequently, in the great scheme of things, it appears likely that if noxious influences can make us sick or depress immune system function, there are opposing emotions or factors that negate such effects or promote good health - what Dr. Selye used to call "eustress" or good stress. A strong faith, sense of control, and pride of accomplishment all appear to fall in this category and may in part account for the power of the placebo effect which is readily acknowledged but poorly understood. What does seem clear, however, from anecdotal reports of the success of faith healing or visitation to shrines is that we have just scratched the surface of our understanding of the individual's ability to influence personal health. Exciting new advances in the emerging discipline of psychoneuroimmunology by Ader and others clearly demonstrates the ability to condition central nervous system influences on immune function that might mimic the effect of pharmacologic agents. If we could discover the pathways whereby such effects are mediated, we could perhaps learn to simulate, stimulate, or emulate them in a naturopathic approach to self healing.

It is one aspect of that search which prompted me to accept Dr. O'Connor's invitation to attend this conference. Sometime late last year, I was approached by a Swiss group to evaluate a "stress reduction device" which achieved its effects through the application of electromagnetic energy by means of an antenna inserted high in the nasopharynx or the soft palate. Its location would obviously provide proximity to structures of the brain vitally concerned with autonomic nervous system function. The electromagnetic energy delivered was in the conventional medical band of 22.2 MH with a power output of approximately 1 milliwatt. Extensive laboratory studies and clinical experience showed no undesirable side effects. Patients did report relief of anxiety, insomnia, and a variety of somatic complaints after only one or two treatments lasting 10 to 15 minutes. Since it is not possible to discern whether the device is on or off by any sensation, it was possible to perform double blind studies which confirmed that these were not placebo effects. Furthermore, I was particularly intrigued by the sophisticated attempt of these investigators to obtain objective parameters to confirm their clinical observations. In this respect, electroencephalograms taken before, during, and after treatment revealed definite diminution in frontalis muscle tension and in most instances, very definite changes in alpha wave activity. Thus, it seemed clear that the device was producing some alteration that could be objectively recorded.

It is known that specific alpha wave patterns are associated with a state of deep relaxation such as that achieved by experienced meditators. Furthermore, EEG biofeedback studies similarly have demonstrated the ability of individuals to alter their own alpha wave activity to conform to such patterns, at which time they also report subjective feelings of tranquility and inner peace, as well as a sense of energy.

Conventional transcutaneous electrical nerve stimulation (TENS) applied transcranially has been reported to relieve headache and depression. Some studies suggest that the efficacy of pain relief by using the TENS device may be predicted by observing its effects on serotonin levels or 5 HIAA excretion patterns. Thus, it seems clear that low level electromagnetic energy can influence both EEG and biochemical parameters of neurobehavioral activity known to be associated with changes in mood, behavior and pain perception. Gaining further insight into more precise pathways of such responses may point the way for our ability to control or mimic them naturally. Dr. Claude Rossel, who is directing this research, and his co-workers have been kind enough to come here from Switzerland to discuss their findings. It is my understanding that Dr. Adey has also had some experience with a Russian device that appears to produce similar effects. Certainly, it seems clear that low level energies can have some effect on behavior, perhaps through stimulation or inhibition of peptide messengers. Deciphering how such effects could be predicted or mediated would significantly advance our understanding of the nature of the stress response in humans.

We spoke previously about health and homeostatic mechanisms and the necessity of maintaining a vital balance. We have also alluded to the fact that we appear to be on the threshold of being able to tap into that vast unknown potential for self healing and individual self design. For the present, it appears that we may need some chemical or mechanical crutches to help us along the path in that quest.

I would like to make a final comment about stress and illness. Our current concept of illness stems largely from the influence of the 17th century French philosopher, Rene Descartes. His mechanistic reductionistic approach was that the body functioned as a machine and that people became ill when the machine broke down, usually from some external influence. Fixing the machine was the province of medicine, and that could best be accomplished by increasing our knowledge of its smallest working parts. Disorders of the mind or spirit, Descartes reasoned, were entirely separate, beyond man's ken, and were entirely matters for the Church to deliberate. The subsequent invention of the microscope, the discovery of microbes and the brilliant investigations of Pasteur and Koch in demonstrating bacterial causes of illness appeared to confirm the impression that we become ill because something attacks us from without. That same attitude prevails today as we read about a host of carcinogens in the air we breathe or foods we consume. Yet, in clinical experiments, it is very hard to "catch" a cold, hepatitis, or tuberculosis. The vast majority of heavy smokers never develop cancer of the lung. What is it that determines "resistance" or susceptibility to illness? In addition to genetic factors, it has become increasingly clear that "stress" can play a major role in lowering immune defenses and heightening other harmful chemical activities.

It is said that on his deathbed, Pasteur, the originator of the germ theory, who engaged in many debates with his celebrated contemporary, Claude Bernard, stated "Bernard avait raison. Le germe n'est rien, c'est le terrain qui est tout." (Bernard was right. The microbe is nothing, the soil is everything).

For the practicing physician, our brief review of stress confirms what every "compleat" physician intuitively knows, namely that "many times it is more important to know what kind of patient has the disease, than what kind of disease the patient has."

Paul J. Rosch, M.D.
President
American Institute of Stress

Clinical Professor of Medicine
New York Medical College

Index

396 / Index

and absolute thresholds of detection of
    irradiation, 238–239
and adventitious acquisition, 256
definitions used in, 235–238
difference, pain, and terminal thresh-
    olds, 241–242
and generality of absolute thresholds,
    241
infrared radiation as negative rein-
    forcer, 245–246
infrared radiation as positive rein-
    forcer, 243–245
and integral dose vs. irradiance
    thresholds, 239–41
and meaning of whole-body reso-
    nance, 237–238
microwave radiation as negative rein-
    forcer, 246–254
microwave radiation as positive rein-
    forcer, 253–254
as motivational stimuli, 242–243
and motivation distinguished from re-
    inforcement, 236–237
as reinforcers, 243–255
and sensory properties, 238–242
Microscopy, light and electron
and morphological changes in micro-
    wave-exposed neonatal rat cere-
    brum, 135–148
of rabbit brain after exposure to power
    frequency electromagnetic fields,
    121–128
Microwave exposure
-drug interactions in cholinergic nervous
    system of mouse, 309–324
and locomotor activity tests, 316–324
and scopolamine effects, 311–324
effects on cardiovascular system, 153–175
cat heart study, 162–166
and industrial exposure of workers,
    156
in isolated heart preparations, 154–161
and maintenance of homeostasis,
    173–174
and partial or whole-body exposure of
    live animals, 155
and ventral exposure of rats, 166–172
effects on fetal development in mice, 136

effects on nervous system, 128–132
effects on thermoregulatory system in
    Saimiri sciureus, 180–199
compared with response to other heat
    sources, 180
and normal thermoregulation,
    179–180
and restricted body exposure, 186–190
role of medial preoptic/anterior hypo-
    thalamic area, 190–197
and thermoregulatory profile, 181–184
in industry, 156
recommendations for, 267–268
and infrared radiations as sensory, moti-
    vational and reinforcement stimuli,
    235–259
and absolute thresholds of detection of
    irradiation, 238–239
and adventitious acquisition, 256
definitions used in, 235–238
difference, pain, and terminal thresh-
    olds, 241–242
and generality of absolute thresholds,
    241
infrared radiation as negative reinfor-
    cer, 245–246
infrared radiation as positive reinfor-
    cer, 243–245
and integral dose vs. irradiance
    thresholds, 239–241
and meaning of whole-body reso-
    nance, 237–238
microwave radiation as negative rein-
    forcer, 246–254
microwave radiation as positive rein-
    forcer, 253–254
as motivational stimuli, 242–243
and motivation distinguished from re-
    inforcement, 236–237
as reinforcers, 243–255
and sensory properties, 238–242
in *Macaca mulatta*
effects on thermoregulatory system at
    frequency near whole-body,
    203–217
as thermal reinforcement, 219–233
prenatal in rats, behavior and, 265–286
and discriminant analysis, 271–275